From Child
Sexual Abuse
to Adult
Sexual Risk

From Child Sexual Abuse to Adult Sexual Risk

Trauma, Revictimization, and Intervention

Edited by

Linda J. Koenig, Lynda S. Doll,
Ann O'Leary, and Willo Pequegnat

American Psychological Association

Washington, DC

First Printing September 2003
Second Printing November 2004

Published by
American Psychological Association
750 First Street, NE
Washington, DC 20002
www.apa.org

To order
APA Order Department
P.O. Box 92984
Washington, DC 20090-2984
Tel: (800) 374-2721; Direct: (202) 336-5510
Fax: (202) 336-5502; TDD/TTY: (202) 336-6123
On-line: www.apa.org/books/
E-mail: order@apa.org

In the U.K., Europe, Africa, and the Middle East, copies may be ordered from
American Psychological Association
3 Henrietta Street
Covent Garden, London
WC2E 8LU England

Typeset in Goudy by Stephen McDougal, Mechanicsville, MD
Printer: United Book Press, Inc., Baltimore, MD
Cover Designer: NiDesign, Baltimore, MD
Technical/Production Editor: Casey Ann Reever

The opinions and statements published are the responsibility of the authors, and such opinions and statements do not necessarily represent the policies of the American Psychological Association. Any views expressed in the introduction, chapter 3, chapter 4, and the conclusion do not necessarily represent the views of the United States government, and the author's participation in the work is not meant to serve as an official endorsement of any statement to the extent that such may conflict with any official position of the United States government.

Library of Congress Cataloging-in-Publication Data

From child sexual abuse to adult sexual risk : trauma, revictimization, and intervention / edited by Linda J. Koenig . . . [et al.].
    p. cm.
Includes bibliographical references and index.
    ISBN 1-59147-030-7 (hardcover : alk. paper)
    1. Adult child sexual abuse victims—Sexual behavior. 2. Adult child sexual abuse victims—Rehabilitation. 3. Hygiene, Sexual. 4. Sexually transmitted diseases—Psychological aspects. 5. AIDS (Disease) —Transmission. 6. Risk-taking (Psychology). I. Koenig, Linda J.

    RC569.5.A28F76 2003   2003012669
    616.85'8369—dc21

British Library Cataloguing-in-Publication Data
A CIP record is available from the British Library.

Printed in the United States of America

To our children—Benjamin, Abby, Jennifer, Sonia, Alexandra, and Geoffrey—who have enriched our lives and strengthened our commitment to creating a safe and healthy world for all children

CONTENTS

CONTRIBUTORS

Lisa Marmelstein Blackwell, PhD, Associate Psychologist, Binghamton
Psychiatric Center, Binghamton, NY

John Briere, PhD, Associate Professor of Psychiatry and Psychology, Keck
School of Medicine, University of Southern California, Los Angeles

Lisa Butler, PhD, Senior Research Scholar, Department of Psychiatry and
Behavioral Sciences, Stanford University School of Medicine,
Stanford, CA

Alex Carballo-Diéguez, PhD, Associate Professor and Research Scientist,
Department of Psychiatry, HIV Center for Clinical and Behavioral
Studies, New York State Psychiatric Institute and Columbia
University, New York

Jennifer Vargas Carmona, PhD, Assistant Research Psychologist,
Codirector, Women's Health Project, Department of Psychiatry and
Biobehavioral Sciences, University of California, Los Angeles

Dorothy Chin, PhD, Assistant Research Psychologist, Department of
Psychiatry and Biobehavioral Sciences, University of California, Los
Angeles

Hollie Clark, MPH, Public Health Analyst, NorthrupGrumann/Centers
for Disease Control and Prevention Information and Technology
Support Contract, Atlanta, GA

Catherine Classen, PhD, Senior Research Scientist, Department of
Psychiatry and Behavioral Sciences, Stanford University School of
Medicine, Stanford, CA

Amy M. Combs-Lane, PhD, Assistant Professor, Department of
Behavioral Medicine and Psychiatry, West Virginia University,
School of Medicine, Morgantown

Curtis Dolezal, PhD, Research Scientist, HIV Center for Clinical and
Behavioral Studies, New York State Psychiatric Institute and
Columbia University, New York

xi

Lynda S. Doll, PhD, Associate Director for Science, National Center for Injury Prevention and Control, Centers for Disease Control and Prevention, Atlanta, GA

Karen Ecklund, MS, Department of Psychology, Binghamton University, Binghamton, NY

Rachael Fite, MS, Department of Psychology, Binghamton University, Binghamton, NY

Jennifer J. Freyd, PhD, Professor, Department of Psychology, University of Oregon, Eugene

Christine Gidycz, PhD, Associate Professor, Department of Psychology, Ohio University, Athens

Lisa L. Harlow, PhD, Professor of Psychology, Department of Psychology, University of Rhode Island, Kingston

T. Robert Harris, PhD, Research Scientist, Green Center for the Study of Science and Society, University of Texas at Dallas

Amy R. Heard-Davison, PhD, Psychologist, Clinical Instructor, Psychiatry and Behavioral Sciences, University of Washington Medical Center, Seattle

Julia R. Heiman, PhD, Professor, Department of Outpatient Psychiatry, University of Washington Medical Center, Seattle

Dean G. Kilpatrick, PhD, Director, National Crime Victims Research and Treatment Center, Department of Psychiatry and Behavioral Sciences, Medical University of South Carolina, Charleston

Linda J. Koenig, PhD, Assistant Chief for Behavioral Science, Mother–Child Transmission and Pediatric/Adolescent Study Section, Epidemiology Branch, Division of HIV/AIDS Prevention, National Center for HIV, STD, and TB prevention, Centers for Disease Control and Prevention, Atlanta, GA

Arlinda F. Kristjanson, PhD, Associate Professor, Department of Neuroscience, School of Medicine and Health Sciences, University of North Dakota, Grand Forks

Tamra Burns Loeb, PhD, Assistant Research Psychologist, Codirector, Women's Health Project, Department of Psychiatry and Biobehavioral Sciences, University of California, Los Angeles

Steven Jay Lynn, PhD, Professor, Department of Psychology, Binghamton University, Binghamton, NY

Robert M. Malow, PhD, Research Professor, Department of Public Health, Florida International University, North Miami

Patricia J. Morokoff, PhD, Professor, Department of Psychology, University of Rhode Island, Kingston

Hector F. Myers, PhD, Professor, Department of Psychology, University of California, Los Angeles

Ann O'Leary, PhD, Senior Behavioral Scientist, Prevention Research Branch, Division of HIV/AIDS Prevention, National Center for HIV, STD, and TB Prevention, Centers for Disease Control and Prevention, Atlanta, GA

James W. Pennebaker, PhD, Professor, Department of Psychology, University of Texas at Austin

Willo Pequegnat, PhD, Associate Director, Prevention, Translational, and International Research, Center for Mental Health Research on AIDS, National Institute of Mental Health, National Institutes of Health, U.S. Department of Health and Human Services, Bethesda, MD

Judith Pintar, PhD, Department of Sociology, University of Illinois, Champaign–Urbana

David W. Purcell, JD, PhD, Chief, Individual and Small Group Intervention Section, Prevention Research Branch, Division of HIV/AIDS Prevention, National Center for HIV, STD, and TB Prevention, Centers for Disease Control and Prevention, Atlanta, GA

Kathryn Quina, PhD, Professor, Department of Psychology and Women's Studies, University of Rhode Island, Kingston

Heidi S. Resnick, PhD, Professor, National Crime Victims Research and Treatment Center, Department of Psychiatry and Behavioral Sciences, Medical University of South Carolina, Charleston

Cindy L. Rich, PhD, Postdoctoral Fellow, Department of Psychology, Ohio University, Athens

David Spiegel, MD, Willson Professor in the School of Medicine, Department of Psychiatry and Behavioral Sciences, Stanford University School of Medicine, Stanford, CA

Jane Stafford, PhD, Department of Psychology, Binghamton University, Binghamton, NY

Lori D. Stone, PhD, Senior Research Associate, Harris Interactive, Inc., Rochester, NY

Elisabeth Thurston, MA, Department of Psychiatry and Behavioral Sciences, Stanford University School of Medicine, Stanford, CA

Holly Vanderhoff, MA, Department of Psychology, Binghamton University, Binghamton, NY

Nancy D. Vogeltanz-Holm, PhD, Associate Professor, Department of Neuroscience, School of Medicine and Health Sciences, University of North Dakota, Grand Forks

Richard W. Wilsnack, PhD, Professor, Department of Neuroscience, School of Medicine and Health Sciences, University of North Dakota, Grand Forks

Sharon C. Wilsnack, PhD, Chester Fritz Distinguished Professor, Department of Neuroscience, School of Medicine and Health Sciences, University of North Dakota, Grand Forks

Gail E. Wyatt, PhD, Professor and Director, Sexual Health Program, Department of Psychiatry and Biobehavioral Sciences, University of California, Los Angeles

Eileen L. Zurbriggen, PhD, Assistant Professor, Department of Psychology, University of California, Santa Cruz

ACKNOWLEDGMENTS

This edited volume has been a collaborative effort of staff from the Centers for Disease Control and Prevention (CDC) and the National Institute of Mental Health (NIMH), U.S. Department of Health and Human Services. The coeditors thank participants at the November 1998, CDC/NIMH meeting on sexual abuse who helped shape our thinking about adult sexual outcomes of sexual abuse. We thank the more than 40 contributors from a variety of universities and disciplines who shared their extensive expertise throughout this book. Finally, we thank the many persons who have shared their sexual abuse experiences with researchers in order to help others. We hope their courage and the work of the many researchers in this volume will encourage clinicians and other practitioners to find new and innovative ways to treat persons who experience child sexual abuse.

I

INTRODUCTION

CHILD SEXUAL ABUSE AND ADULT SEXUAL RISK: WHERE ARE WE NOW?

LYNDA S. DOLL, LINDA J. KOENIG, AND DAVID W. PURCELL

Child sexual abuse (CSA), while not a new problem, has only received significant attention in both academic and public arenas within the last two decades. Heightened awareness of the problem may stem from a growing societal concern over child maltreatment in general, an increased comfort level in discussing sexual violence, or perhaps even the publicity surrounding several recent cases. Whatever the source, this attention has been accompanied by a growing recognition that children who experience sexual violence may be vulnerable to many negative life outcomes in the years following abuse.

Much of the research about abuse sequelae has addressed psychiatric morbidity and mental health. However, an emerging body of literature suggests that children who are abused also face increased risk of physical health problems in adulthood, including negative sexual and reproductive health consequences such as unwanted pregnancy, sexually transmitted diseases including HIV infection, and adult sexual violence. In this book, we bridge the current scientific literature about CSA, basic trauma research, and clinical practice to help practitioners and researchers meet the needs of this vulnerable population. We review evidence about the link between CSA and adult outcomes and draw on both theory and data to begin translating that knowledge into interventions for people who have experienced CSA.

This chapter was authored or coauthored by an employee of the United States government as part of official duty and is considered to be in the public domain. Any views expressed herein do not necessarily represent the views of the United States government.

3

Considerable effort has recently gone into determining the number of children who have experienced CSA (Haugaard, 2000). Even the most conservative estimates from these studies indicate that these rates have reached alarming proportions in the United States.

Overall, data from large or nationally representative samples suggest that 12% to 53% of girls and 3% to 16% of boys experience some form of sexual abuse during childhood (Finkelhor, Hotaling, Lewis, & Smith, 1990; Holmes & Slap, 1998; Molnar, Buka, & Kessler, 2001; Rind & Tromovitch, 1997). Rates appear higher when samples are gathered from convenience or other selected populations. For example, in their report, Holmes and Slap (1998) noted that prevalence rates among boys vary dramatically from 4% to 76% across studies. In a systematic review of data derived from 16 U.S. and Canadian studies published over 25 years, Gorey and Leslie (1997) estimated unadjusted prevalence rates of 23% among girls and 9% among boys across all studies. Twelve of the studies used random samples derived from the general population; four used convenience samples from captive audiences such as college students. More than two thirds of the aggregate sample from all studies was female.

Prevalence rates for girls are usually three to five times higher than for boys. However, cases among boys may be less likely to be reported, perhaps because such cases usually involve same-sex behavior that is more stigmatized by society (Boney-McCoy & Finkelhor, 1995). Sexual orientation is a key variable to consider when examining retrospective reports of CSA among adult men. Generally, men who have sex with men report a much higher prevalence than do heterosexual men (Doll et al., 1992; Lenderking et al., 1997; Paul, Catania, Pollack, & Stall, 2001). Rates typically range from 20% to 39%, similar to or only slightly higher than those reported in studies of general population women. Whereas most of the research showing elevated prevalence rates among men who have sex with men has used convenience samples, work by Paul et al. (2001) that used a more representative sample of this population recruited in four urban areas found similarly elevated rates. With a relatively stringent definition that included actual sexual contact as well as coercion, the prevalence rate was 21%.

Few studies have examined racial or ethnic differences in prevalence rates. Among those that have, some suggest that CSA is equally prevalent among Black and White girls (Cappelleri, Eckenrode, & Powers, 1993; Wyatt, 1985; Wyatt, Loeb, Solis, & Carmona, 1999); some studies show lower rates for girls from other racial and ethnic backgrounds (Cappelleri et al., 1993), whereas others show no differences (Romero, Wyatt, Loeb, Carmona, & Solis, 1999). In their review, Holmes and Slap (1998) found that more men of color reported experiencing CSA than did White men. Additional data suggest that gay men of color may be particularly likely to report such experiences during their childhood (Carballo-Diéguez & Dolezal, 1995; Doll et al., 1992).

Prevalence rates may also differ depending on the methodological rigor and the definition used for CSA in the studies. Gorey and Leslie (1997) estimated that prevalence rates were inversely associated with participant response rates. In the aggregated female sample derived from the studies Gorey and Leslie reviewed, estimated prevalence rates were two thirds higher (27.8%) in studies with responses rates below 60% than in studies with response rates of 60% or more (16.8%). Estimated rates were 15% and 7% for girls and boys, respectively, when a broad, noncontact definition of abuse was excluded from the calculations. After excluding noncontact abuse from the definition and taking into account the effect of differences in response rates, Gorey and Leslie provided general population prevalence estimates of 12% to 17% for girls and 5% to 8% for boys.

ADULT SEQUELAE OF CHILD SEXUAL ABUSE

The number of children experiencing sexual violence during childhood or adolescence is clearly alarming. Primary prevention efforts that focus on child safety, family functioning, and the characteristics of perpetrators must be enhanced to address these disturbing figures. Also important, and the primary focus of this book, is the number of children and adults who experience heightened vulnerability to a range of negative life outcomes, linked in part to these early sexual experiences. Increased rates of sexual revictimization (e.g., rape), sexual risk (e.g., multiple sexual partners, commercial sex work), and other forms of maltreatment (e.g., physical assault, crime victimization) have been found among people reporting CSA, as compared with those who have not reported such experiences (see chap. 2, this volume; Tjaden & Thoennes, 2000).

Moreover, research has consistently shown that CSA is one of the strongest predictors of adult sexual assault (chap. 2, this volume; Coid et al., 2001). The National Violence Against Women Survey found that 18% of the women raped before age 18 were also raped after the age of 18, compared with only 9% of women who did not report being raped when they were young (Tjaden & Thoennes, 2000). Data from 8,000 men ages 18 and older collected during this same survey showed that men who reported being sexually abused as children were nearly five times more likely to be sexually revictimized by a nonintimate partner than were those who did not report being sexually abused (Desai, Arias, Thompson, & Basile, 2002). Similarly, in a study of college students, Gidycz and colleagues (Gidycz, Coble, Latham, & Layman, 1993) found that 30% of female victims of childhood rape and 32% of female victims of attempted childhood rape were revictimized in adulthood. By comparison, only 14% of women with no history of CSA reported being raped during adulthood.

Also disturbing are the high rates of negative psychological, reproductive, and other health outcomes experienced by those reporting CSA. These negative outcomes include posttraumatic stress symptoms, drug abuse and dependency, unintended pregnancy, gynecological complications, and sexually transmitted diseases such as HIV infection (Bartholow et al., 1994; Bensley, Van Eenwyk, & Simmons, 2000; Doll et al., 1992; Molnar et al., 2001; Thompson, Arias, Basile, & Desai, 2002; see also chaps. 1 & 8, this volume). Such data confirm the argument that child, adolescent, and adult victims of sexual violence urgently need greater medical, psychological, and public health attention.

INTRODUCTION TO THE BOOK

The first goal of this book is to synthesize and bring attention to the growing scientific literature about sequelae of CSA, particularly sexual revictimization (e.g., experiencing sexual violence or rape with another person) and sexual risk (e.g., having multiple sexual partners, unprotected sexual intercourse). Toward this end, we bring together research from a variety of disciplines, including epidemiology, traumatology, and prevention science, to better understand the relationship between CSA and adult sexual risk and to explore opportunities for prevention. The book contains information that will be helpful to those working with people who have a history of CSA; however, overall, the book does not concentrate on clinical applications.

The book has three major parts, as well as an introduction and conclusion. Part II, Child Sexual Abuse and Sexual Risk in Adulthood, provides a foundation for the remaining two sections of the book by summarizing research about the relationship between CSA and a range of social, psychological, behavioral, and health outcomes. In chapter 1, Heiman and Heard-Davison summarize the association between CSA and adult sexual functioning and relationship problems. In chapter 2, Rich, Combs-Lane, Resnick, and Kilpatrick assess the complex relationship between CSA and adult sexual violence or revictimization. In chapter 3, Koenig and Clark explore the link between CSA and HIV infection in women. Finally, in chapter 4, Purcell, Malow, Dolezal, and Carballo-Diéguez describe the link between CSA of boys and adult functioning, including sexual risk behaviors.

Part III, Theoretical Bases for Adult Risk and Revictimization, describes cognitive, social, and behavioral processes that may mediate and potentially mitigate the relation between these child experiences and adult outcomes. Quina, Morokoff, Harlow, and Zurbriggen begin this section in chapter 5 with a focus on cognitive and attitudinal consequences of abuse and their role in adult risk behavior. In chapter 6, Zurbriggen and Freyd take a cognitive processing approach to the relation between CSA and adult sexual risk, focusing on the role of dissociative tendencies, information-processing effects, and consensual sex decision mechanisms. In chapter 7, Lynn, Pintar, Fite, Ecklund, and Stafford describe a social narrative model in which they argue that the key to revictimization is the social contexts in which the children lived and in which they continue to live as adults. In chapter 8, Wilsnack, Wilsnack, Kristjanson, Vogeltanz-Holm, and Harris explore alcohol use as a mediator between CSA and adult sexual risk. The section ends with chapter 9, by Pennebaker and Stone, who describe the importance of linguistic processing, such as occurs when traumatic experiences are translated into words and stories, in managing the effect associated with traumatic events such as CSA.

Part IV, Interventions to Promote Healthier Sexual Outcomes Among Child Sexual Abuse Survivors, describes a variety of therapeutic issues and interventions for adults. In chapter 10, Briere describes how HIV prevention can be incorporated into traditional psychotherapeutic treatment of sexual abuse trauma. Chin, Wyatt, Vargas Carmona, Loeb, and Myers then describe in chapter 11 preliminary qualitative findings from an evaluation of an integrative risk-reduction approach for HIV-seropositive women with CSA histories. In chapter 12, Spiegel, Classen, Thurston, and Butler describe two psychotherapeutic models that may ameliorate negative sequelae—one that focuses on memories of past abuse and another that focuses on present emotional and interpersonal experiences. Finally, in chapter 13, Blackwell, Lynn, Vanderhoff, and Gidycz review outcomes of sexual assault risk reduction programs, both for general population women and for women with histories of CSA. This book concludes with a chapter by O'Leary, Koenig, and Doll identifying future research directions.

As the book was being planned, the editors made several decisions about its focus. For example, until recently, research has generally investigated sexual abuse of girls. While researchers have broadened their work to include sexual abuse of boys, many of these studies have lacked methodological rigor (Holmes & Slap, 1998; Rind, Tromovitch, & Bauserman, 1998). Even today, some studies continue to combine data on girls and boys for analysis, despite growing evidence that gender differences may be particularly important in assessing outcomes (Rind et al., 1998). In this book we include a separate chapter about CSA and its sequelae among men and discuss limited data on men throughout other chapters. However, given the state of the science, this book emphasizes experiences of women, among whom prevalence rates are higher (Djeddah, Facchin, Ranzato, & Romer, 2000; chap. 2, this volume).

The body of well-designed studies on sexual abuse is growing. However, as readers will note throughout the book, the authors struggled with the variety of terms and methods used to assess the experiences (Goldman & Padayachi, 2000). For example, little consensus exists about how to define sexual abuse (Haugaard, 2000; Holmes & Slap, 1998; Neumann, Houskamp,

Pollock, & Briere, 1996; Rind & Tromovitch, 1997; Rind et al., 1998; Romano & De Luca, 2001). Definitions typically involve, to varying degrees, a focus on (a) the ages of the child and the perpetrator; (b) the behaviors of both, including the presence of force or coercion; and (c) the perception of the person that he or she was abused. Childhood may be defined as the period before puberty or before the age of 18. Abuse may include only penetrative or contact sexual experiences or may encompass a much broader set of behaviors. Additionally, study samples vary; they may include large, nationally representative samples, clinical samples, or samples drawn from law enforcement or social service agencies. Any one of these variations in definitions or samples may affect estimates of the prevalence of CSA and negative sequelae.

The Centers for Disease Control and Prevention (CDC) is leading an effort to define sexual violence to improve measurement of CSA (Basile & Saltzman, 2002). This should enhance our ability to assess outcomes of CSA and to monitor trends in prevalence rates (Saltzman, Fanslow, McMahon, & Shelley, 1999). For now, we encourage readers to conceptualize CSA on a continuum rather than in the typical dichotomous form (abused versus not). We also encourage readers to consider the relationship between adult sequelae and various components of the definition separately (e.g., age of child, whether force was used), where such data are available. Together these factors will allow readers to explore which aspects of the violence may be associated with subsequent outcomes.

As in many fields of research, there has been insufficient research looking at the nexus of risk faced by children who are sexually abused. Many of these children and youths are at risk for a range of negative events in their families and communities that independently, or along with the sexual abuse, may influence subsequent outcomes. Where studies are available, the authors in this book describe research that has attempted to parse out some of these relationships. However, readers are encouraged to remember these multiple influences as they consider the evidence provided in this book.

The methodological issues we have noted deserve further research attention. However, the urgency of the problem demands that we draw upon the research literature that exists today. This literature can yield initial recommendations for developing therapeutic treatments for those experiencing CSA. Suggestions for improving definitions and research designs should also emerge as the authors identify gaps in the literature or in their ability to interpret findings.

REFERENCES

Bartholow, B., Doll, L., Joy, D., Douglas, J., Bolan, G., Harrison, J., et al. (1994). Emotional, behavioral, and HIV risks associated with sexual abuse among adult homosexual and bisexual men. *Child Abuse and Neglect, 18,* 747–761.

Basile, K. C., & Saltzman, L. E. (2002). *Sexual violence surveillance: Uniform defini-tions and recommended data elements*. Atlanta, GA: National Center for Injury Prevention and Control, Centers for Disease Control and Prevention.

Bensley, L. S., Van Eenwyk, J., & Simmons, K. W. (2000). Self-reported childhood sexual and physical abuse and adult HIV-risk behaviors and heavy drinking. *American Journal of Preventive Medicine, 18,* 151–158.

Boney-McCoy, S., & Finkelhor, D. (1995). Prior victimization: A risk factor for child sexual abuse and for PTSD-related symptomatology among sexually abused youth. *Child Abuse and Neglect, 19,* 1401–1421.

Cappelleri, J. C., Eckenrode, J., & Powers, J. L. (1993). The epidemiology of child abuse: Findings from the Second National Incidence and Prevalence Study of Child Abuse and Neglect. *American Journal of Public Health, 83,* 1622–1624.

Carballo-Diéguez, A., & Dolezal, C. (1995). Association between history of child-hood sexual abuse and adult HIV-risk sexual behavior in Puerto Rican men who have sex with men. *Child Abuse and Neglect, 19,* 595–605.

Coid, J., Petruckevitch, A., Feder, G., Chung, W., Richardson, J., & Moorey, S. (2001). Relation between childhood sexual and physical abuse and risk of revictimization in women: A cross-sectional survey. *Lancet, 358,* 450–454.

Desai, S., Arias, I., Thompson, M. P., & Basile, K. C. (2002). Childhood victimiza-tion and subsequent adult revictimization assessed in a nationally representa-tive sample of women and men. *Violence and Victims, 17,* 639–653.

Djeddah, C., Facchin, P., Ranzato, C., & Romer, C. (2000). Child abuse: Current problems and key public health challenges. *Social Science and Medicine, 51,* 905–915.

Doll, L., Joy, D., Bartholow, B., Harrison, J., Bolan, G., Douglas, J., et al. (1992). Self-reported childhood and adolescent sexual abuse among adult homosexual and bisexual men. *Child Abuse and Neglect, 16,* 855–864.

Finkelhor, D., Hotaling, G., Lewis, I., & Smith, C. (1990). Sexual abuse in a na-tional survey of adult men and women: Prevalence, characteristics, and risk factors. *Child Abuse and Neglect, 14,* 19–28.

Gidycz, C. A., Coble, C. N., Latham, L., & Layman, M. J. (1993). Sexual assault experiences in adulthood and prior victimization experiences. *Psychology of Women Quarterly, 17,* 151–168.

Goldman, J. D., & Padayachi, U. K. (2000). Some methodological problems in esti-mating incidence and prevalence in child sexual abuse research. *Journal of Sex Research, 37,* 305–314.

Gorey, K. M., & Leslie, D. R (1997). The prevalence of child sexual abuse: Integra-tive review adjustment for potential response and measurement biases. *Child Abuse and Neglect, 21,* 391–398.

Haugaard, J. (2000). The challenge of defining child sexual abuse. *American Psy-chologist, 55,* 1036–1039.

Holmes, W. C., & Slap, G. B. (1998). Sexual abuse of boys: Definition, prevalence, correlates, sequelae, and management. *Journal of the American Medical Associa-tion, 280,* 1855–1862.

Lenderking, W. R., Wold, C., Mayer, K. H., Goldstein, R., Losina, E., & Seage, G. R. (1997). Childhood sexual abuse among homosexual men: Prevalence and association with unsafe sex. *Journal of General Internal Medicine, 12,* 250–253.

Molnar, B. E., Buka, S. L., & Kessler, R. C. (2001). Child sexual abuse and subsequent psychopathology: Results from the National Comorbidity Survey. *American Journal of Public Health, 91,* 753–760.

Neumann, D. A., Houskamp, B. M., Pollock, V. E., & Briere, J. (1996). The long-term sequelae of childhood sexual abuse in women: A meta-analytic review. *Child Maltreatment, 1,* 6–16.

Paul, J. P., Catania, J., Pollack, L., & Stall, R. (2001). Understanding childhood sexual abuse as a predictor of sexual risk-taking among men who have sex with men: The Urban Men's Health Study. *Child Abuse and Neglect, 25,* 557–584.

Rind, B., & Tromovitch, P. (1997). A meta-analytic review of findings from national samples on psychological correlates of child sexual abuse. *Journal of Sex Research, 34,* 237–255.

Rind, B., Tromovitch, P., & Bauserman, R. (1998). A meta-analytic examination of assumed properties of child sexual abuse using college samples. *Psychological Bulletin, 124,* 22–53.

Romano, E., & De Luca, R. V. (2001). Male sexual abuse: A review of effects, abuse characteristics, and links with later psychological functioning. *Aggression and Violent Behavior, 6,* 55–78.

Romero, G. J., Wyatt, G. E., Loeb, T. B., Carmona, H. V., & Solis, B. M. (1999). The prevalence and circumstances of child sexual abuse among Latina women. *Hispanic Journal of Behavioral Sciences, 21,* 351–365.

Saltzman, L. E., Fanslow, J. L., McMahon, P. M., & Shelley, G. A. (1999). *Intimate partner violence surveillance.* Atlanta, GA: Centers for Disease Control and Prevention.

Thompson, M. P., Arias, I., Basile, K. C., & Desai, S. (2002). The association between childhood physical and sexual victimization and health problems in adulthood in a nationally representative sample of women. *Journal of Interpersonal Violence, 17,* 1115–1129.

Tjaden, P., & Thoennes, N. (2000). *Full report of the prevalence, incidence, and consequences of violence against women* (Research Report No. NCJ 183781). Washington, DC: U.S. Department of Justice.

Wyatt, G. E. (1985). The sexual abuse of Afro-American and White-American women in childhood. *Child Abuse and Neglect, 9,* 507–519.

Wyatt, G. E., Loeb, T. B., Solis, B., & Carmona, J. V. (1999). The prevalence and circumstances of child sexual abuse: Changes across a decade. *Child Abuse and Neglect, 23,* 45–60.

II

CHILD SEXUAL ABUSE AND SEXUAL RISK IN ADULTHOOD

1

CHILD SEXUAL ABUSE AND ADULT SEXUAL RELATIONSHIPS: REVIEW AND PERSPECTIVE

JULIA R. HEIMAN AND AMY R. HEARD-DAVISON

Sexual behavior is integral to the experience of child sexual abuse (CSA). However, subsequent sexuality has been less commonly studied than other aspects of psychological, physical, and social functioning. Methodological factors, funding priorities, cultural sensitivities, and political exigencies all contribute to the uneven knowledge distribution. This chapter summarizes the research that has attempted to deal with the correlation between CSA and later sexual function, adjustment, satisfaction, and relationship problems and to place these findings in a perspective of a past and future research agenda.

The sources for this review are English-language articles found through Medline and PsycLIT, plus a review of several journals not included on these search engines, with a particular focus on research since 1985. Search words included *sexual abuse-dysfunction, sexuality, adult function, pain, pelvic pain,* and *arousal.* In addition, reference lists from review articles were examined for relevant articles. Twenty-six articles with information about adult sexual functioning were included. Because the focus was on sexual functioning, we did not include studies that exclusively presented data on the outcome variables of prostitution, sexual risk-taking, or revictimization.

We summarize issues raised in this literature regarding theory, methods, and results. Our primary emphasis is on the results of those studies that are based on representative sampling techniques or that included comparison groups. We also discuss some sexual relationship factors such as relationship durability and pregnancy. Although we focus primarily on adult sexual functioning and satisfaction, we comment briefly on child and adolescent sexuality because we view sexuality and adjustment as requiring a developmental framework. We also focus on women because of the limited data for men on this topic and studies indicating that reactions by men are more frequently neutral or positive (Bauserman & Rind, 1997). Where there are comparisons with men in the same study, we discuss them. Human sexuality happens in the context of being human. Although we do not have the space here to provide a more integrated look at how psychosocial and physical functioning interact with sexual adjustment, they are present to an extent that interpretations of results from studies attempting to isolate sexual functioning are often inconclusive. Some illustrations of this are presented.

The chapter begins by presenting terminology and methodological issues across both CSA and sexuality. We then discuss several theoretical frameworks, review studies that have examined correlations between CSA and adult sexual health, and examine contextual variables affecting sexuality. We have organized the research in both the text and a table (see later) by study method and sampling, beginning with meta-analyses, and then national probability, college, self-selected, and clinical and forensic samples.

TERMINOLOGY AND METHODOLOGICAL CAVEATS

We distinguish CSA from child sexual behavior. Child sexual abuse is defined according to the key elements identified in research studies. Although a standard definition is lacking, and some researchers have included noncontact sexual activity and verbal comments, the more common elements of CSA are coercive or manipulative sexual contact, during the period when a victim is legally considered a child and the perpetrator occupying a position of relative power with respect to the child (Paolucci, Genuis, & Violato, 2001; Rind, Tromovich, & Bauserman, 1998). Child sexual behavior is defined as developmentally appropriate (clearly subject to different interpretations), noncoercive, between individuals of similar ages or incidental nudity between family members. However, some of the literature collapses all child sexual behaviors into "abuse," suspected precursors of abuse, or evidence of abuse proneness (e.g., young children taking showers with adult family members). This is part of the confusion of the current epoch of research in this area. Definitional disagreements are reflective of strong personal–cultural opinions regarding what constitutes normative, healthy childhood sexuality. We can expect these definitions to change over time as well as across cultures. Current definitional imprecision limits our ability to form firm conclusions about the universality, pervasiveness, and durability of CSA correlates for women and men (Goldman & Padayachi, 2000; Roosa, Reyes, Reinholtz, & Angelini, 1998).

Methodological challenges beyond definitional consistency of CSA and normal child sexuality have been noted in general and in studies on adult adjustment more specifically (Briere, 1992; Rind & Tromovitch, 1997; Rind et al., 1998). Of note to the area of CSA and adult sexuality are several particularly troublesome issues: (a) the definition of normative sexual functioning, behavior, and relationships; (b) sampling strategies; (c) the availability of reliable or standardized measures of CSA, physical abuse, and particularly sexual behavior and functioning; and (d) the enduring problem of a reliance on the correlational nature of the data.

Thus, although we cite background prevalence rates, we do so cautiously as the range of rates may be the most accurate indicator. As one can see from Goldman and Padayachi (2000, Table 1, pp. 308–309), rates of CSA depend on the sample selected, gender, definitions of CSA, and type of abuse. With definitional caveats in mind, a few background comments regarding prevalence establish a basis for examining the sexuality data. Between 4% and 50% of children and adolescents have been reported to have experienced CSA, with an average prevalence of 15% to 20% (Goldman & Padayachi, 2000; Violato & Genuis, 1993). Contact sexual abuse is always reported at lower frequencies, and males are consistently reported to be less often the objects of CSA (Goldman & Padayachi, 2000).

Sexual health can include sexual behavior, sexual functioning, sexual satisfaction, and reproduction. We focus on sexual functioning and satisfaction, with less attention to sexual behavior and reproduction. In this chapter, sexual behavior refers to specific sexual activities, whereas sexual functioning is used to describe the experience of sexual desire, sexual responsiveness, or genital pain. Sexual satisfaction is a subjective term that generally indicates whether an individual is happy with his or her sexual activity and response.

Clinically, sexual dysfunction and sexual problems are not synonymous because problems are subjectively defined by the person experiencing them and dysfunction indicates that a specific sexual diagnosis has been identified, as defined by the *Diagnostic and Statistical Manual of Mental Disorders* (4th ed., Text Revision; *DSM–IV–TR*; American Psychiatric Association, 2000) or the International Consensus Committee (Basson et al., 2000). It is important to note that in order for a diagnosis to be assigned, a person must report dissatisfaction with her or his sexual functioning. Sexual dysfunction and sexual problem prevalence estimates have also been problematic to define and determine. Recent research indicates that sexual problems are highly prevalent in both sexes, with community samples estimating ranges from 10% to 52% of men and 25% to 63% of women (Feldman, Goldstein, Hatzichristou, Krane, & McKinlay, 1994; Frank, Anderson, & Rubenstein, 1978; Rosen, Taylor, Leiblum, & Bachmann, 1993; Spector & Carey, 1990). The National Health and Social Life Survey, a 1992 national probability sample of 1,410 men and 1,749 women between the ages of 18 and 59 years living in U.S. households, comprises our best estimate of sexual problems in the United States (Laumann, Gagnon, Michael, & Michaels, 1994; Laumann, Paik, & Rosen, 1999). In the analyses that included only those individuals who reported any sexual activity with a partner in the prior 12-month period, the prevalence of sexual dysfunction was 43% for women and 31% for men (Laumann et al., 1999). Although this study did not use the *DSM* criteria (American Psychiatric Association, 1994, 2000), and thus does not connote clinical dysfunction, it provides an estimate of potential sexual dysfunction. Nevertheless, because these are not formal clinical diagnostic categories they may overestimate prevalence (e.g., Simons & Carey, 2001), or, because the Laumann et al. (1999) figures exclude the 139 men and 238 women who were sexually inactive in the past year, these estimates could also be conservative.

THEORETICAL MODELS

Although researchers have struggled to create models that might explain the impact of abuse, an encompassing theoretical structure is lacking. This is particularly the case in the area of sexual functioning and satisfaction. Here we briefly summarize the theoretical positions and comment as they relate to sexuality.

The most prevalent, one could say the dominant, theoretical position in the CSA literature is a *trauma model*. This model takes the CSA experience and looks for the traumatic elements and evidence that fit the outcomes of a trauma experience. The majority of the posttraumatic stress disorder (PTSD) literature is a result of this view. In a recent meta-analysis of risk factors for PTSD in trauma-exposed adults, Brewin, Andrews, and Valentine (2000) noted that family psychiatric history and child abuse had more uniform predictive effects on adult response to trauma, but the effect sizes were small. Although their analyses were based on adult trauma, their conclusions may be relevant to CSA. They suggested that pretrauma factors either are mediated by responses to the trauma or interact with trauma severity or trauma response to increase the risk of PTSD. Indeed there is a body of research suggesting that the environment of the child who experiences CSA may be troubled by family stress, parental dysfunction, parent–child conflict, and other types of abuse that could serve as pretrauma factors that increase the risk for symptoms (e.g., Wind & Silvern, 1994). The advantage to the trauma model is that the literature is substantial and includes links to mechanisms of emotion, conditioning, and memory that can be informed by cognitive neuroscience methods (e.g., Pitman, Shalev, & Orr, 2000). The disadvantage of the trauma model is that it does not clearly explain the CSA that is not at the time experienced as traumatic or cases in which PTSD symptoms do not result. CSA seems to be a more heterogeneous experience than witnessing murder or battle violence and involves sexuality that has different biological underpinnings and demands for individuals.

There has been some attempt to use an *attachment model* to examine CSA effects. The capacity for a child to develop a secure attachment to an adult may be impaired in an environment in which CSA occurs and remains hidden. Howes, Cicchetti, Toth, and Rogosch (2000) located attachment concepts in a family systems perspective and found that sexual abuse families had more difficulty regulating anger, were more chaotic with less role clarity, and relied less on adaptive and flexible styles of relating than did families without CSA. Attachment is a conceptualization of how individuals form "internal working models" of themselves in relationship to others. Learning about sexuality as a child, if it includes the elements of coercion, fear, threat of unwanted exposure, disloyalty, and even pain, could be seen as contributing to disrupted, neglectful, or abusive adult relationships. Even without these elements one can imagine early sexual exposure in the context of the family environment contributing to the ease of earlier and more frequent sexual experiences noted in the data above. An attachment model has the advantage of being both biological and interpersonal and, unlike the trauma model, is not a pathology-based system. However, the methods for measurement are somewhat limited, and we could locate no research on attachment, adult sexuality, and CSA.

A *developmental perspective* is implied in the attachment and systems approach. It is also suggested by the limited but intriguing data on brain development from developmental neuroscience (Thompson & Nelson, 2001). Yet there is almost no information on the course of normal childhood sexual development. An understanding of possible impacts of CSA, as well as of consensual and desired sexual activity such as sex play, on attachment and relationship choices requires a consideration of the content of the sexual experience, its frequency, the relationship between the individuals involved, the family context, and the subsequent experiences that have further shaped a child's development. We are missing this information as it applies to sexual development, in part because of the sociocultural hesitancy, particularly in the United States, to believe children can be sexual and to ask questions of them about their sexuality.

Elsewhere, we have suggested a more general model based on *evolutionary theory* (Heiman, Verhulst, & Heard-Davison, in press) to attempt to begin to conceptualize the wide range in sexual outcomes associated with a CSA history. One can assume that evolution will select for *effective sexual functioning* as an adaptive outcome because sexual functioning fosters reproduction and may even contribute to stability in the nurturance of the offspring. The question is: What are the means that were selected by evolution to ensure that effective sexual functioning is a likely outcome of sexual development? Indeed, development is the result of extremely complex and continuous interactions among genetic, epigenetic, and environmental factors, and there must be numerous pathways and variables that affect the outcome. Genetically determined propensities, such as arousal ease, orgasmic ease, and latency, or sexual desire, are probably distributed according to a bell-shaped curve. Developmental experiences may either complement or interfere with these propensities. However, effective sexual functioning is an outcome that tends to override developmental experiences and cultural proscriptions that interfere with it, as has been demonstrated by the variable effectiveness of restricted religious teachings and legal barriers. Thus the multiple pathways of development toward an outcome of effective sexual functioning help to ensure that sexual abuse will not necessarily lead to impaired sexual desire and response.

Each of these perspectives could be used to attempt to deal with the variability in the data on adult sexuality and to inform effective treatment. It is unlikely that these models are mutually exclusive, therefore early, multimodal intervention (both individual and systemic) is likely to be the most helpful in managing symptoms and altering long-term response. Assessment of family functioning and medical and psychiatric history may facilitate detection of children at risk for more negative outcomes (sexually, physically, psychosocially, and psychologically). For children and adolescents, effective cognitive–behavioral treatments for PTSD provide education about abuse, skills training in relaxation, assertiveness and self-talk, and graded exposure using a variety of modalities (King et al., 2000). This method is consistent with a trauma model in that it would provide them with exposure to any traumatic elements of the experience and reduce PTSD symptoms. For children whose response was neutral or even positive, a similar process could develop skills that may be helpful for dealing with subsequent issues and should enable them to express and assimilate their feelings without creating negative associations retrospectively. Family and broader system interventions could address some of the attachment issues (even if the abuse was extrafamilial) by clearly defining boundaries and role expectations for family members and other authority figures and by giving children appropriate power in relationships with adults to make requests and express their feelings. Each of the models indicate that intervention at intermittent time points would allow for an assessment of symptoms specific to subsequent developmental stages and an exploration of how the CSA experience is influencing functioning. It also would potentially provide normalization of developmental experiences and foster realistic expectations that may help to increase relationship and sexual satisfaction.

A QUANTITATIVE OVERVIEW: META-ANALYTIC REVIEWS

From the three more recent meta-analytic reviews of adult correlates of CSA, we find evidence of small effect sizes for sexual variables. One of them, Rind and Tromovitch (1997), only included seven national samples, and little was discussed relevant to specific sexual adjustment.

In their review of 59 college samples, including 36 published studies, 21 unpublished doctoral dissertations, and 2 unpublished master's theses, Rind et al. (1998) were able to locate 20 study samples ($N = 7,723$) that measured sexual adjustment variables. Studies selected spanned 1966 to 1995. Their variable of sexual adjustment was a composite of a range of measures used across studies (see Rind et al., 1998, p. 28). The effect sizes for sexual adjustment were $r_u = .09$; 95% confidence interval (CI) = .07–.11, in the small range according to Cohen's (1988) guidelines (r_u = unbiased effect size estimate). These effect sizes were similar to those for the 17 other symptoms (e.g., anxiety, depression, alcohol abuse, dissociation) reviewed. In addition, Rind et al. found gender differences. Female participants were more likely than male participants to evaluate their CSA experiences as negative (72% vs. 33%), current reflections on CSA experiences were more often reported as negative for female (59%) than male (26%) participants, and self-reported negative effects on current sex lives or attitudes were (unweighted means) 13.5% for female and 8.5% for male participants. (The latter two analyses used relatively small samples to estimate effects.) Thus, by self-report, the effects on current sexual lives are reported modest by both sexes but higher for women. Another important finding was the correlation of CSA with problems in the home environment, with family environment emerging as a more important predictor of symptoms than CSA. In the case of sexual adjustment as a function of family environment, $r = .23$; 95% CI = .15–.29 (based on three samples and 653 participants). In addition to gender, level of consent and the occurrence of incest each moderated symptoms, but force, penetration, duration, frequency, and contact versus noncontact did not. However, the lack of moderator variable effects may be a reflection of the small sample sizes available for these subanalyses or the imprecision of the measures.

Paolucci and colleagues (Paolucci et al., 2001) examined 37 studies published between 1981 and 1995 and tested two types of sexual variables: sexual promiscuity and sexual acts toward others (which they called the *victim–perpetrator cycle*). Sexual promiscuity was defined as early involvement in sexual activity or prostitution and included 14 studies ($N = 4,386$), and sexual acts toward others was defined as acts of sexual victimization directed against others following CSA. Average weighted effect sizes, using Glass's delta, were .29 (95% CI = .25–.32) for sexual promiscuity and .16 (95% CI = .11–.21) for sexual acts toward others. These correspond to medium to small effect sizes, respectively, and were lower than the deltas for depression (.44), suicide (.44), and PTSD (.40). Paolucci et al. estimated that a CSA history added a minimum of 14% increase in sexual promiscuity and 8% increase in the victim–perpetrator cycle. Unlike Rind et al. (1998), they found no mediating effects of gender, socioeconomic status, abuse type, age of abuse occurrence, relationship to abuser, and number of incidents of abuse on the above symptoms. Paolucci et al. suggested that the failure to find significant differences may be a reflection of crudeness and imprecision of the data.

In summary, from a meta-analytic point of view, variously defined adult sexual "symptoms" (problems) or "adjustment" (functioning) are correlated with CSA histories, showing modest effect sizes. Discrepancies in meta-analytic findings could be accounted for by selection criteria and by samples used, with Rind et al. (1998) using what we presume to be the more homogeneous and higher functioning college samples. Yet we have little information about the specific sexual issues or problems that might make up the composite variable markers used in these studies. Differences in the operational definitions for sexual problems and functioning between studies may affect results and make identification of relationships more challenging. We turn now to look at sexual correlates in greater specificity.

CHILD SEXUAL ABUSE AND SEXUAL PROBLEMS, FUNCTIONING, AND DISSATISFACTION

Summary of Child Sexual Abuse and Childhood Sexuality

Researchers comparing sexually abused children with nonabused comparison samples have found that abused children are more symptomatic on many variables, including fear, PTSD, mental illness, cruelty, tantrums, enuresis, encopresis, self-injurious behavior, low self-esteem, and inappropriate sexual behavior (Beitchman, Zucker, Hood, daCosta, & Akman, 1991; Conte & Schuerman, 1987; Friedrich, Urquiza, & Beilke, 1986; Kendall-Tackett, Williams, & Finkelhor, 1993). When comparisons have been made between sexually abused children and other clinical nonabused samples, sexually abused children were less symptomatic than clinical samples in most of the studies. However, in their review of 45 studies, Kendall-Tackett et al. (1993) found that the abused children consistently showed more sexual behavior problems and greater levels of PTSD symptoms, although there was no specific syndrome and no single traumatizing process. These authors noted that the most commonly studied symptom among preschool-age and school-age children was sexualized behavior. Sexual abuse status accounted for 43% of the variance of sexualized behavior and, along with aggression, had the highest effect size (to be viewed with caution because only 5–6 studies were available for effect size calculations).

Because of developmental differences in sexuality, sexual outcomes of CSA have been found to differ by age group (Kendall-Tackett et al., 1993).

However, this finding may be due in part to differences in the types of behaviors that are measured for younger children and adolescents. In their review, none of the studies reported on promiscuity in school-age children, and only one reported on inappropriate sexual behavior in adolescents. Another factor that may affect measured symptoms and may vary between children and adolescents is time from abuse. Whereas most symptoms improved over time, sexual preoccupation has been shown to increase (Kendall-Tackett et al., 1993). Sexualized behavior has mostly been identified in preschool-age samples and typically included excessive or public masturbation, seductive behavior, sexualized play with dolls, placing objects in vaginas or anuses, requesting sexual stimulation, and age-inappropriate sexual knowledge (Beitchman et al., 1991). In adolescence, sexualized behavior was expressed in the forms of promiscuity, sexual aggression, or prostitution.

The study of CSA in children is hampered by the lack of consensus regarding definitions of CSA, report reliability checks, and consistent measures of individual and family functioning. With these limitations in mind, we can briefly summarize several patterns noted in the literature (Kendall-Tackett et al., 1993; Rind et al., 1998): (a) Psychiatric symptoms may be related to the presence of penetration, force, duration, and frequency of abuse; the perpetrator's relationship to the child; and maternal support. (b) Sexual behavior problems occurred in 26%–38% of children and adolescents; about two thirds show no evidence of sexual problems. (c) About one third of victims are generally asymptomatic. (d) About two thirds of victims show recovery within 12–18 months; approximately 10%–25% may get worse. (e) There is no evidence of a specific syndrome or traumatizing process from CSA.

Child Sexual Abuse and Adult Sexuality

Table 1.1 presents a summary of relevant empirical studies, including the type of sample used, characteristics of the CSA and control groups studied, measures administered, and relevant findings. These factors are subsequently discussed by type of population studied.

National Probability Samples

Of the national probability sample studies not including exclusively college samples, only two have included specific *sexual problems* (Laumann et al., 1999; Mullen, Martin, Anderson, Romans, & Herbison, 1994). These studies show that a greater incidence of some sexual problems is correlated with a CSA history. Specifically, Laumann et al. (1999) found that women who were touched before puberty were more likely to report sexual arousal (including orgasm) problems in the past year. It is interesting to note that men with the same history were more likely to report premature ejaculation, erectile dysfunction, or low sexual desire over the past year. Data from Mullen

TABLE 1.1

Summary of Research of Child Sexual Abuse and Adult Sexual and Relationship Functioning in Women

Study	Sample	Group (CSA & CG)	Measure	Sexual dysfunction/Relationships
			National probability	
Laumann, Paik, and Rosen (1999)	National probability Female = 1,749 Male = 1,410 Ages 18–59	CSA: N varied depending on dysfunction and risk factor measured. CG: Female = 58% no sexual problems Male = 70% no sexual problems	CSA: In-person interview Sexual Fx: 7 dichotomous response items	Women with a history of sexual touching before puberty had an increased likelihood of arousal disorders [OR* = 1.73 (1.11–2.71)]. Women with a history of being sexually forced by a man had an increased likelihood of low desire [OR* = 1.45 (0.98–2.12)] and arousal disorders [OR* = 1.31 (1.31–3.07)]. Men reporting prepubertal sexual touching had an increased likelihood of premature ejaculation [OR* = 1.80 (1.12–2.90)], erectile dysfunction [OR* = 3.13 (1.49–6.59)], and low desire [OR* = 2.23 (1.10–4.56)].
Fergusson, Horwood, and Lynskey (1997)	National probability Longitudinal N = 520 female Age 18	CSA: 90 female 22 = noncontact 39 = contact 29 = SI CG: 430 Female no report of CSA	CSA: Interview at age 18 Sexual Fx: Interview (longitudinal)	The relationship between pregnancy, sexually transmitted infections, and sexual assault history was accounted for by other family characteristics. Greater severity of CSA (contact, intercourse) related to multiple sexual behaviors (>5 partners, unprotected SI, first SI before 16, and revictimization. CSA–sexual behavior relationship mediated by age at first consensual SI.

| Mullen, Martin, Anderson, Romans, and Herbison (1994) | National probability $N = 1,376$ UK-representative of population except for Ages 18–20 | CSA: 248 female
CSA prior to age 16
CG: 248 female Randomly selected from 716 without CSA | CSA and sexual Fx: Interview |

Sexual Functioning

NSD in mean age of first intercourse, sexual activity in the previous 6 months or in frequency of SI.

NSD in attribution of sexual problems to physical complaints.

CSA with SI cases were more likely to engage in consensual intercourse under age 16 (23.3% vs. 4.4% controls and 8.4 % all CSA cases).

CSA cases were more likely to report one or more current sexual problem (47.2% vs. 28.4%), 67.8% among CSA with SI cases.

CSA cases were less satisfied with their sexual lives and with frequency of SI, and were more likely to believe their own or their partners' attitudes about sex would cause problems than were controls.

CSA with SI cases were more likely to complain of too much sexual activity but not too little.

CSA, especially CSA with SI, was associated with increased odds for a number of social/relationship and sexual problems including decreased satisfaction with sexual activity and relationships.

Sexual Relationships

NSD between controls and CSA for involvement in close relationships, marriage, or cohabitating.

CSA with SI cases were less likely to be living with a partner (53.1% vs. 73.3%). CSA cases were more likely to cohabitate before age 20 (27.8% vs. 14.7%) and to separate or divorce (11.9% vs. 4.0%), to

continues

TABLE 1.1 (Continued)

Study	Sample	Group (CSA & CG)	Measure	Sexual dysfunction/ Relationships
				become pregnant prior to age 19 (15.9% vs. 6.7%) with 31.3% of CSA with SI pregnant prior to age 19 and 26.9% pregnant prior to marriage. Relationship satisfaction was high among 72.4% of controls and 54.7% of CSA cases (lowest for CSA with INT). CSA cases also saw their partners as less caring and more controlling than controls.
Finkelhor, Hotaling, Lewis, and Smith (1989)	National probability $N = 2,630$ Female = 1,485 Male = 1,145 Ages 18+	CSA: Female = 27% of sample Male = 16% of sample CG: No report of CSA	CSA and sexual Fx: Phone interview	Victims who had experienced abuse involving SI reported significantly more marital disruption (23% male, 35% female) and decreased relationship satisfaction compared with individuals with no history of abuse or abuse that did not involve actual or attempted SI. Discriminant analyses indicated CSA SI predicted sexual dissatisfaction in women (not men) and of marital disruption in men and women.
Russell (1986)	National probability $N = 930$ female Ages 18–85+	CSA: 260 female (incest) 479 female (nonfamily) 297 = prior to age 18 CG: 191 female No report of CSA	CSA and sexual Fx: In-person interview	Incest cases: younger age at first child and > to be divorced or separated. Severity of abuse predicted marital and reproductive health (single mother, separation/divorce, early childbearing-19 or younger). Incest duration predicted revictimization. 2% incest cases were described as positive or neutral, but not all women reported negative long-term effects and not all instances of abuse were perceived as traumatic.

College

Study	Sample	Measures	Findings
Meston, Heiman, Trapnell, and Carlin (1999)	College $N = 1,032$ Female = 656 Male = 376 Asian and non-Asian Ages 18–30	Abuse not limited to CSA (also physical/emotional abuse) Female = 65% of sample Male = 22% of sample CG: No report of abuse	CSA and sexual Fx: Standardized and specialized questionnaires	CSA in women was significantly positively correlated with intercourse, frequency of intercourse, variety of sexual experience, unrestricted sexual behavior, frequency of masturbation, variety of sexual fantasy, liberal sexual attitudes, unrestricted sexual attitudes, and fantasies. CSA was negatively correlated with sexual drive. CSA in women was unrelated to sexual satisfaction and orientation. CSA in men was unrelated to any of the sexuality variables.
Jackson, Calhoun, Amick, Maddever, and Habif (1990)	College $N = 40$	CSA: 22 female Age $M = 23.14$ CG: 18 female Age $M = 21.94$ No report of CSA	CSA and sexual Fx: 1-Standardized questionnaires 2-Semistructured interview	CSA victims had poorer body images: Derogatis Sexual function inventory Body Image Scale, $F(1, 32) = 6.97, p < .01$. CSA reported less satisfaction with sexual functioning: Sexual Satisfaction Scale, $F(1, 32) = 10.49, p < .01$; Global Sexual Satisfaction Index, $F(1, 32) = 8.35, p < .01$. 65% of CSA victims met *DSM–III* criteria for Female Sexual Dysfunction: 50% inhibited desire, 45% inhibited orgasm, 35% inhibited sexual excitement, 25% dyspareunia, 10% vaginismus.
Fromuth (1986)	College $N = 383$ (complete questionnaires of 482)	CSA: 106 female CG: 376 female (of original 482)	CSA: 1-Standardized questionnaires 2-Rating scale Sexual Fx:	NSD between CSA and no-CSA groups for age began dating; pregnancy, abortion, age first intercourse, intercourse frequency, sexual self-esteem, and sexual adjustment.

continues

TABLE 1.1 (Continued)

Study	Sample	Group (CSA & CG)	Measure	Sexual dysfunction/ Relationships
	Age $M = 19.41$	No report of CSA	1-Specialized questionnaire 2-Rating scale	Low/high extremes in dating orgasmic capacity and sexual desire were not related to CSA. CSA did not provide additional prediction beyond the measure of family background for whether participants had engaged in SI. CSA predicted more than 10 incidents of noncoital sexual behavior in past month, $r(383) = .13$, $p < .01$. CSA victims were more likely to describe themselves as promiscuous, $r(383) = .13$, $p < .01$, despite no differences in number of partners. Masturbation was correlated with history CSA, $r(383) = .14$, $p < .01$. Homosexual experience was related to CSA, $r(383) = .12$, $p < .05$. CSA predicted an increased likelihood of being raped over and above what was predicted by the Parental Support Scale, $F(1, 380) = 7.72$, $p < .01$.
Finkelhor (1984)	College $N = 806$ Age NR	CSA: $N = 121$ (104 female; 17 male) CG: $N = 685$ (243 female; 432 male) No report of CSA	CSA: Specialized questionnaire Sexual Fx: Standardized questionnaire	Both female and male CSA cases scored lower on Sexual Self-Esteem Scale. Men who were abused in childhood by much older men were more likely to report homosexual experiences. A trend was found for the relationship between CSA < 13 and revictimization (32% vs. 22% if CSA ≥ 13, $p = .07$).

Study	Population	Sample	Measures	Findings
Fritz, Stoll, and Wagner (1981)	College N = 952 Age NR	CSA: N = 62 (42 female; 20 male) CG: N = 890 (498 female; 392 male) No report of CSA	CSA and sexual Fx: Specialized questionnaire	Women reported their experiences as more negative whereas men were neutral or positive. Adult female victims were less likely to achieve orgasm with SI and to have their first postpubescent sexual experience in a serious relationship than adult male victims.
Finkelhor (1979)	College N = 796 Female = 530 Male = 266 Age 75% ≤ 21	CSA: N = 264 (19% female; 8.6% male) CG: N = 532 No report of CSA	CSA and sexual Fx: Questionnaire	CSA cases scored lower on the Sexual Self-Esteem Scale.
Self-selected				
Meston and Heiman (2000)	Self-selected N = 118	CSA: 61 female Age 20–40 CG: N = 57 female Age 21–38	CSA: Standardized questionnaires Sexual Fx: Card sort task (to determine association networks)	Network averages among sexuality-relevant words were different between CSA cases and non-CSA cases. CSA cases viewed the concepts of intercourse and lovemaking as less related than non-CSA cases. Findings are discussed in terms of information-processing theory and differences in how sexual information may be organized between women with and without a history of CSA.

continues

TABLE 1.1 (Continued)

Study	Sample	Group (CSA & CG)	Measure	Sexual dysfunction/ Relationships
Pistorello and Follette (1998)	Self-selected (for 12-week therapy groups) $N = 55$	CSA: 55 female (82% incest) Ages 19–52 No CG	CSA: Standardized questionnaires Sexual Fx: Interview	(Qualitative/descriptive study) Videotapes were coded into 23 categories of themes with the following content: sex-related (history guilt, avoidance, control), survivor-specific (lack of boundaries, blaming survivor's history, excess/lack of control), partner-specific (partner personal difficulties, partner reaction to treatment), relationship-specific (abusive style, difficulties with emotional communication/intimacy), and attitudinal (negative attitudes). Trauma symptoms were correlated with sex avoidance ($r = .44$) and sex history guilt ($r = .42$). The Sexual Abuse Trauma Index was correlated with the total number of couples' issues brought up in the course of group therapy ($r = .48$). Longer duration ($r = .57$) and earlier onset ($r = -.39$) of CSA were both correlated with the total number of problems with emotion/intimacy, and issues of control (excess or lack) were correlated with believing the nonoffending parent was aware of but did nothing to stop the abuse ($r = .43$).

Study	Sample	Measures	Findings
Wenninger and Heiman (1998)	Self-selected $N = 104$ Age $M = 31$	CSA: 57 female CG: 47 female No report of CSA	CSA: Specialized questionnaires Sexual Fx and body image: Standardized questionnaires	CSA cases rated themselves as lower on sexual attractiveness and reported more sexual aversion, less subjective arousal, and fewer signs of physiological sexual arousal and more lifetime sexual partners. There also was a trend toward more pain during sexual activity ($p = .06$).
Greenwald, Leitenberg, Cado, and Tarran (1990)	Self-selected (nurses) $N = 108$ (Low response rate)	CSA (<15 years old): 54 female Ages 23–61 CG: 54 female (of 113) Ages 22–59 No report of CSA	CSA and sexual Fx: Standardized and specialized questionnaires	No differences were found between participants with and without a history of CSA on measures of sexual satisfaction or dysfunction (including differences in sexual desire and sexual aversion, arousal problems, pain, and orgasm difficulties).
Feinauer (1989)	Self-selected $N = 57$	CSA: 57 female Age $M = 37$ No CG	CSA and sexual Fx: Specialized questionnaire (also $N = 25$ interviewed)	62% = married 63% = orgasmic 30% sex with women; 9% lesbian/bisexual 5% asexual pain/physical discomfort with SI 36% desire for sex therapy; 36% prior therapy Adjustment and sexual self-esteem contributed to variance in orgasmic capacity.
Gold (1986)	Self-selected $N = 191$	CSA: 103 female Age $M = 30.4$ CG: 88 female Age $M = 29.8$	CSA and sexual Fx: Standardized questionnaires	CSA victims reported more negative sexual symptoms, $F(1, 164) = 11.16$, $p < .001$; less sexual responsiveness, $F(1, 164) = 7.70$, $p < .01$); less satisfaction with current sexual relationships, $F(1, 164) = 5.11$, $p < .05$.

continues

TABLE 1.1 (Continued)

Study	Sample	Group (CSA & CG)	Measure	Sexual dysfunction/ Relationships
Courtois (1979)	Self-selected $N = 31$	CSA: 31 female Ages 21–50 CSA = incest No CG	CSA and sexual Fx: Interview	Short-term effects on sexual Fx = no difference if CSA onset pre vs. post puberty. Long-term effects on relation to men/sense of self greater for CSA pre vs. post puberty.
Gundlach (1977)	Self-selected $N = 458$ female (225 lesbians 233 heterosexual) Age NR	CSA/sexual assault (SA): 35 female SA < 16 years old; 69 F SA > 16 years old No CG	CSA: Qualitative questionnaire Sexual Fx: Orientation	94% (16/17) women who were raped by friends or relatives before age 17 were lesbians. 56% (10/18) women age 16 or younger raped by strangers were lesbians. 49% (34/69) women raped over age 17 were lesbians. Qualitative data indicating feelings of fear, anger, distrust, disgust (often toward men in general).
Clinical/Forensic				
Drauker (1995)	Clinical $N = 146$ Ages 19–56	CSA: 146 female No CG	CSA and sexual Fx: Standardized questionnaires	Sexual self-esteem not included as outcome in final model due to lack of internal reliability.
Fisher, Winne, and Ley (1993)	Clinical $N = 54$	CSA: 32 female therapy completers (TC); Age $M = 31.5$ 22 female therapy dropouts (TD); Age $M = 33.4$ No CG	CSA and sexual Fx: Clinical data	High levels of physical abuse within relationships (TC = 82%, TD = 84%) and sexual assault as adults (TC = 87%, TD = 95%).

Study	Sample	CSA/CG	Measures	Results
Brown and Garrison (1990)	Clinical N = 432 Ages 19–52	CSA: 132 female CG: 300 female (college students without CSA)	CSA and sexual Fx: Clinical records review CG = questionnaire	Sexual dysfunction: 37% CSA, 1.2% controls "promiscuity": 10% CSA. 1.6% controls
de Young (1982)	Clinical/forensic N = 80	CSA: 72 female; 8 male Ages 4–53 CSA = incest No CG	CSA and sexual Fx: Semistructured interviews by author	28% and 15% reported "promiscuity" during adolescence and adulthood, respectively. 38% were victims of CSA by someone else in addition to their fathers or stepfathers, and 29% were sexually victimized as adults. 83% reported complete or partial "frigidity" (lack of sexual response or feeling). 10% of the sample were lesbians. 8% of the sample had engaged in prostitution.
Herman and Hirschman (1981)	Clinical N = 60 Ages 20s–30s	CSA: 40 female CSA = incest CG: 20 female with "seductive fathers"	CSA and sexual Fx: Semistructured interview	CSA cases were significantly more likely to become pregnant as adolescents. 35% of CSA cases described themselves as having been sexually promiscuous at some point. 55% of the victims complained of impaired sexual functioning (decreased pleasure), but this was not significantly different from controls. Qualitative information was reported indicating that CSA cases perceived their relationships with men as poor.

continues

TABLE 1.1 (Continued)

Study	Sample	Group (CSA & CG)	Measure	Sexual dysfunction/ Relationships
Tsai, Feldman-Summers, and Edgar (1979)	Clinical N = 90 Ages 18-65	CSA: 60 female (30 clinical; 30 nonclinical) CG: 30 female No report of CSA	CSA and sexual Fx: Specialized questionnaire	NSD between clinical CSA, nonclinical CSA, and control groups on childhood sexual experiences that were not abuse. The clinical CSA group reported less frequent orgasms during SI, had more individuals who reported over 15 partners (43%) than either of the other two groups (17% nonclinical, 9% control), reported less sexual responsiveness to their current partner, were less satisfied with their sexual relationships, and were less satisfied with their relationships with men.
Meiselman (1978)	Clinical N = 158	CSA: N = 58 (47 female; 11 male) Age M = 27.6 CG N = 100 patients Age M = 31.1 No report of CSA	CSA and sexual Fx: 1-Chart review 2-Interview	24% of 26 female patients with CSA vs. 8% of 50 female patients without CSA presented with sexual problems and 64% vs. 40% with partner conflict. 4% of patients with CSA vs. no patients without CSA were diagnosed with "sexual deviation." 87% of CSA patients (62% during intake) reported some form of sexual problem (anorgasmia 74%, "promiscuity" 19%, confusion regarding orientation, sexual masochism) at some time since the abuse vs. 20% of patients without CSA.

Note. CSA = childhood sexual abuse; CG = comparison group; NR = not reported; SI = sexual intercourse; Fx = function; OR = odds ratio; CI = confidence interval; NSD = no significant difference; DSM–III = *Diagnostiic and Statistical Manual of Mental Disorders* (3rd ed.). *Numbers indicate adjusted odds rations with 95% CI.

et al.'s (1994) U.K. female sample indicated that CSA cases were considerably more likely to report current sexual problems, especially those who had experienced sexual intercourse (SI) during CSA (67.8% for SI-CSA vs. 28.4% for non-CSA). When *sexual dissatisfaction* was measured, it was greater in CSA groups (Finkelhor, Hotaling, Lewis, & Smith, 1989; Mullen et al., 1994) than in control groups, although Finkelhor et al. found this was only true for women, not men. Other *sexual and relationship health* variables studied indicated that women with a CSA history were more likely to cohabitate before age 20, become pregnant before age 19, separate or divorce, be less satisfied with their relationship, and view their partners as more controlling and less caring (Finkelhor et al., 1989; Mullen et al., 1994; Russell, 1986).

Fergusson, Horwood, and Lynskey (1997) interviewed 18-year-old women as part of a longitudinal study. Greater severity of CSA was related to behaviors categorized as risky: more than 5 sexual partners, unprotected sexual intercourse, first sexual intercourse before 16, and revictimization. They noted that family characteristics such as low family stability, limited maternal education, and parental adjustment and substance abuse were associated with CSA. They also found statistical support for two models that provide information about how CSA may affect sexual outcomes in (female) adolescence: (a) CSA was more prevalent in children from households with family instability, parent adjustment problems, impaired parent–child relationships, and social disadvantage, and these factors accounted for pregnancy and sexually transmitted diseases (STDs); and (b) the early onset of sexual activity associated with victims of CSA (especially consensual intercourse) accounted for multiple partners and unprotected sex. The only sexual outcome for victims of CSA that did not appear to be mediated by other factors was subsequent rape or attempted rape. Thus, although this study addresses behaviors rather than sexual functioning, it is a useful basis from which to consider why sexual problems might emerge for a subgroup of women with CSA histories.

If we summarize the factors from the national probability sample studies, variables that increased the differences between individuals with and without CSA are being female and the CSA including sexual intercourse. Family characteristics were convincingly important in the Fergusson et al. (1997) longitudinal study, but the other national probability sample studies did not examine these variables.

College Samples

Although the college samples have a less heterogeneous population and almost always use self-selection rather than random selection of participants, they offer an opportunity to study large samples of women and men and examine patterns to test in other samples. Specific sexual dysfunctions are rarely examined (Jackson, Calhoun, Amick, Maddever, & Habif, 1990) in this age group. Rind et al.'s (1998) meta-analysis summarizes the general results; here we point out some of the more specific details and add one study not available to the Rind analysis. All of the studies cited here used comparison non-CSA groups.

Perhaps one of the reasons the small effect sizes were found is that there are contradictory findings both within and across data sets. There is evidence that CSA participants report more sexual problems, including less satisfaction and less sexual drive, and show an increased likelihood of subsequent sexual assault (Fritz, Stoll, & Wagner, 1981; Fromuth, 1986; Jackson et al., 1990; Meston, Heiman, Trapnell, & Carlin, 1999). In addition, a history of CSA in college women has been demonstrated to correlate with more frequent and more varied sexual behavior, including age at first intercourse, intercourse frequency, unrestricted sexual behavior (defined by items that included number of sexual partners, one-time-only encounters, more than one concurrent sexual relationship, openness to a brief affair), unrestricted sexual attitudes and fantasies, and masturbation frequency (Fromuth, 1986; Meston et al., 1999). However, these same studies have failed to identify a relationship between CSA and other sexual outcomes, such as sexual adjustment (Meston et al., 1999), female orgasmic response, pregnancy, abortion, or sexual satisfaction (Fromuth, 1986). Findings regarding how CSA affects sexual orientation are also contradictory, with some studies identifying no relationship (Meston et al., 1999) and others indicating a correlation with homosexual experiences (Fromuth, 1986) or a high proportion of abuse among self-selected lesbian women (not a college sample; Gundlach, 1977). Thus, the college samples highlight the apparent contradictions in the data, showing on the one hand impairments in sexual satisfaction and on the other a higher level and broader range of sexual behavior.

Several related issues emerge from these studies. One is that even if CSA and non-CSA individuals have apparently similar later sexual experiences, they may view them differently. This is nicely illustrated by the finding that women with a CSA history were more likely to describe themselves as promiscuous even though there was no difference in the number of sexual partners between themselves and non-CSA women. A second issue is that there are repeatedly more effects for women than men. For example, in Meston et al.'s (1999) study, CSA was related to none of the sexuality variables in men and most of the sexuality variables in women. For men, there were correlations between child physical and emotional abuse and adult sexuality items. In another study, Fromuth and Burkhart (1987) found that men responded differently to experiences of sexual abuse and often regarded them less negatively than women did. A third emerging factor is the role that other types of abuse might have on sexuality; in a sample of 1,032 students, a history of child physical abuse was correlated with unrestricted sexual behavior in women and variety of sexual fantasies in women and men (Meston et al., 1999). Histories of emotional abuse also showed correlations with variety of sexual fantasies in women.

The college studies show more modest connections between CSA and sexuality variables than did the (typically older except for Fergusson et al., 1997) national probability sample studies cited earlier. Both types of studies indicate that the adult sexual lives of individuals with a history of CSA vary, with one trajectory being greater sexual activity and exploration. In adolescence, this early trajectory may incur risks because of the outcomes of early sexuality, such as more partners, earlier intercourse, earlier pregnancy, as well as exposure to the health risks of pregnancy, STDs, and sexual coercion. Until HIV, most of these risks were less costly to men, because more partners, earlier and more sexual activity, and even pregnancy are not necessarily personal risks and in fact may be markers of sexual success for young men. The finding that CSA is related to decreased sexual satisfaction may be independent of greater exploration but is not necessarily mutually exclusive.

Self-Selected Samples

We located four studies that used self-selected samples of individuals with CSA and a non-CSA comparison group (Gold, 1986; Greenwald, Leitenberg, Cado, & Tarran, 1990; Meston & Heiman, 2000; Wenninger & Heiman, 1998). All of the samples used women, for a total sample size of 521. Mean ages of the samples ranged between 28 and 35 years. CSA individuals reported more negative sexual symptoms, such as less sexual responsiveness, less satisfaction with current sexual relationship in Gold's (1986) study; more sexual aversion, less subjective sexual arousal, and fewer signs of physiological arousal in the Wenninger and Heiman (1998) sample; but no differences in sexual satisfaction and specific sexual problems in the matched samples of nurses of Greenwald et al. (1990). The negative findings of Greenwald et al. may be accounted for by a low return rate (22% for non-CSA) with only 54 of 1,000 questionnaires returned by women with a history of CSA compared with 22% for non-CSA. These rates suggest that only women who were functioning relatively well chose to respond. Although there were differences between women with and without CSA on measures of psychological distress, the mean score for each group failed to fall within the clinical range on the Global Severity Index of the Brief Symptom Inventory (Derogatis & Spencer, 1982). Greenwald et al.'s findings are consistent with other representative samples that have noted a broad range of responses that are characteristic of those with a CSA history.

Meston and Heiman (2000) used an implicit methods experimental paradigm to examine how sexual information may be organized for women with different CSA histories. They examined network differences between word clusters and found that the word *lovemaking* was unrelated to any of the positive affect words for CSA women but was related to *desirable* and *enjoyable* for non-CSA women. Relatedly, *clitoris* was linked to *pleasurable* for non-CSA women and not linked to any affect words for the CSA women. *Intercourse* and *lovemaking* were both directly linked to female genitalia words for

CSA women only. We should note that other studies have pursued cognitive style differences but without including sexual variables (see review by Spaccarelli, 1994). For example, Wenninger and Ehlers (1998) compared 43 CSA and 29 non-CSA women and found that a global attribution style for negative events was significantly related to the severity of adult PTSD symptoms.

Clinical and Forensic Samples

Research on individuals who are seeking treatment or legal help provides information on a more selective subset of CSA individuals, usually biased toward having more problems (Tsai, Feldman-Summers, & Edgar, 1979). Most of the studies with comparison groups found that patients with CSA were more likely to have sexual problems, including less sexual responsiveness and satisfaction (Herman & Hirschman, 1981; Meiselman, 1978; Tsai et al., 1979). A common theme in addition to sexual problems was the report of more partner conflict and less satisfaction in their relationships with men.

CONTEXTUAL VARIABLES AND SEXUALITY

Nonsexual variables associated with CSA such as psychological and medical problems in adulthood also may affect a person's sexual functioning and relationships. As noted in other chapters of this volume, long-term correlates associated with CSA include depression (e.g., Saunders, Villeponteaux, Lipovsky, Kilpatrick, & Veronen, 1992; Sedney & Brooks, 1984; Wenniger & Heiman, 1998), anxiety (e.g., Bryer, Nelson, Miller, & Krol, 1987; Cole, 1986), PTSD (e.g., Brewin et al., 2000; Orr et al., 1998; Rowan & Foy, 1993), borderline personality disorder (e.g., Briere & Zaidi, 1989; Shearer, Peters, Quaytman, & Ogden, 1990; Wagner & Linehan, 1994), and self-destructive behavior (e.g., Brown & Anderson, 1991; Herman & Hirschman, 1981; Saunders et al., 1992). Other symptoms have included dissociation, eating disorders, hostility, low self-esteem, somatization, and social maladjustment (see reviews by Bauserman & Rind, 1997; Beitchman et al., 1992; Briere & Runtz, 1993; Rind et al., 1998) as well as more self-report of symptom-related distress and physician-coded diagnoses (Walker et al., 1999).

To the extent that CSA is an impactful event, either by itself or in combination with coexisting family environment variables, the above symptoms may influence the ability to form or maintain sexual relationships in the following ways. Depression may decrease sexual interest, one's sense of self-worth, communication, and positive experiencing. In addition, couples in which one person is depressed report more relationship discord and unhappiness (Fincham, Beach, Harold, & Osborne, 1997; Kurdek, 1998). Borderline personality disorder, a relatively rare diagnosis sometimes associated with CSA, is marked by features such as volatile instability of interpersonal relationships, body endangerment, and sexual impulsivity (e.g., Wagner & Linehan, 1994). Anxiety disorders including PTSD may also impair sexual function. The full effects of anxiety on sexual response are still not fully understood (lower levels can facilitate genital vasocongestion), but it is generally accepted that clinically significant anxiety and fear can interfere with the parasympathetic–sympathetic balance necessary for sexual arousal and orgasm (Bartlik & Goldberg, 2000).

Similarly, pain and medical problems can affect sexuality and relationship patterns, although almost all of these data are on female patients. Medical disorders that have been associated with a history of sexual assault include chronic pain (Finestone et al., 2000), gastrointestinal problems, somatization, and premenstrual symptoms (Berkowitz, 1998; Golding, Taylor, Menard, & King, 2000; Golding, Wilsnack, & Learman, 1998; Koss & Heslet, 1992; Laws, 1993). Chronic pelvic pain (CPP) is a diagnosis that often is without clear organic findings and is treatment refractory. Although it is not synonymous with dyspareunia (pain with intercourse), it generally impairs sexual functioning and has been associated with an increased prevalence of CSA (for reviews, see Fry, Crisp, & Beard, 1997; Savidge & Slade, 1997). Increased pelvic symptoms, including vaginal discharge and chronic abdominal pain, also have been documented in sexually abused children and adolescents (Rimsza, Berg, & Locke, 1988).

The range and heterogeneity among types of pelvic pain may complicate the association of gynecological pain syndromes with CSA. Medical research examining the association of CPP and CSA typically involves a different method than studies examining sexual and emotional problems associated with CSA and therefore should be interpreted differently. Rather than a comparison of symptom profiles between groups with and without CSA, the prevalence of CSA in women with a particular set of symptoms (e.g., pelvic pain) are compared with women without pain or with a different pain condition (e.g., headache). Findings from early studies on women with CPP indicated a high prevalence of sexual abuse and psychiatric symptoms (Gross, Doerr, Caldirola, Guzinski, & Ripley, 1980; Toomey, Hernandez, Gittelman, & Hulka, 1993), but they were limited by the lack of comparison groups. Subsequent research identified a higher prevalence of child physical and sexual abuse for CPP participants compared with control participants (Collett, Cordle, Stewart, & Jagger, 1998; Ehlert, Heim, & Hellhammer, 1999; Harrop-Griffiths et al., 1988; Walker et al., 1992; Walker et al., 1995).

Similar to the data on sexual outcomes, there are inconsistencies among the findings. In the 1992 national probability study, Laumann et al. (1999) found no relationship between sexual pain and a history of CSA in women, and sexual pain as an outcome of psychosocial variables was not reported for men. Other studies that failed to find a relationship between sexual abuse and pelvic pain did find a higher prevalence of physical abuse among CPP patients compared with control participants (Rapkin, Kames, Darke, Stampler, & Naliboff, 1990). In a series of studies, Walling, O'Hara, et al. (1994) and Walling, Reiter, et al. (1994) found higher rates of both physical and sexual abuse among CPP patients but identified physical and not sexual abuse as a predictor of depression, anxiety, and somatization in CPP patients. Thus, consistent with data from Fergusson et al. (1997) on sexual outcomes, the relationship often observed between sexual abuse and somatization may be accounted for by other familial factors (in this case physical abuse).

Although no clear association exists between CSA and pain, distinguishing between different pain syndromes may increase our understanding of the relationship found in some studies. One type of localized pelvic pain, vulvar vestibulitis, does not appear to be related to CSA (Bornstein, Zarfati, Goldik, & Abramovici, 1999; Danielsson, Sjoberg, & Wikman, 2000). Women with localized vulvar pain were more similar to no-pain control participants, whereas those with CPP were more likely to have a history of physical and sexual abuse (Bodden-Heidrich, Kuppers, Beckmann, Rechenberger, & Bender, 1999; Reed et al., 2000). The distinction between localized and diffuse or chronic pain, however, does not account for all of the relationship with CSA. Although some CPP patients with pelvic venous congestion (Fry, Beard, Crisp, & McGuigan, 1997) or a lack of somatic markers for pain (Reiter, Shakerin, Gambone, & Milburn, 1991) showed trends toward more sexual abuse and greater general somatization than control participants, another comparison study found that patients with and without objective findings had similar histories of CSA and somatization (Ehlert et al., 1999).

In part, the relationship between CSA and pelvic pain is poorly understood because of limitations in the research design and methods used to date, such as small sample sizes, lack of standardized definitions for chronicity of pain, and lack of appropriate control groups (Berkowitz, 1998). Further research designed to understand the mechanism for this association, examining psychological factors such as somatization, biological factors associated with autonomic arousal, or behavioral factors including increased sexual risk-taking (Berkowitz, 1998) is necessary before we can better identify which CSA individuals are at risk for developing medical symptoms. Recent studies have begun to propose endocrinological factors that may help to explain the relationship between CSA and medical disorders. In one small sample of 16 patients and 14 control participants, women with CPP were found to have more abuse experiences and PTSD symptoms along with diminished functioning of the hypothalamic-pituitary-adrenal axis characterized by lowered activity in the adrenal gland (Heim, Ehlert, Hanker, & Hellhammer, 1998). A similar explanation citing the ability of early stressful experiences to increase subsequent corticotrophin-releasing hormone production in fear-provoking situations that may be associated with pregnancy has been suggested for the association of CSA with preterm labor (Horan, Hill, & Schulkin, 2000).

Several researchers have advocated for the classification of sexual pain as a pain disorder and for a decrease in the distinction between organic and nonorganic pain (Binik, Pukall, Reissing, & Khalife, 2001; Grace, 1998; Meana & Binik, 1994; Meana, Binik, Khalife, & Cohen, 1997). This integrated model for understanding pelvic and coital pain and their relationship to sexuality may ultimately be informative for understanding these disorders in women with a history of CSA (Savidge & Slade, 1997).

CONCLUSION

There are several directions for future research indicated by the discrepant findings in the current literature. The first involves information about how CSA is perceived and what leads an experience to be labeled as traumatic. Second, the interaction of familial factors, physical abuse, and CSA could potentially provide information about individuals at greater risk (using statistical procedures alone to accomplish this task should be done with caution; Briere & Elliott, 1993). Third, precisely specifying sexual outcomes would allow for differentiation among behavior, function, and satisfaction. Fourth, clarifying definitions of sexual problems in terms of whether they conform to current diagnostic categories and symptom profiles will allow for increased information about the prevalence of sexual dysfunction in women with a history of CSA. And, finally, including sexuality questions in longitudinal designs of human development, though difficult for sociocultural and methods reasons, would be a tremendous advantage for understanding normal childhood sexual development.

In addition, the role of ethnic and cultural factors deserves more attention. Although few ethnic differences have been identified between African American, Latina, and European American women with CSA histories (e.g., Roosa, Reinholtz, & Angelini, 1999; Wyatt, 1985), we would benefit from more details about how CSA might interact with ethnicity to produce different sexual health and relationship outcomes. The data from men, typically focused on gay and bisexual men, do find important CSA differences by ethnicity. For example, Doll et al. (1992) found that Latino and African American gay and bisexual men were more likely than European American men to report child–adolescent (median age 10) sexual contact with older partners (mean age 11 years older), 51% of which involved force. Nevertheless, we have little data on adult sexual functioning and relationships with regards to ethnicity and CSA in either gender.

At this time we are still left with the observations that the CSA experience itself varies in intensity and emotional valence, and its correlational relationship to later sexuality varies in the effects on functioning and satisfaction. It is unlikely that women with CSA histories are more satisfied with their adult sexual relationships, but they may not differ from non-CSA in their sexual responsiveness and may even be responsive earlier. They tend to have more sexual partners, which may be a sign that they find it easier to make a relationship sexual, are more easily pressured into a sexual relationship, pick partners for the short term, or find ongoing relationships less desirable than seeking new relationships. In other words, more sexual partnerships may say more about a woman's relationship choices than her sexual choices (to the extent that she indeed has choices). These possibilities are relevant to sexual risk as well as sexual health.

REFERENCES

American Psychiatric Association. (1994). *Diagnostic and statistical manual of mental disorders* (4th ed.). Washington, DC: Author.

American Psychiatric Association. (2000). *Diagnostic and statistical manual of mental disorders* (4th ed., Text Revision). Washington, DC: Author.

Bartlik, B., & Goldberg, J. (2000). Female sexual arousal disorder. In S. R. Leiblum & R. C. Rosen (Eds.), *Principles and practice of sex therapy* (pp. 85–177). New York: Guilford Press.

Basson, R., Berman, J., Burnett, A., Derogatis, L., Ferguson, D., Fourcroy, J., et al. (2000). Report of the international consensus development conference on female sexual dysfunction: Definitions and classifications. *Journal of Urology, 163,* 888–893.

Bauserman, R., & Rind, B. (1997). Psychological correlates of male child and adolescent sexual experiences with adults: A review of the nonclinical literature. *Archives of Sexual Behavior, 26,* 105–141.

Beitchman, J. H., Zucker, K. J., Hood, J. E., daCosta, G. A., & Akman, D. (1991). A review of the short-term effects of child sexual abuse. *Child Abuse and Neglect, 15,* 537–556.

Beitchman, J. H., Zucker, K. J., Hood, J. E., daCosta, G. A., Akman, D., & Cassavia, E. (1992). A review of the long-term effects of child sexual abuse. *Child Abuse and Neglect, 16,* 101–118.

Berkowitz, C. D. (1998). Medical consequences of child sexual abuse. *Child Abuse and Neglect, 22,* 541–550.

Binik, Y. M., Pukall, C. F., Reissing, E. D., & Khalife, S. (2001). The sexual pain disorders: A desexualized approach. *Journal of Sex and Marital Therapy, 27,* 113–116.

Bodden-Heidrich, R., Kuppers, V., Beckman, M. W., Rechenberger, I., & Bender, H. G. (1999). Chronic pelvic pain syndrome (CPPS) and chronic vulvar pain syndrome (CVPS): Evaluation of psychosomatic aspects. *Psychosomatic Obstetrics, 20,* 145–151.

Bornstein, J., Zarfati, D., Goldik, Z., & Abramovici, H. (1999). Vulvar vestibulitis: Physical or psychosexual problem? *Obstetrics and Gynecology, 93,* 876–880.

Brewin, C. R., Andrews, B., & Valentine, J. D. (2000). Meta-analysis of risk factors for posttraumatic stress disorder in trauma-exposed adults. *Journal of Consulting and Clinical Psychology, 68,* 748–766.

Briere, J. (1992). Long-term impacts of child abuse: II. Behaviors and relationships. In J. Briere (Ed.), *Child abuse trauma: Theory and treatment of the lasting effects* (pp. 48–77). Thousand Oaks, CA: Sage.

Briere, J., & Elliott, D. (1993). Sexual abuse, family environment, and psychological symptoms: On the validity of statistical control. *Journal of Consulting and Clinical Psychology, 61,* 284–288.

Briere, J., & Runtz, M. (1993). Childhood sexual abuse: Long-term sequelae and implications for psychological assessment. *Journal of Interpersonal Violence, 8,* 312–330.

Briere, J., & Zaidi, L. Y. (1989). Sexual abuse histories and sequelae in female psychiatric emergency room patients. *American Journal of Psychiatry, 146,* 1602–1606.

Brown B. E., & Garrison C. J. (1990). Patterns of symptomatology of adult women incest survivors. *Western Journal of Nursing Research, 12,* 587–596.

Brown, G. R., & Anderson, B. (1991). Psychiatric morbidity in adult inpatients with childhood histories of sexual and physical abuse. *American Journal of Psychiatry, 148,* 55–61.

Bryer, J. B., Nelson, B. A., Miller, J. B., & Krol, P. A. (1987). Childhood sexual and physical abuse as factors in adult psychiatric illness. *American Journal of Psychiatry, 144,* 1082–1083.

Cohen, J. (1988). *Statistical power analyses for the behavioral sciences* (2nd ed.). Hillsdale, NJ: Erlbaum.

Cole, M. (1986). Socio-sexual characteristics of men with sexual problems. *Sexual and Marital Therapy, 1,* 89–108.

Collett, B. J., Cordle, C. J., Stewart, C. R., & Jagger, C. (1998). A comparative study of women with chronic pelvic pain, chronic nonpelvic pain and those with no history of pain attending general practitioners. *British Journal of Obstetrics and Gynaecology, 105,* 87–92.

Conte, J. R., & Schuerman, J. R. (1987). Factors associated with an increased impact of child sexual abuse. *Child Abuse and Neglect, 11,* 201–211.

Courtois, C. A. (1979). The incest experience and its aftermath. *Victimology: An International Journal, 4,* 337–347.

Danielsson, I., Sjoberg, I., & Wikman, M. (2000). Vulvar vestibulitis: Medical, psychosexual and psychosocial aspects, a case-control study. *Acta Obstetricia et Gynecologica Scandinavica, 79,* 872–878.

Derogatis, L. R., & Spencer, P. M. (1982). *The Brief Symptom Inventory: Administration scoring and procedures manual.* Baltimore: Clinical Psychometric Research.

de Young, M. (1982). *The sexual victimization of children.* Jefferson, NC: McFarland.

Doll, L. S., Joy, D., Bartholow, B. N., Harrison, J. S., Bolan, G., Douglas, J. N., et al. (1992). Self-reported childhood and adolescent sexual abuse among adult homosexual and bisexual men. *Child Abuse and Neglect, 16,* 855–864.

Drauker, C. B. (1995). A coping model for adult survivors of childhood sexual abuse. *Journal of Interpersonal Violence, 10,* 159–175.

Ehlert, U., Heim, C., & Hellhammer, D. H. (1999). Chronic pelvic pain as a somatoform disorder. *Psychotherapy and Psychosomatics, 68,* 87–94.

Feinauer, L. L. (1989). Sexual dysfunction in women sexually abused as children. *Contemporary Family Therapy: An International Journal, 11,* 299–309.

Feldman, H. A., Goldstein, I., Hatzichristou, D. G., Krane, R. J., & McKinlay, J. B. (1994). Construction of a surrogate variable for impotence in the Massachusetts Male Aging Study. *Journal of Clinical Epidemiology, 47,* 457–467.

Fergusson, D. M., Horwood, J. L., & Lynskey, M. T. (1997). Childhood sexual abuse, adolescent sexual behaviors and sexual revictimization. *Child Abuse and Neglect, 21,* 789–803.

Fincham, F. D., Beach, S. R. H., Harold, G. T., & Osborne, L. N. (1997). Marital satisfaction and depression: Different causal relationships for men and women? *Psychological Science, 8,* 351–357.

Finestone, H. M., Stenn, P., Davies, F., Stalker, C., Fry, R., & Koumanis, J. (2000). Chronic pain and health care utilization in women with a history of childhood sexual abuse. *Child Abuse and Neglect, 24,* 547–556.

Finkelhor, D. (1979). *Sexually victimized children.* New York: Free Press.

Finkelhor, D. (1984). *Child sexual abuse: New theory and research.* New York: Free Press.

Finkelhor, D., Hotaling, G. T., Lewis, I. A., & Smith, C. (1989). Sexual abuse and its relationship to later sexual satisfaction, marital status, religion, and attitudes. *Journal of Interpersonal Violence, 4,* 379–399.

Fisher, P. M., Winne, P. H., & Ley, R. G. (1993). Group therapy for adult women survivors of child sexual abuse: Differentiation of completers versus dropouts. *Psychotherapy, 30,* 616–624.

Frank, E., Anderson, C., & Rubinstein, D. N. (1978). Frequency of sexual dysfunction in normal couples. *New England Journal of Medicine, 299,* 111–115.

Friedrich, W. N., Urquiza, A. J., & Beilke, R. L. (1986). Behavior problems in sexually abused young children. *Journal of Pediatric Psychology, 11,* 47–57.

Fritz, G. S., Stoll, K., & Wagner, N. N. (1981). A comparison of males and females who were sexually molested as children. *Journal of Sex and Marital Therapy, 7,* 54–59.

Fromuth, M. E. (1986). The relationship of childhood sexual abuse with later psychological and sexual adjustment in a sample of college women. *Child Abuse and Neglect, 10,* 5–15.

Fromuth, M. E., & Burkhart, B. R. (1987). Sexual victimization among college men: Definitional and methodological issues. *Violence Victims, 2,* 241–253.

Fry, R. P. W., Beard, R. W., Crisp, A. H., & McGuigan, S. (1997). Sociopsychological factors in women with chronic pelvic pain with and without pelvic venous congestion. *Journal of Psychosomatic Research, 42,* 71–85.

Fry, R. P. W., Crisp, A. H., & Beard, R. W. (1997). Sociopsychological factors in chronic pelvic pain: A review. *Journal of Psychosomatic Research, 42,* 1–15.

Gold, E. R. (1986). Long-term effects of sexual victimization in childhood: An attributional approach. *Journal of Consulting and Clinical Psychology, 54,* 471–475.

Golding, J. M., Taylor, D. L., Menard, L., & King, M. J. (2000). Prevalence of sexual abuse history in a sample of women seeking treatment for premenstrual syndrome. *Journal of Psychosomatic Obstetrics and Gynecology, 21,* 69–80.

Golding, J. M., Wilsnack, S. C., & Learman, L. A. (1998). Prevalence of sexual assault history among women with common gynecologic symptoms. *American Journal of Obstetrics and Gynecology, 179,* 1013–1019.

Goldman, J. D. G., & Padayachi, U. K. (2000). Some methodological problems in estimating incidence and prevalence in child sexual abuse research. *Journal of Sex Research, 37,* 305–314.

Grace, V. M. (1998). Mind/body dualism in medicine: The case of chronic pelvic pain without organic pathology: A critical review of the literature. *International Journal of Health Services, 28,* 127–151.

Greenwald, E., Leitenberg, H., Cado, S., & Tarran, M. J. (1990). Childhood sexual abuse: Long-term effects on psychological and sexual functioning in a nonclinical and nonstudent sample of adult women. *Child Abuse and Neglect, 14,* 503–513.

Gross, R. J., Doerr, H., Caldirola, D., Guzinski, G. M., & Ripley, H. S. (1980). Borderline syndrome and incest in chronic pelvic pain patients. *International Journal of Psychiatry in Medicine, 10,* 79–96.

Gundlach, R. H. (1977). Sexual molestation and rape reported by homosexual and heterosexual women. *Journal of Homosexuality, 2,* 367–384.

Harrop-Griffiths, J., Katon, W., Walker, E., Holm, L., Russo, J., & Hickok, L. (1988). The association between chronic pelvic pain, psychiatric diagnoses, and childhood sexual abuse. *Obstetrics and Gynecology, 71,* 589–594.

Heim, C., Ehlert, U., Hanker, J. P., & Hellhammer, D. H. (1998). Abuse-related posttraumatic stress disorder and alterations of the hypothalamic-pituitary-adrenal axis in women with chronic pelvic pain. *Psychosomatic Medicine, 60,* 309–318.

Heiman, J. R., Verhulst, J., & Heard-Davison, A. R. (in press). Childhood sexuality and adult sexual relationships: How are they connected by data and by theory? In J. Bancroft (Ed.), *Sexual development.* Bloomington: Indiana University Press.

Herman, J. L., & Hirschman, L. (1981). *Father–daughter incest.* Cambridge, MA: Harvard University Press.

Horan, D. L., Hill, L. D., & Schulkin, J. (2000). Childhood sexual abuse and preterm labor in adulthood: An endocrinological hypothesis. *Women's Health Issues, 10,* 27–33.

Howes, P. W., Cicchetti, D., Toth, S. L., & Rogosch, F. A. (2000). Affective, organizational, and relational characteristics of maltreating families: A systems perspective. *Journal of Family Psychology, 14,* 95–110.

Jackson, J. L., Calhoun, K. S., Amick, A. E., Maddever, H. M., & Habif, V. L. (1990). Young adult women who report childhood intrafamilial sexual abuse: Subsequent adjustment. *Archives of Sexual Behavior, 19*, 211–221.

Kendall-Tackett, K. A., Williams, L. M., & Finkelhor, D. (1993). Impact of sexual abuse on children: A review and synthesis of recent empirical studies. *Psychological Bulletin, 113*, 164–180.

King, N. J., Tonge, B. J., Mullen, P., Myerson, N., Heyne, D., Rollings, S., et al. (2000). Treating sexually abused children with posttraumatic stress symptoms: A randomized clinical trail. *Journal of the American Academy of Child and Adolescent Psychiatry, 39*, 1347–1355.

Koss, M. P., & Heslet, L. (1992). Somatic consequences of violence against women. *Archives of Family Medicine, 1*, 53–59.

Kurdek, L. A. (1998). The nature and predictors of the trajectory of change in marital quality over the first 4 years of marriage for first-married husbands and wives. *Journal of Family Psychology, 12*, 494–510.

Laumann, E. O., Gagnon, J. H., Michael, R. T., & Michaels, S. (1994). *The social organization of sexuality: Sexual practices in the United States.* Chicago: University of Chicago Press.

Laumann, E. O., Paik, A., & Rosen, R. C. (1999). Sexual dysfunction in the United States: Prevalence and predictors. *Journal of the American Medical Association, 281*, 537–544.

Laws, A. (1993). Does a history of sexual abuse in childhood play a role in women's medical problems? A review. *Journal of Women's Health, 2*, 165–171.

Meana, M., & Binik, Y. M. (1994). Painful coitus: A review of female dyspareunia. *Journal of Nervous and Mental Disease, 182*, 264–272.

Meana, M., Binik, Y. M., Khalife, S., & Cohen, D. R. (1997). Dyspareunia: Sexual dysfunction or pain syndrome? *Journal of Nervous and Mental Disease, 185*, 561–569.

Meiselman, K. C. (1978). *Incest: A psychological study of causes and effects with treatment recommendations.* San Francisco: Jossey-Bass.

Meston, C. M., & Heiman, J. R. (2000). Sexual abuse and sexual function: An examination of sexually relevant cognitive processes. *Journal of Consulting and Clinical Psychology, 68*, 399–406.

Meston, C. M., Heiman, J. R., Trapnell, P. D., & Carlin, A. S. (1999). Ethnicity, desirable responding, and self-reports of abuse: A comparison of European- and Asian-ancestry undergraduates. *Journal of Consulting and Clinical Psychology, 67*, 139–144.

Mullen, P. E., Martin, J. L., Anderson, J. C., Romans, S. E., & Herbison, G. P. (1994). The effect of child sexual abuse on social, interpersonal and sexual function in adult life. *British Journal of Psychiatry, 165*, 35–47.

Orr, S. P., Lasko, N. B., Metzger, L. J., Berry, N. J., Ahern, C. E., & Pitman, R. K. (1998). Psychophysiologic assessment of women with posttraumatic stress disorder resulting from childhood sexual abuse. *Journal of Consulting and Clinical Psychology, 66*, 906–913.

Paolucci, E. O., Genuis, M. L., & Violato, C. (2001). A meta-analysis of the published research on the effects of child sexual abuse. *Journal of Psychology, 135,* 17–36.

Pistorello, J., & Follette, V. M. (1998). Childhood sexual abuse and couples' relationships: Female survivors' reports in therapy groups. *Journal of Marital and Family Therapy, 24,* 473–485.

Pitman, R. K., Shalev, A. Y., & Orr, S. P. (2000). Posttraumatic stress disorder: Emotion, conditioning, and memory. In M. S. Gazzaniger (Ed.), *The new cognitive neurosciences* (pp. 1133–1147). Cambridge, MA: MIT Press.

Rapkin, A. J., Kames, L. D., Darke, L. L., Stampler, F. M., & Naliboff, B. D. (1990). History of physical and sexual abuse in women with chronic pelvic pain. *Obstetrics and Gynecology, 76,* 92–96.

Reed, B. D., Haefner, H. K., Punch, M. R., Roth, R. S., Gorenflo, D. W., & Gillespie, G. W. (2000). Psychosocial and sexual functioning in women with vulvodynia and chronic pelvic pain: A comparative evaluation. *Journal of Reproductive Medicine, 45,* 624–632.

Reiter, R. C., Shakerin, L. R., Gambone, J. C., & Milburn, A. K. (1991). Correlation between sexual abuse and somatization in women with somatic and nonsomatic chronic pelvic pain. *American Journal of Obstetrics and Gynecology, 165,* 104–109.

Rimsza, M. E., Berg, R. A., & Locke, C. (1988). Sexual abuse: Somatic and emotional reactions. *Child Abuse and Neglect, 12,* 201–208.

Rind, B., & Tromovitch, P. (1997). A meta-analytic review of findings from national samples on psychological correlates of child sexual abuse. *Journal of Sex Research, 34,* 237–255.

Rind, B., Tromovitch, P., & Bauserman, R. (1998). A meta-analytic examination of assumed properties of child sexual abuse using college samples. *Psychological Bulletin, 124,* 22–53.

Roosa, M. W., Reinholtz, C., & Angelini, P. J. (1999). The relation of child sexual abuse and depression in young women: Comparisons across four ethnic groups. *Journal of Abnormal Child Psychology, 27,* 65–76.

Roosa, M. W., Reyes, L., Reinholtz, C., & Angelini, P. J. (1998). Measurement of women's child sexual abuse experiences: An empirical demonstration of the impact of choice of measure on estimates of incidence rates and of relationships with pathology. *Journal of Sex Research, 35,* 225–233.

Rosen, R. C., Taylor, J. F., Leiblum, S. R., & Bachmann, G. A. (1993). Prevalence of sexual dysfunction in women: Results of a survey study of 329 women in an outpatient gynecological clinic. *Journal of Sex and Marital Therapy, 19,* 171–188.

Rowan, A. B., & Foy, D. W. (1993). Post-traumatic stress disorder in child sexual abuse survivors: A literature review. *Journal of Traumatic Stress, 6,* 3–20.

Russell, D. E. H. (1986). *The secret trauma: Incest in the lives of girls and women.* New York: Basic Books.

Saunders, B. E., Villeponteaux, L. A., Lipovsky, J. A., Kilpatrick, D. G., & Veronen, L. J. (1992). Child sexual assault as a risk factor for mental disorders among women: A community survey. *Journal of Interpersonal Violence, 7,* 189–204.

Savidge, C. J., & Slade, P. (1997). Psychological aspects of chronic pelvic pain. *Journal of Psychosomatic Research, 42,* 433–444.

Sedney, M. A., & Brooks, B. (1984). Factors associated with a history of childhood sexual experience in a nonclinical female population. *Journal of the American Academy of Child and Adolescent Psychiatry, 23,* 215–218.

Shearer, S. L., Peters, C. P., Quaytman, M. S., & Ogden, R. L. (1990). Frequency and correlates of childhood sexual and physical abuse histories in adult female borderline inpatients. *American Journal of Psychiatry, 147,* 214–216.

Simons, J. S., & Carey, M. P. (2001). Prevalence of sexual dysfunctions: Results from a decade of research. *Archives of Sexual Behavior, 30,* 177–219.

Spaccarelli, S. (1994). Stress, appraisal, and coping in child sexual abuse: A theoretical and empirical review. *Psychological Bulletin, 116,* 340–362.

Spector, I. P., & Carey, M. P. (1990). Incidence and prevalence of the sexual dysfunctions: A critical review of the empirical literature. *Archives of Sexual Behavior, 19,* 389–408.

Thompson, R. A., & Nelson, C. A. (2001). Developmental science and the media. *American Psychologist, 56,* 5–15.

Toomey, T. C., Hernandez, J. T., Gittelman, D. F., & Hulka, J. F. (1993). Relationship of sexual and physical abuse to pain and psychological assessment variables in chronic pelvic pain patients. *Pain, 53,* 105–109.

Tsai, M., Feldman-Summers, S., & Edgar, M. (1979). Childhood molestation: Variables related to differential impacts on psychosexual functioning in adult women. *Journal of Abnormal Psychology, 88,* 407–417.

Violato, C., & Genuis, M. L. (1993). Problems of research in male child sexual abuse: A review. *Journal of Child Sexual Abuse, 2,* 33–54.

Wagner, N. N., & Linehan, M. M. (1994). Relationship between childhood sexual abuse and topography of parasuicide among women with borderline personality disorders. *Journal of Personality Disorders, 8,* 1–9.

Walker, E. A., Gelfand, A. N., Katon, W. J., Koss, M. P., Von Korff, M., Bernstein, D., & Russo, J. (1999). Adult health status of women with histories of childhood abuse and neglect. *American Journal of Medicine, 107,* 332–339.

Walker, E. A., Katon, W., Hansom, J., Harrop-Griffiths, J., Holm, L., Jones, M. L., et al. (1995). Psychiatric diagnoses and sexual victimization in women with chronic pelvic pain. *Psychosomatics, 36,* 531–540.

Walker, E. A., Katon, W., Neraas, K., Jemelka, R. P., & Massoth, D. (1992). Dissociation in women with chronic pelvic pain. *American Journal of Psychiatry, 149,* 534–537.

Walling, M. K., O'Hara, M. W., Reiter, R. C., Milburn, A. K., Lilly, G., & Vincent, S. D. (1994). Abuse history and chronic pain in women: II. A multivariate analysis of abuse and pyschological morbidity. *Obstetrics and Gynecology, 84,* 200–206.

Walling, M. K., Reiter, R. C., O'Hara, M. W., Milburn, A. K., Lilly, G., & Vincent, S. D. (1994). Abuse history and chronic pain in women: I. Prevalences of sexual abuse and physical abuse. *Obstetrics and Gynecology, 84,* 193–199.

Wenninger, K., & Ehlers, A. (1998). Dysfunctional cognitions and adult psychological functioning in child sexual abuse survivors. *Journal of Traumatic Stress, 11,* 281–300.

Wenninger, K., & Heiman, J. R. (1998). Relating body image to psychological and sexual functioning in child sexual abuse survivors. *Journal of Traumatic Stress, 11,* 543–562.

Wind, T. W., & Silvern, L. E. (1994). Parenting and family stress as mediators of the long-term effects of child abuse. *Child Abuse and Neglect, 18,* 439–453.

Wyatt, G. E. (1985). The sexual abuse of Afro-American and White women in childhood. *Child Abuse and Neglect, 9,* 507–519.

2

CHILD SEXUAL ABUSE AND ADULT SEXUAL REVICTIMIZATION

CINDY L. RICH, AMY M. COMBS-LANE, HEIDI S. RESNICK,
AND DEAN G. KILPATRICK

Research indicates that a range of factors are associated with an increased risk for adult sexual assault (ASA) among women, including alcohol use (Harrington & Leitenberg, 1994), illicit drug use (Kilpatrick, Acierno, Resnick, Saunders, & Best, 1997), psychological distress related to past exposure to traumatic events (Koss & Dinero, 1989), sexual behaviors (Arata, 2000), and impaired risk recognition (Wilson, Calhoun, & Bernat, 1999). However, a history of child sexual abuse (CSA), which has been associated with these potential mediating risk factors, has been identified as the strongest predictor of ASA (Gidycz, Coble, Latham, & Layman, 1993; Gidycz, Hanson, & Layman, 1995; Koss & Dinero, 1989; Messman & Long, 1996). Across various samples, the phenomenon of sexual revictimization has been demonstrated, including research with national probability samples and col-

This study was supported by Centers for Disease Control and Prevention (CDC) Grant No. U49/CCU415877-0, titled "National Violence Against Women Prevention Research Center"; CDC Grant No. R49/CCR419810–01, titled "Child Violence, Adult Victimization, Injury, and Health"; National Institute on Drug Abuse Grant No. R01 DA11158, titled "Prevention of Post Rape Psychopathology and Drug Abuse"; and National Institutes of Health–sponsored Medical University of South Carolina General Clinical Research Center Supported Study No. 5M01 RR01070.

lege, community, and clinical samples. In a recent meta-analysis that included 19 revictimization studies (Roodman & Clum, 2001), researchers found a moderate overall effect size of .59, indicating a significant relationship between CSA and ASA. These findings have motivated researchers to investigate the possible relationships between child and adult sexual victimization experiences in an effort to better understand the factors that are associated with risk for revictimization. It is important to note that most studies addressing sexual revictimization have investigated predictor variables in isolation or those found to be associated with sexual assault in general (e.g., alcohol and drug use, risky sexual behavior, and trauma symptoms). Very few researchers have used theoretical models to guide their research. However, a few researchers have begun to develop and test integrated theoretically driven models designed to investigate sexual revictimization (e.g., Gold, Sinclair, & Balge, 1999; Grauerholz, 2000; Maker, Kemmelmeier, & Peterson, 2001).

In the present chapter, we focus on research that has investigated the relationship between CSA and ASA, beginning with a review and critique of several studies. We then evaluate some of the limitations of previous research and discuss ways to advance the current state of knowledge. The chapter concludes with a discussion of implications for clinical interventions with CSA survivors and risk-reduction programming, as well as suggestions for future research directions.

The studies reviewed here differed in some parameters that may be critical in evaluating the validity and generalizability of findings related to associations between rape in childhood and rape in adulthood. In Table 2.1, we highlight some of the methodological differences that are a focus of this review. A major difference across epidemiological studies of revictimization was the age criterion used to determine what constituted childhood assault. For example, some studies defined childhood abuse as experiences that occur prior to the age of 14 years old, whereas other studies included experiences that occur until the age of 18 years old as childhood incidents. Therefore, adolescent assaults may have been included with either child cases or adult cases depending on definitions of the age ranges for childhood and adult victimization experiences. In addition, the age difference between the perpetrator and victim may or may not have been specified in a given study. In some cases, sexual interactions between consenting individuals of the same age could be inadvertently counted as sexual abuse. Thus, the age difference between the victim and perpetrator could be especially important for studies that use broader definitions of CSA.

Definitions also differed in a manner that may have influenced prevalence rates. The definitions of both CSA and ASA might influence prevalence rates such that broader definitions would be associated with higher victimization prevalence. For example, some studies included experiences ranging from unwanted touching to unwanted sexual intercourse as sexual assault, whereas other studies included only unwanted, forced sexual inter-

TABLE 2.1

Assault Characteristics for Studies Included in Review

Study	N	Developmental period[a]	Age cut-off[b]	CSA definition[c]	ASA definition[c]	Design[d]	Estimated increased risk of ASA given history of CSA
Probability samples							
Koss and Dinero (1989)	3,187	C, A	14	1,2,3,4	2,3,4	CS, P	3.3[e]
Kilpatrick, Acierno, Resnick, Saunders, and Best (1997)	4,009	C, A	18	3,4,	3,4	L, P	4.4[f]
Tjaden and Thoennes (2000)	16,005	C, A	18	3,4	3,4	CS, P	> 2.0[e]
College samples							
Gidycz, Coble, Latham, and Layman (1993)	927	C, Ad, A	14	1,2,3,4	2,3,4	L, C	> 2.0[e]
Gidycz, Hanson, and Layman (1995)	796	C, Ad, A	14	1,2,3,4	2,3,4	L, C	> 2.0[e]
Mayall and Gold (1995)	654	C, A	15	1,2,4	1,2,4	CS, C	—
Messman-Moore, Long, and Siegfried (2000)	648	C, A	17	1,2,3,4	2,3,4	CS, C	—
Community samples							
Russell (1986)	930	C, A	14	2,3,4	3,4	CS	> 2.0[e]
Wyatt, Guthrie, and Notgrass (1992)	161	C, A	18	1,2,3,4	1,3,4	CS	2.4[e]

Note. CSA = child sexual abuse; ASA = adult sexual assault. [a]C = child; A = adult; Ad = adolescent. [b]Age shown is the cutoff age (in years) for childhood sexual abuse. [c]1 = noncontact; 2 = contact with no attempt to penetrate; 3 = attempted rape; 4 = rape. [d]CS = cross-sectional; P = probability; L = longitudinal; C = convenience. [e]These values were estimated from data given in the original studies. [f]This value refers to an odds ratio.

course as sexual assault. Additionally, behaviorally phrased questions may more accurately assess actual victimization, as opposed to questions that include labels or legal terms. Studies under review varied in terms of the specific definitions used. This is especially important when considering that women may not identify or label their experiences as rape even though they meet the legal definition of rape (e.g., Layman, Gidycz, & Lynn, 1996). Thus, studies using labels such as rape or sexual assault may have underestimated true prevalence of child and adult incidents of rape, molestation, or attempted sexual assault. Some studies required that the assault incidents include force or threat of force as a necessary element to be included as assault, whereas others did not specify the element of force. Additionally, some studies included information about assault characteristics such as relationship to the perpetrator or reactions to victimization that might mediate associations between CSA and ASA (e.g., psychological distress, mental health outcomes noted above), whereas other studies did not. Finally, design characteristics also differed across studies. Longitudinal designs have advantages over cross-sectional designs because they allow for the examination of the temporal relationships among variables, whereas probability samples are more representative of women in the general population, resulting in better generalizability of findings.

SELECTION CRITERIA FOR LITERATURE REVIEW

Studies have examined relationships between sexual victimization experiences occurring within (e.g., childhood) and between (e.g., childhood and adulthood) developmental periods, and with various forms of repeat victimization, including physical assault and psychological maltreatment. In the present review, however, we have restricted our focus to studies pertaining to the association between CSA and ASA. We have chosen to restrict our discussion to CSA as a predictor of ASA because the preponderance of extant studies have focused on this form of revictimization.

In addition, for the purpose of the review, we selected studies that were conducted with college or community samples. Thus, we did not review studies that involved clinical samples because findings from clinical samples may not generalize to women in the general population. We also selected studies that included relatively large, representative samples. We incorporated studies that used behaviorally defined methods for assessing a history of interpersonal violence. Finally, it should be noted that the present review focuses on women and is therefore only generalizable to women. We have not addressed the phenomenon of sexual revictimization among boys and men. Research has indicated that the preponderance of sexual assaults in adulthood occurs to women (Tjaden & Thoennes, 2000) and the majority of studies addressing sexual revictimization have been conducted on women participants.

Therefore, data on the prevalence rates or possible mediating factors that may be specific to sexual revictimization among men are lacking. Because the factors associated with the sexual assault of men in adulthood may be different from those of women, it is not clear whether findings that pertain to populations of women are generalizable to men.

REVIEWED SAMPLES

Probability Studies

We identified three studies that used a sophisticated research design to obtain large nationally representative samples (Kilpatrick et al., 1997; Koss & Dinero, 1989; Tjaden & Thoennes, 2000). One study used a sampling procedure that surveyed a representative sample of college students in the United States, and the others used random-digit dialing methods to recruit and interview a representative sample of adults in the United States.

The first study, conducted by Koss and Dinero (1989), investigated the incidence of sexual assault among college women and examined a number of proposed mediating variables associated with interpersonal victimization. The researchers used enrollment data for all U.S. colleges and sorted the colleges into geographical regions by proximity to metropolitan areas, ethnic enrollment, type of institutions, and size of the student population. Of the 92 schools that were contacted, 32 agreed to participate, resulting in a total of 3,187 college women who completed the study.

Anonymous questionnaires were administered that assessed sexual victimization experiences and three sets of potential mediating variables: (a) potential vulnerability-creating traumatic experiences (e.g., divorce, physical abuse, domestic violence), (b) social-psychological characteristics (e.g., personality traits and attitudes), and (c) vulnerability-enhancing situation variables (e.g., alcohol use, number of sexual partners). CSA was defined as experiences ranging from exhibitionism to rape that occurred before the age of 14 (Finkelhor, 1979). ASA included experiences ranging from sexual contact to rape that occurred after the age of 14 (Koss & Oros, 1982).

Findings indicated a significant relationship between CSA and ASA. Specifically, 66% of the adult rape victims had a history of CSA, compared with only 20% of the women with no history of adult victimization. Therefore, adult victims were over three times more likely to have a history of CSA compared with adult nonvictims. Analyses did not include an examination of differences based on racial or ethnic differences. Several variables were found to effectively differentiate rape victims and nonvictims, including CSA, sexual attitudes, level of sexual activity, and alcohol use.

Strengths of this study included a large representative sample of college women and the exploration of a large number of predictor variables that were based on a proposed theory. The limitations of this study related to the use of a cross-sectional design, a lack of consideration of racial differences, and definitional issues. The age range for ASA was defined as experiences since age 14, meaning that adolescent sexual assaults were incorporated into the ASA category. Therefore, it is not clear whether the phenomenon of revictimization in this study reflected a relationship between CSA and adolescent or adult experiences.

A second study, the National Women's Study (Kilpatrick et al., 1997), used a stratified sample random-digit dialing procedure to recruit a representative sample of U.S. women. A structured telephone interview was conducted to assess demographic characteristics, a history of physical and sexual assault, assault-related characteristics, and a variety of psychological symptoms. Women completed an initial assessment (Wave 1) and were contacted at 1- and 2-year follow-ups, labeled Waves 2 and 3, respectively. There were 4,009 women who participated in the study.

Kilpatrick et al. (1997) examined risk factors for revictimization among a subsample of 3,006 women who completed the Wave 3 follow-up assessment. Rape was defined as unwanted experiences of oral, vaginal, or anal penetration in which the perpetrator used force or threats of force. Physical assault was defined as being physically attacked by another person with a gun, knife, or other weapon, or without a weapon but with the intent to kill or seriously injure. At the Wave 1 assessment, 14.5% of women reported a history of rape. A majority of prior lifetime rape incidents assessed at Wave 1 (62%) occurred prior to age 18. Eleven percent of women reported a history of physical assault, and 21.8% reported having experienced rape or physical assault. At the Wave 3 assessment, 1.6% of women reported a new rape since the initial interview, 3.4% reported a new physical assault, and 4.8% reported a new assault of either type.

Results indicated a strong relationship between a prior history of victimization at Wave 1 and subsequent assault. Furthermore, findings suggested that substance abuse was an important mediator of revictimization. Controlling for sociodemographic variables, both a history of rape or physical assault and a history of alcohol abuse or illicit drug use were significant predictors of new rape and physical assault. Specifically, a history of interpersonal victimization was associated with an odds ratio of 4.99 (confidence interval [CI] = 3.51–7.53), and substance abuse was associated with an odds ratio of 1.68 (CI = 1.09–2.59). For a report of separate predictors of new incidents of rape and physical assault, see Acierno, Resnick, Kilpatrick, Saunders, and Best (1999).

Major strengths of this study were its use of a longitudinal design and a nationally representative sample of women. In addition, the researchers investigated multiple types of victimization experiences. Therefore, data were collected about baseline history of lifetime experiences, and assessments were repeated over a 2-year period of time for both victimization experiences and symptom measures. A limitation of the study with respect to examining risk factors for revictimization was that the assessment of initial victimization experiences was not restricted to assaults occurring prior to a specific age cutoff. Thus, although the majority of prior rapes reportedly occurred prior to age 18, this study did not specifically examine CSA alone as a predictor of ASA.

The National Violence Against Women Study (Tjaden & Thoennes, 2000) provides data from another nationally representative sample, consisting of 8,000 women and 8,005 men, ages 18 and older. Participants were recruited by use of a random-digit dialing system that included all 50 states and the District of Columbia. Interviews assessed a range of child and adult victimization experiences, including stalking, physical assault, and sexual assault. Rape was defined as nonconsensual penetration of the victim's vagina or anus by penis, tongue, fingers, or object, or the victim's mouth by penis, involving force or threats of force. Physical assault included events that threatened, attempted to inflict, or actually caused physical harm to an individual. Stalking was defined as events that were directed at a specific person and included behaviors involving repeated visual or physical proximity, nonconsensual communication, or a combination of experiences that produced fear in the victim.

Descriptive analysis of the data indicated that 17.6% of the women and 3% of the men in the study reported a rape or attempted rape at some time in their life. Approximately 52% of the women and 66% of the men reported a physical assault at some time in their life. Physical assault was reported during the most recent rape in 41.4% of women and 33.9% of the men who were raped since the age of 18. Additionally, 8.1% of the women and 2.2% of the men reported being stalked at some time in their life. Finally, 40% of women and 53.8% of men reported being physically abused as children, and 9% of the women and 1.9% of the men reported being the victim of CSA.

Data indicated that 18.3% of the women who reported CSA before age 18 also reported ASA, whereas only 8.7% of the women who were not sexually abused as children reported ASA. Therefore, CSA victims were more than twice as likely as nonvictims to be sexually assaulted in adulthood. Rates of revictimization were not calculated for the men based on the low prevalence of sexual victimization experiences. A significant relationship between history of childhood physical abuse and subsequent adult physical assault was also observed. Over 46% of women and 60% of men who reported a history of child physical abuse also reported a physical assault in adulthood, whereas only 19.8% of the women and 27.3% of the men without a history of child physical abuse reported an adult physical assault. Similar to sexual assault revictimization rates, both men and women with a child physical abuse history were twice as likely to be physically assaulted as an adult when compared with individuals without a childhood physical abuse history.

Strengths of this study included a large nationally representative sample of women and men, the use of behaviorally specific questions, and the gathering of contextual information on victimization events, including the rate of injury and use of medical services. Thus, data from representative samples indicated that women with prior histories of CSA were at least two to three times more likely to experience sexual assault as adults. Kilpatrick et al. (1997) reported an odds ratio of nearly 5.0 associated with the likelihood of experiencing a new assault during the 2-year follow-up period among individuals with a history of either physical or sexual assault.

College Studies

The majority of studies that have examined revictimization have been conducted with college student populations. The reliance on data gathered from college student populations has been criticized in that college students are not believed to be representative of the general population. There is evidence to suggest that college women are twice as likely to report a sexual assault compared with women in the general population (Koss & Dinero, 1989). A number of factors, including increased use of alcohol, a rape-supportive environment, and lack of parental supervision, have been posited to account for increased vulnerability for sexual assault among college women (Warshaw, 1988). In contrast, some researchers propose that college women are less likely to have been revictimized in "adulthood" by virtue of their young age, meaning they have limited time frames in which revictimization may occur.

We identified a total of four college studies for inclusion in the present review. The first one, conducted by Gidycz et al. (1993), examined the rates of sexual assault and revictimization using a mixed retrospective and prospective research design. Participants completed a survey that assessed sexual victimization experiences and psychological functioning at the beginning of the college quarter and 9 weeks later. CSA included experiences of exhibitionism, fondling, attempted rape, and rape occurring prior to age 14. Adolescent and adult sexual assault focused on events that occurred since the age of 14. Responses to adult victimization questions were coded as sexual contact, sexual coercion, attempted rape, or rape. Victims were classified on the basis of the most severe type of sexual victimization they endorsed.

A significant relationship was found between CSA and ASA, such that 29.5% of the child rape victims and 32.1% of the child attempted rape victims were sexually revictimized during the 9-week assessment interval. Of the women with no history of childhood rape, only 13.6% reported an adult rape. Thus, those with a history of CSA were more than twice as likely to be revictimized. It is important to note that these rates of revictimization reflect events that occurred during a brief 9-week follow-up period. Thus, the incidence of assault may have been higher if assessed over a longer period of time. Results also indicated a significant relationship between child and adolescent victimizations, and between adolescent and adult victimizations. Furthermore, women who were victimized in both childhood and adulthood reported significantly more psychological symptoms than nonvictims, childhood-only victims, and adulthood-only victims, suggesting that revictimization is associated with cumulative psychological effects.

In an extension of this study, Gidycz and colleagues (Gidycz et al., 1995) surveyed 677 women, using the same research design and survey instruments that were used in the 1993 study. Women were evaluated for sexual victimization history at Time 1. In addition to anxiety and depression, several other potential mediating variables were assessed, such as alcohol use, family adjustment, psychological adjustment, interpersonal functioning, and sexual behavior. Three follow-up sessions were conducted at 3-month, 5–6-month, and 9-month intervals.

CSA, adolescent sexual assault, and ASA were divided into five categories (none, contact, coercion, attempted rape, and penetration) of increasing severity. A significant relationship between a prior history of sexual victimization and a recent victimization was indicated during the follow-up period. Women with a prior sexual victimization history were 1.5 to 2 times more likely than nonvictims to report a new victimization. In addition, the severity of prior sexual assaults was strongly associated with the severity of subsequent assaults. Psychological adjustment, interpersonal functioning, number of sexual partners, and alcohol use were found to be mediators of the relationship between CSA and adolescent sexual assault. However, none of these mediating variables predicted a future adult victimization. Therefore, across all time periods and follow-up periods, the strongest predictor of sexual victimization was a previous sexual victimization.

Gidycz et al.'s (1993, 1995) studies are innovative in that they used a prospective design, providing information regarding abuse history and psychological functioning prior to a new sexual assault. In addition, the design allowed for the examination of how child and adolescent sexual experiences may psychologically affect women who have recently experienced ASA. In Gidycz et al.'s (1995) study, results demonstrated a relationship between child and adolescent victimization and between adolescent and adult victimization, but not between child and adult victimizations. Thus, only the categories contiguous by age ranges (most proximal in terms of age or initial and subsequent victimization) demonstrated the increased risk for revictimization pattern. These findings are extremely important when considering the differing cutoff ages across various studies. Weaknesses of the study included limited generalizability associated with a college student sample and retrospective reporting of child and adolescent abuse events.

In another college sample, Mayall and Gold (1995) explored the relationship between CSA and ASA and examined the manner in which abuse definitions relate to different outcomes. First, they manipulated the definitions of both CSA and ASA, hypothesizing that more restrictive definitions of child and adult abuse experiences (e.g., requiring physical contact or penetration) would be associated with higher rates of revictimization. Second, they hypothesized that mediating variables such as nonexpressive coping styles, lack of parental support, severity of abuse, negative attributions about the abuse, and a lack of disclosure to a helping professional would be associated with higher rates of sexual revictimization. Finally, they hypothesized that victims of ASA would report a greater use of alcohol and larger number of sexual partners than women who were not sexually assaulted in adulthood.

Participants included 654 college women. CSA was defined as sexual contact before the age of 15 that involved a perpetrator 5 or more years older than the victim. Mayall and Gold (1995) also measured contextual variables associated with the assault, such as frequency and duration of the abuse and use of force. In addition, coping styles, attributions about the assault, parental support, and treatment history were assessed. The child and adult victimization experiences were grouped into three categories of increasing severity. For child abuse experiences, the "Child 1" group consisted of noncontact CSA experiences, the "Child 2" group included CSA experiences that involved physical contact but no penetration, and the "Child 3" group included childhood rape experiences. Adult victimizations were grouped in a similar fashion, with experiences categorized into three levels of increasing severity ranging from noncontact sexual experiences (e.g., exhibitionism) to rape.

Participants with CSA histories that were more severe reported a higher prevalence of ASA. In contrast, analyses based on less restrictive abuse definitions were not significant. Next, a discriminant analysis was conducted to identify variables that discriminated between CSA victims who were and were not revictimized as adults. The only significant finding was that revictimization was inversely related to the participant's involvement in treatment. Finally, number of sexual partners was also significantly related to revictimization, whereas alcohol use was not.

A primary strength of this study was the examination of different definitions of sexual victimization and the impact that definitions have on observed outcomes. This study shows that narrower definitions are associated with higher rates of revictimization, indicating that more severe sexual assault experiences may predispose one to subsequent victimization. In addition, Mayall and Gold (1995) investigated a large number of contextual variables, allowing for the examination of possible mediating factors. Weaknesses of the study included the retrospective methodology, inclusion of adolescent experiences in the adult category, and the use of a college sample that potentially limits the generalizability of findings.

Messman-Moore, Long, and Siegfried (2000) conducted a study involving 648 college women that was designed to examine multiple types of assault, including CSA and adult sexual and physical assaults. CSA was defined as involuntary sexual experiences before the age of 17, ranging from noncontact abuse to rape, that were perpetrated by someone 5 or more years older than the victim, or involved the use of force or threats of force. Adult experiences included events that occurred after the age of 17 that involved unwanted vaginal or anal intercourse.

Women were grouped into five categories of abuse that included a revictimization group (CSA and adult physical or sexual assault). Results indicated that 20.1% of the participants reported CSA experiences, and over half of the CSA victims also reported an adult physical or sexual assault. Revictimized women reported more somatic complaints, depression, anxiety, interpersonal sensitivity, hostility, and posttraumatic stress symptoms than women with no abuse history and women with only child abuse experiences. In addition, women with multiple types of adult victimizations but no CSA history reported higher symptoms than women with no abuse and women with only one type of ASA experience but no CSA history.

A significant contribution of this study was the assessment of both sexual and physical assault. Past research has typically focused on one type of victimization and has neglected to investigate the cumulative effects of violence over time. Limitations of the study relate to the use of a retrospective design and reliance on a college student sample.

Community Studies

In addition to college studies, researchers have investigated sexual revictimization among community samples. A number of these studies have demonstrated a relationship between CSA and ASA. These studies have recruited women with greater age ranges and racial diversity, which may make their findings somewhat more generalizable to the general population than findings from college samples.

We identified two community studies for inclusion in the present review. In an early study, Russell (1986) recruited 930 women from the community who were interviewed by trained individuals. Although recruitment for the study was limited to the San Francisco area, with a focus on incest survivors, a marketing and research firm used a probability sampling method to obtain a random list of addresses for the study. The interview used both behaviorally phrased questions and labeled terms to assess for a history of sexual assault. Age 14 was used as the cutoff for defining CSA, and ages 14 to 18 defined adolescent experiences. The definitions for CSA experiences distinguished between incest and extrafamilial experiences. The definition of incestuous abuse included any contact or attempted contact with a child prior to age 18 by a relative. Extrafamilial CSA was defined as experiences ranging from molestation to rape with a child up to age 14, and completed or attempted rape with a child from the ages between 14 and 18 years by a nonrelative. Rape was further defined for participants as penile–vaginal intercourse with force or threats of force, or when the woman was rendered unable to physically resist (e.g., drugged, unconscious).

Findings revealed a significant relationship between CSA and ASA. Specifically, 65% of the women who experienced incest and 61% who experienced extrafamilial CSA were revictimized after the age of 14, compared with 35% of women who were never sexually abused in childhood but were victimized after age 14. Therefore, incest survivors and extrafamilial CSA survivors were nearly two times more likely to report an ASA compared with women who were not sexually abused in childhood. Finally, incest victims were significantly more likely to be subsequent victims of "wife rape" and domestic violence. The risk for wife rape was nearly three times greater for incest victims (19%) than for women who were not victims of incest (7%). Incest victims were more than twice as likely (27%) to be victims of domestic violence than women who were not victims of incest (12%).

Strengths of this study were the large sample size and the attempt to recruit a random sample. Also, this is one of the few studies that attempted to classify child and adult assaults on the basis of the victim's relationship to the perpetrator. A potential limitation of the study was the use of legal terms, which may have resulted in underreporting of cases. Research has demonstrated that women may have experienced incidents that meet the legal definition for rape but do not label them as such (Layman et al., 1996).

Wyatt, Guthrie, and Notgrass (1992) investigated the relationship between CSA and ASA and attempted to address the discrepancies among rates of revictimization that have been reported in previous studies. Women between the ages of 18 and 36 years old were recruited from Los Angeles, California, using a random-digit dialing procedure. The first 248 women meeting the criteria were interviewed, resulting in a sample of 126 Black and 122 White participants. CSA included experiences ranging from noncontact abuse to rape occurring with someone at least 5 years older than the victim or involving coercion. An adult sexual victimization was defined as an event that occurred after the age of 18 and included a range of experiences from "flashing" to rape.

Of the 248 women in the study, 176 reported at least one incident of sexual victimization sometime in their lives. One hundred fifty-four participants reported sexual assault in childhood, of which 121 involved contact. CSA victims were 2.4 times more likely to be victimized in adulthood compared with non-CSA victims. None of the mediating variables that were examined were statistically significant when analyzed based on assault severity. However, CSA victims who were revictimized in adulthood were significantly more likely to experience unintended pregnancies and abortions. In addition, women who had two or more sexual victimizations in childhood and two or more sexual victimizations in adulthood reported a higher number of sexual partners, engaged in more types of sexual experiences, and had more unintended pregnancies and abortions.

Strengths of this study included an attempt to recruit a representative sample and investigation of a large number of possible mediating variables.

A limitation of this study was that labeled terms were used to assess for abuse experiences and, as previously mentioned, this may have omitted women from the victimization categories who experienced an assault and did not label it as such. In addition, the study did not have a nonvictim control group for comparison on symptom measures.

SUMMARY

We examined nine studies that investigated the relationship between CSA and ASA. Studies were selected on the basis of their use of large, representative community and college samples. All studies found support for the phenomenon of revictimization. In each study, women with a history of CSA were significantly more likely than nonvictims to have experienced a subsequent sexual assault. Across these studies, victims of CSA were generally two to three times more likely to have experienced ASA compared with non-CSA victims. Therefore, simply having a prior assault history increased a woman's risk for later sexual assault in adolescence or adulthood.

Across studies, potential mediating variables that might shed more light on specifically why those with a history of CSA are at greater risk for later revictimization were rarely examined. Of the few studies that assessed mediating variables, findings indicated that revictimization was associated with participants reporting a higher number of sexual partners (Mayall & Gold, 1995), more unintended pregnancies and abortions (Wyatt et al., 1992), greater alcohol use (Koss & Dinero, 1989), and use of illicit drugs (Kilpatrick et al., 1997).

LIMITATIONS IN CURRENT LITERATURE

As noted in this chapter and in Table 2.1, studies differed on a number of critical methodological and definitional characteristics. Regardless of the limitations across studies, a significant relationship between child and adult sexual victimization experiences was observed. In addition, several mediating variables such as drug and alcohol use and number of sex partners were found to be associated with sexual revictimization. However, the significance of mediating variables was inconsistent across studies. Study differences and limitations may have prohibited researchers from identifying variables that may put a woman at risk for a sexual revictimization. Subsequently, knowledge that might guide effective programs designed to prevent sexual revictimization is limited. For example, across studies, different definitions of abuse were used. Some researchers used a narrower definition, assessing for either attempted or completed rape experiences involving force or threats of force (e.g., Kilpatrick et al., 1997). Other researchers used a broader definition and assessed for experiences such as being exposed to another person's genitals (e.g., Wyatt et al., 1992) or being assaulted in the context of alcohol or drug use (Gidcyz et al., 1993, 1995). Mayall and Gold's (1995) findings indicated that the relationship between CSA and ASA was strongest when sexual assault was more narrowly defined. Studies that used definitions pertaining to severe assault experiences in childhood, such as attempted and completed rape, observed stronger associations with subsequent victimization, compared with definitions involving broader or less clearly specified definitions of sexual assault. Attempts should be made to standardize both definitions of child and adult sexual assault as well as to create measures that will adequately represent these definitions.

Another major limitation of past studies has been the sampling methodology that has been used. With the exception of a few large-scale probability studies, the bulk of research has been conducted with small, select samples, such as college students and volunteers from the community. Although convenience samples provide valuable information, particularly in the initial stages of research when pilot data are needed, the findings may not generalize to other groups. For example, college women have routinely been used to study interpersonal victimization phenomena. Researchers have proposed that college students are an appropriate target group because they represent an age group at high risk for experiencing interpersonal violence. However, factors that may be unique to college participants, such as their birth cohort, life circumstances, and their willingness to volunteer to participate in research studies, may differentiate them from the general population. It is also noteworthy that college students, by virtue of being enrolled in an institution of higher learning, may possess characteristics that differentiate them from the general population. Consequently, it is essential for researchers to use representative samples, as much as possible, to maximize the likelihood that findings are generalizable to a larger segment of the population.

Varying definitions of age cutoffs determining child, adolescent, and adult assaults may be associated with different patterns of findings related to risk of revictimization, because the recency of a previous assault may be an important risk factor. Gidcyz et al. (1995) found that risk for assault within a particular developmental period (i.e., adolescent or adult) was predicted by an assault within the most recent preceding developmental period, as opposed to an assault occurring within a more distant developmental period. Thus, an assault in adolescence was predictive of adult victimization, whereas an assault in childhood was not. Therefore, researchers must attend to the time frame in which prior victimization experiences occur. Thus, there is a need to recognize multiple developmental periods and to assess for a range of assault characteristics that may be pertinent to each developmental stage.

Another limitation related to sampling methodology has been the over-reliance on demographically homogeneous groups. Specifically, research examining victimization and revictimization has relied primarily on data gathered from Caucasian women. Given the strong reliance on convenience sampling methodology, little effort has been devoted to recruiting heterogeneous samples. As a result, there is a paucity of research examining the interrelationships among race, gender, socioeconomic status, and victimization or revictimization. Research has indicated that girls and women are significantly more likely than boys and men to be victims of sexual assault (Boney-McCoy & Finkelhor, 1995; Burnam et al., 1988; Finkelhor, Hotaling, Lewis, & Smith, 1990; Silverman, Reinherz, & Giaconia, 1996; Tjaden & Thoennes, 2000).

There are limitations of the present review that should be acknowledged. The process for identifying studies for inclusion in this review was not meant to be comprehensive. We selected studies on the basis of several criteria, including studies that used large, representative samples, recruited from either college or community populations, and investigated the relationship between CSA and ASA. Therefore, we may have overlooked some important studies. Despite these restrictions, the findings of the review point to the importance of recognizing CSA as a risk factor for subsequent victimization and suggest the need for additional research examining revictimization phenomena.

FUTURE DIRECTIONS

Despite the previously noted methodological differences, studies have consistently found that CSA increases a woman's risk for future victimization. Data are lacking regarding whether this phenomenon is true for men. In addition, a few studies have identified variables that may mediate the relationship between a past sexual victimization and a future sexual victimization. In many respects, this line of research is in its infancy because the majority of studies have merely documented the association between childhood victimization and later victimization experiences. Additional research is needed to understand how and why revictimization occurs. Unfortunately, the limitations that have plagued the child abuse literature, such as methodological and definitional differences across studies, also plague revictimization research. Therefore, clarifying definitional issues and standardizing assessment instruments must first be accomplished to advance research into the phenomenon of sexual revictimization.

Future research will require a greater emphasis on theoretical explanations to better understand the mechanisms for why individuals are revictimized. There is a need to develop testable theories, especially those that attend to potential mediating and moderating variables. With the use of theory, findings are more easily synthesized, and the interrelationships among variables can be taken into account. At this point, we have limited understanding of the potential factors that may mediate or moderate the effects of CSA in association with revictimization. It is possible that something unique about CSA creates the vulnerability. Alternatively, susceptibility may be increased by some factor that is common to traumatic events more generally, such as the development of posttraumatic stress disorder (PTSD) or other trauma-related sequelae following a traumatic incident or incidents that may occur at varying points across the life span.

Future research must also address prevention efforts. Much may be learned about the phenomenon of revictimization by successfully reducing its occurrence. With regard to primary prevention efforts, preliminary findings suggest that risky sexual behaviors (Mayall & Gold, 1995; Wyatt et al., 1992), alcohol abuse (Koss & Dinero, 1989), use of illicit drugs (Kilpatrick et al., 1997), low income (Byrne, Resnick, Kilpatrick, Best, & Saunders, 1999), PTSD (Acierno et al., 1999), other psychological symptoms (Gidycz et al., 1993; Messman-Moore et al., 2000), and risk recognition processes (Combs-Lane & Smith, 2002; Wilson et al., 1999) may mediate the relationship between CSA and ASA. Thus, clinicians may be able to address these factors with clients and perhaps help individuals to lower their risk for revictimization. Prevention of revictimization will require improving on traditional sexual assault risk reduction programs, which have been ineffective for women with a previous victimization history (Hanson & Gidycz, 1993). For a review of sexual assault prevention programs, see Gidycz, Rich, and Marioni (2002) and chapter 13, this volume. Recently, two studies have assessed the effectiveness of a sexual assault risk reduction program designed especially for women with a previous sexual victimization history (Calhoun et al., 2001; Marx, Calhoun, Wilson, & Meyerson, 2001). The program focused on enhancing risk recognition and problem solving, as well as teaching coping and assertion skills. Results from the Calhoun et al. (2001) study indicated that women victims who completed the prevention program reported increased self-efficacy, increased psychological functioning, and significantly lower rates of severe sexual victimizations compared with the control group. These results suggest that prevention efforts must focus on risk factors that are most relevant for previously victimized women in order to design more effective risk reduction programs.

Future studies also need to consider contextual factors that may lead to an increased risk for revictimization. Factors such as race, relationship to the perpetrator, the use of force, and socioeconomic status should be systematically investigated to assess their impact on psychological functioning, availability of resources and social support, as well as their mediating effects on sexual revictimizaion. There is also a need to investigate revictimization among men, because almost all research to date has focused on women. Among women, research suggests that assault characteristics, such as the relationship to the perpetrator, may affect the risk for revictimization. For instance, Maker et al. (2001) found that sexual abuse by a peer was not associated with adult sexual revictimization, whereas sexual abuse by an older perpetrator (5 years or more older) was related. The prevalence of CSA has not been found to differ between White and Black women (Urquiza & Goodlin-Jones, 1994; Wyatt, 1985). However, poverty and being a member of a racial minority group have been associated with higher rates of revictimization in some samples (Kilpatrick, Resnick, Saunders, & Best, 1998). Other studies have indicated no differences in rates of revictimization based on race (Wyatt et al., 1992). Data from the National Violence Against Women study (Tjaden & Thoennes, 2000) reveal the importance of racial status in assessing for victimization history. Comparisons of White and non-White women (a group comprising African American, American Indian or Alaska Native, Asian or Pacific Islander, and mixed-race women) indicated no significant differences in the prevalence of rape, physical assault, stalking, or childhood physical assault. However, American Indian or Alaska Native women were significantly more likely than other groups to report rape or stalking, women of mixed race were more likely to report history of rape than White women, and Hispanic women were less likely to report rape than non-Hispanic women.

Several studies have found that lower socioeconomic status is associated with increased risk of assault. For instance, Byrne et al. (1999) found that women with incomes below poverty level and newly divorced women were at a significant increased risk of new or repeat future victimization. Consistent with these findings, Bassuk et al. (1996) found substantially elevated prevalence of sexual or physical assault histories among homeless (92%) and low-income housed women (82%). Clearly, there is a need for additional research to examine associations among demographic factors, different types of assault, and different categories of perpetrators. In addition, potential mediating variables should be included in such studies to gain a better understanding of potential mechanisms by which demographic variables may relate to victimization.

A final area of future research is to examine the interactions between violent incidents that an individual may experience over time. At this point most researchers have narrowly focused on specific types of violence, excluding all others. The majority of studies have examined either sexual or physical assault, resulting in separate, disjointed bodies of literature. With respect to revictimization, studies have focused almost exclusively on the relationship between CSA and ASA. Consequently, relatively little is known about the potential for child physical abuse to be associated with increased risk for revictimization. There are a number of childhood or early traumatic experiences that may also contribute to increased risk of assault as an adult. Similarly, there are few studies that have examined revictimization by physical assault and sexual assault in adolescence or adulthood classified on the basis of relationship to the perpetrator (intimate partner, stranger, acquaintance). It is highly likely that risk factors for assaults by strangers, intimate partners, or acquaintances may differ. Thus, failure to distinguish between different types of assault and to comprehensively assess multiple types of assault by multiple categories of perpetrators limits our understanding of specific risk factors for revictimization.

As the study of sexual victimization is a relatively new endeavor, the study of revictimization is in its infancy. The investigation into the phenomenon of sexual revictimization has thus far been pursued without theoretical guidance and has often been conducted in an unsystematic manner. What is known is that a woman who is sexually victimized during childhood has an increased vulnerability to experience another sexual victimization in the future. What is not understood is the manner in which a victimization history creates this vulnerability. Nor is it known how to effectively intervene with rape victims in a way that will reduce their vulnerability for experiencing a subsequent sexual victimization. Therefore, the study of this devastating phenomenon affords researchers a unique and intriguing challenge. This challenge includes, first, the development of statistically sound measures, innovative research methods, and testable theoretical models. Second, it will be necessary to identify mediating variables, especially contextual variables related to assault, the effects of subsequent trauma symptoms, and the availability of personal and financial resources after an assault experience. And finally, the field requires the systematic development and evaluation of effective CSA and ASA prevention programs that explicitly address prior victimization experiences and the factors that render women and children vulnerable to future victimization.

REFERENCES

Acierno, R., Resnick, H., Kilpatrick, D. G., Saunders, B., & Best, C. L. (1999). Risk factors for rape, physical assault, and posttraumatic stress disorder in women: Examination of differential multivariate relationships. *Journal of Anxiety Disorders, 13*, 541–563.

Arata, C. (2000). From child victim to adult victim: A model for predicting sexual revictimization. *Child Maltreatment, 5*, 28–38.

Bassuk, E. L., Weinreb, L. F., Buckner, J. C., Browne, A., Salomon, A., & Bassuk, S. S. (1996). The characteristics and needs of sheltered homeless and low-income housed mothers. *Journal of the American Medical Association, 276*, 640–646.

Boney-McCoy, S., & Finkelhor, D. (1995). Prior victimization: A risk factor for child sexual abuse and for PTSD-related symptomatology among sexually abused youth. *Child Abuse and Neglect, 19*, 1401–1421.

Burnam, M. A., Stein, J. A., Golding, J. M., Siegel, J. M., Sorenson, S. B., Forsythe, A. B., & Tellas, C. A. (1988). Sexual assault and mental disorders in a community population. *Journal of Consulting and Clinical Psychology, 56*, 843–850.

Byrne, C. A., Resnick, H. S., Kilpatrick, D. G., Best, C. L., & Saunders, B. E. (1999). The socioeconomic impact of interpersonal violence on women. *Journal of Consulting and Clinical Psychology, 67*, 362–366.

Calhoun, K. S., Gidycz, C. A., Loh, C., Wilson, A., Lueken, M., Outman, R. C., & Marioni, N. L. (2001, November). *Sexual assault prevention in high-risk women*. Poster presented at the meeting of the Association for the Advancement of Behavior Therapy, Philadelphia, PA.

Combs-Lane, A. M., & Smith, D. W. (2002). Risk of sexual victimization in college women: The role of behavioral intentions and risk-taking behaviors. *Journal of Interpersonal Violence, 17*, 165–183.

Finkelhor, D. (1979). *Sexually victimized children*. New York: Macmillian.

Finkelhor, D., Hotaling, G., Lewis, I. A., & Smith, C. (1990). Sexual abuse in a national survey of adult men and women: Prevalence, characteristics, and risk factors. *Child Abuse and Neglect, 14*, 19–28.

Gidycz, C. A., Coble, C. N., Latham, L., & Layman, M. J. (1993). Sexual assault experiences in adulthood and prior victimization experiences. *Psychology of Women Quarterly, 17*, 151–168.

Gidycz, C. A., Hanson, K., & Layman, M. (1995). A prospective analysis of the relationships among sexual assault experiences. *Psychology of Women Quarterly, 19*, 5–29.

Gidycz, C. A., Rich, C. L., & Marioni, N. L. (2002). Interventions to prevent rape and sexual assault. In J. Petrak & B. Hedge (Eds.), *The trauma of adult sexual assault: Treatment, prevention, and policy* (pp. 235–260). New York: Wiley.

Gold, S. R., Sinclair, B. B., & Balge, K. A. (1999). Risk of sexual revictimization: A theoretical model. *Aggression and Violent Behavior, 4*, 457–470.

Grauerholz, L. (2000). An ecological approach to understanding sexual revictimzation: Linking personal, interpersonal, and sociocultural factors and processes. *Child Maltreatment, 5*, 5–17.

Hanson, K. A., & Gidycz, C. A. (1993). Evaluation of a sexual assault prevention program. *Journal of Consulting and Clinical Psychology, 61*, 1046–1052.

Harrington, N. T., & Leitenberg, H. (1994). Relationship between alcohol consumption and victim behaviors immediately preceding sexual aggression by an acquaintance. *Violence and Victims, 4*, 315–324.

Kilpatrick, D. G., Acierno, R., Resnick, H. S., Saunders, B. E., & Best, C. L. (1997). A 2-year longitudinal analysis of the relationship between violent assault and substance use in women. *Journal of Consulting and Clinical Psychology, 65*, 834–847.

Kilpatrick, D. G., Resnick, H. S., Saunders, B. E., & Best, C. L. (1998). Rape, other violence against women, and posttraumatic stress disorder. In B. P. Dohrenwend (Ed.). *Adversity, stress, and psychopathology* (pp. 161–176). New York: Oxford University Press.

Koss, M. P., & Dinero, T. (1989). Discriminant analysis of risk factors for sexual victimization among a national sample of college women. *Journal of Consulting and Clinical Psychology, 57*, 242–250.

Koss, M. P., & Oros, C. J. (1982). Sexual Experiences Survey: A research instrument investigating sexual aggression and victimization. *Journal of Consulting and Clinical Psychology, 50*, 455–457.

Layman, M. J., Gidycz, C. A., & Lynn, S. J. (1996). Unacknowledged versus acknowledged rape victims: Situational factors and posttraumatic stress. *Journal of Abnormal Psychology, 105*, 124–131.

Maker, A. H., Kemmelmeier, M., & Peterson, C. (2001). Child sexual abuse, peer sexual abuse, and sexual assault in adulthood: A multi-risk model of revictimization. *Journal of Traumatic Stress, 14*, 351–368.

Marx, B. P., Calhoun, K. S., Wilson, A. E., & Meyerson, L. A. (2001). Sexual revictimization prevention: An outcome evaluation. *Journal of Consulting and Clinical Psychology, 69*, 25–32.

Mayall, A., & Gold, S. R. (1995). Definitional issues and mediating variables in the sexual revictimization of women sexually abused as children. *Journal of Interpersonal Violence, 10*, 26–42.

Messman, T. L., & Long, P. J. (1996). Child sexual abuse and its relationship to revictimization in adult women: A review. *Clinical Psychology Review, 16*, 397–420.

Messman-Moore, T. L., Long, P. J., & Siegfried, N. J. (2000). The revictimization of child sexual abuse survivors: An examination of the adjustment of college women with child sexual abuse, adult sexual assault, and adult physical abuse. *Child Maltreatment, 5*, 18–27.

Roodman, A. A., & Clum, G. A. (2001). Revictimization rates and method variance: A meta-analysis. *Clinical Psychology Review, 21*, 183–204.

Russell, D. E. H. (1986). *The secret trauma: Incest in the lives of girls and women*. New York: Basic Books.

Silverman, A. B., Reinherz, H. Z., & Giaconia, R. M. (1996). The long-term sequelae of child and adolescent abuse: A longitudinal community study. *Child Abuse and Neglect, 20*, 709–723.

Tjaden, P., & Thoennes, N. (2000). *Full report of the prevalence, incidence, and consequences of violence against women* (Research Report No. NCJ 183781). Washington, DC: U.S. Department of Justice.

Urquiza, A. J., & Goodlin-Jones, B. L. (1994). Child sexual abuse and adult revictimization with women of color. *Violence and Victims, 9*, 223–232.

Warshaw, R. (1988). *I never called it rape: The "Ms." report on recognizing, fighting, and surviving date and acquaintance rape*. New York: Harper & Row.

Wilson, A. E., Calhoun, K. S., & Bernat, J. A. (1999). Risk recognition and trauma-related symptoms among sexually revictimized women. *Journal of Consulting and Clinical Psychology, 67*, 705–710.

Wyatt, G. E. (1985). The sexual abuse of Afro-American and White-American women in childhood. *Child Abuse and Neglect, 9*, 507–519.

Wyatt, G. E., Guthrie, D., & Notgrass, C. M. (1992). Differential effects of women's child sexual abuse and subsequent sexual revictimization. *Journal of Consulting and Clinical Psychology, 60*, 167–173.

3

SEXUAL ABUSE OF GIRLS AND HIV INFECTION AMONG WOMEN: ARE THEY RELATED?

LINDA J. KOENIG AND HOLLIE CLARK

Among the many negative health outcomes that can be associated with sexual behavior, infection with the human immunodeficiency virus (HIV) is certainly the most life threatening. More than 440,000 people in the United States have died of AIDS, and nearly 1 million have been infected with HIV (Centers for Disease Control and Prevention [CDC], 2001a, 2001b). Identification of behaviors that place individuals at risk of acquiring HIV and the behavioral interventions designed to decrease those risks have constituted a critical component of the public health response to the prevention of HIV/AIDS. Focused on education, risk assessment, and skills training (e.g., condom use and negotiation), these approaches have been decidedly here and now, targeting the most proximal causes of risk behavior. Although these behavioral interventions are critical for containing the spread of HIV/AIDS, 40,000 new infections occur in the United States every year (CDC, 2001a), and it is widely recognized that many people do not respond to prevention messages.

This chapter was authored or coauthored by an employee of the United States government as part of official duty and is considered to be in the public domain. Any views expressed herein do not necessarily represent the views of the United States government.

Identifying those in need of more specific prevention and understanding the factors that maintain risk behaviors in the face of potential health consequences are critical tasks for the next wave of HIV prevention researchers.

Child sexual abuse (CSA) and its traumatizing effects, previously unrecognized as an experience related to HIV, may be one such factor. Anecdotal and scientific research are beginning to suggest a possible link between CSA and HIV—specifically, that people who were sexually victimized as children are at increased risk of acquiring HIV as adults. Whereas much of this research has focused on the relation between CSA and various behaviors that increase the risk of acquiring HIV (see, e.g., National Institute of Mental Health [NIMH] Multisite HIV Prevention Trial, 2001), relatively few studies have investigated whether CSA is overrepresented among people with HIV/AIDS, and this literature had not been systematically reviewed. Toward this end, our goals in this chapter are to review and to examine the epidemiologic evidence for such a link, particularly as it relates to women. (See chap. 4, this volume, for an examination of this issue among men.)

We begin by considering the epidemiology of CSA and of HIV/AIDS in the United States, noting characteristics that may bear relevance for a potential association between the two epidemics. Next, we consider the first step toward evidence for this link, that is, studies on the prevalence of CSA among HIV-infected women and studies that report the prevalence of CSA among women in populations considered at high risk for HIV infection (sexually transmitted disease [STD] clinic patients, sex workers, and injection drug users). We include studies that examine historical factors related to these risk groups (i.e., a history of sexually transmitted infection, injection drug use, or bartering of sex for money, drugs, or shelter) among women with or without a history of CSA. To evaluate the association, we consider (a) the prevalence of CSA among members of these groups in relation to that of the general population; (b) the prevalence of CSA among women with HIV infection versus HIV-negative comparison women, and women in high-risk groups versus nonrisk group comparison women; and (c) the prevalence of related risk factors among women with and women without a history of CSA. We integrate and summarize the findings from these research areas with respect to CSA as a risk for HIV infection and conclude with implications for HIV prevention.

DEMOGRAPHICS OF CHILD SEXUAL ABUSE AND THE HIV/AIDS EPIDEMIC IN THE UNITED STATES

Child Sexual Abuse

In the United States, CSA affects girls of all racial and ethnic backgrounds equally (Sedlak & Broadhurst, 1996; Wyatt, Loeb, Solis, & Carmona,

1999) and constitutes a significant public health problem (McMahon & Puett, 1999). Because of inconsistencies in definitions, measures, and samples, as well as the private and stigmatized nature of CSA, prevalence estimates have varied widely, but they indicate that girls are at three times the risk that boys are (Sedlak & Broadhurst, 1996). Although prevalence estimates range from 8% to 62% for women and 3% to 29% for men (Fergusson & Mullen, 1999), more conservative estimates obtained from representative samples of U.S. women suggest that 8% to 27% of women have experienced contact or noncontact forms of sexual abuse before the age of 18 (Elliott & Briere, 1992; Finkelhor, Hotaling, Lewis, & Smith, 1990; Kilpatrick et al., 2000; Molnar, Buka, & Kessler, 2001; Moore, Nord, & Peterson, 1989; Wilsnack, Vogeltanz, Klassen, & Harris, 1997).

HIV/AIDS

Since HIV was identified more than two decades ago, significant shifts have occurred in the demographics of the domestic HIV/AIDS epidemic, and these shifts are critical for understanding whether and how CSA may relate to HIV infection. Once a disease primarily affecting White gay men, AIDS affects an increasingly larger proportion of women: Cumulative AIDS cases in women increased from 6.7% in 1986 to 18% in 1999 (Hader, Smith, Moore, & Holmberg, 2001). In 2000, women accounted for 25% of AIDS cases reported that year and 31% of new infections (CDC, 2001b). Corresponding to the growing epidemic among women has been the increasing proportion of infections attributable to heterosexual sex. Although needle sharing accounted for 53% of AIDS cases in women through 1988, by 1995 heterosexual transmission surpassed injection drug use as the leading mode of transmission (Hader et al., 2001). Using data from several AIDS reporting surveys, Hader et al. (2001) estimated that 54% of women newly reported with AIDS in 1998 had acquired HIV infection heterosexually. Within this emerging epidemic are a disproportionate number of minority women. Whereas Black and Hispanic women together represent less than one fourth of all U.S. women, they account for more than three fourths of the cumulative AIDS cases among women (CDC, 2001c). Moreover, Black women are more likely than White women to have become infected through heterosexual transmission or a risk that was not known or reported (Hader et al., 2001; Neal, Fleming, Green, & Ward, 1997). Finally, young women are at greatest risk: It has been estimated that 26% to 50% of women who acquire HIV heterosexually do so when they are in their teens or early 20s (Hader et al., 2001; Neal et al., 1997).

As the AIDS epidemic moves into communities of color and HIV is increasingly transmitted to young women through their heterosexual relationships, women who engage in HIV risk behaviors have a greater chance of becoming infected. Women who have experienced sexual abuse as children, particularly those with psychological and behavioral characteristics often identified as sequelae of CSA, may be the women least able to protect themselves and at greatest risk for infection.

REVIEW OF LITERATURE

Method

To locate relevant studies, we searched six databases: PubMed, CINAHL, Medline, PsycINFO, AIDSLINE, and OVID. The search terms entered were combined with either *child sexual abuse* or *sexual abuse* and included a variety of terms related to HIV/AIDS, STD, prostitution, substance abuse, and unprotected sex. Additionally, a search was conducted using the heading *violence and HIV*. Finally, we also used Porpoise (a service of the Institute for Scientific Information, which retrieves articles from the Science Citation Index Expanded Database) to gather recent publications. As articles were reviewed, relevant citations that had not been identified through earlier literature searches were retrieved.

Prevalence of Child Sexual Abuse Among Women With HIV Infection

One way to begin to examine whether a history of CSA is related to later HIV infection is to consider whether CSA is more common among HIV-infected women than would be expected from the national prevalence data. We found 14 studies with data on the prevalence of sexual abuse among women infected with HIV. Of these, 1 study reported only on abuse during childhood, that is, at 11 years or younger (Lynch, Kranz, Russell, Hornberger, & VanNess, 2000); 3 studies did not distinguish abuse during childhood and abuse during adulthood (Bedimo, Kissinger, & Bessinger, 1997; Kimerling, Armistead, & Forehand, 1999; Liebschutz, Feinman, Sullivan, Stein, & Samet, 2000); and 1 study of women with, or at risk for, HIV infection did not report prevalence of CSA separately for HIV-infected and HIV-negative women (Zierler et al., 1991). According to the 9 remaining studies from which CSA (i.e., sexual abuse during childhood or adolescence) among HIV-infected women could be ascertained (Cohen et al., 2000; Gielen, McDonnell, Wu, O'Campo, & Faden, 2001; Hein, Dell, Futterman, Rotheram-Borus, & Shaffer, 1995; Kirkham & Lobb, 1998; Lyon, Richmond, & D'Angelo, 1995; Simoni & Ng, 2000; Stevens et al., 1995; Vlahov et al., 1998; Wyatt et al., 2002), the proportion of HIV-infected women who had a history of CSA ranged from 31% to 53% (see Table 3.1). This is higher than would be expected from national prevalence data. Although studies differed in sample size (from 16 to 1,288), age of study participants (2 studies of older teens and 7 studies of adults), and operational definition of sexual abuse (ranging from a self-reported response on a single item to a history of abuse in the medical record),

TABLE 3.1
Prevalence of Child Sexual Abuse Among HIV-Infected Women

Study/year	Sample HIV-positive No. (% CSA)	Sample HIV-negative No. (% CSA)	Different by statistical test?	Sample Characteristics HIV-positive	Sample Characteristics HIV-negative	CSA definition/measure
Cohen et al. (2000)	1,288 (31)	357 (27)	No	6 states; clinical consortia	Risk behavior matched	Before age 18; ever pressured or forced to touch sexual parts of, or have intercourse with another person
Vlahov et al. (1998)	764 (41)	367 (45.8)	No	4 states; HIV clinics	Risk behavior matched	Sexually abused or raped as a child
Wyatt et al. (2002)	299 (52)	158 (43)	No	Southern CA[a]; health and social service agencies	Demographically and geographically matched	Wyatt Sex History: Nonconsensual sex before age 18 with adult, consensual sex, with someone ≥ 5 years older
Stevens et al. (1995)	61 (49)	27 (26)	Yes	MA[b]; ID[c] prison clinic	ID and GYN[d] prison clinics; older, more Hispanics	Before age 18; forced sex
Hein et al. (1995)	25 (32)	453 (28)	Not tested	NY[e]; adolescent care unit or hospital	Sexually active unit/hospital patients	History of sexual abuse
Gielen et al. (2001)	287 (41)	0	NA[f]	MD[g]; clinic and community sites	NA	As a child; sexual abuse or rape
Simoni and Ng (2000)	220 (38)	0	NA	NY; ages 25–61	NA	Before age 16; sexual abuse or rape
Lyon et al. (1995)	16 (53)	0	NA	DC[h]; teens; HIV clinic	NA	Sexual abuse history documented in medical record
Kirkham and Lobb (1998)	81 (43.2)	0	NA	BC[i], Canada; in care or from AIDS orgs.[j]	NA	As a child; sexual abuse

Note. [a]CA = California. [b]MA = Massachusetts. [c]ID = infectious disease. [d]GYN = gynecology. [e]NY = New York. [f]NA = Not applicable. [g]MD = Maryland. [h]DC = Washington, DC. [i]BC = British Columbia. [j]Organizations.

the proportion of participants in each sample who had a history of CSA did not seem to vary systematically according to these study characteristics.

Of these nine studies, findings from the five that included an HIV-negative comparison group (Cohen et al., 2000; Hein et al., 1995; Stevens et al., 1995; Vlahov et al., 1998; Wyatt et al., 2002) further addressed an association between CSA and HIV infection in two ways. In addition to indicating whether the proportion of CSA survivors was higher among HIV-infected women relative to an HIV-negative comparison sample assessed similarly, the nature of the comparison group, that is, whether or not they also engaged in HIV risk behavior, also speaks to the role of HIV risk behavior as a mediator of the CSA–HIV connection. Of the five studies with HIV-negative comparison groups (Cohen et al., 2000; Hein et al., 1995; Stevens et al., 1995; Vlahov et al., 1998; Wyatt et al., 2002), only one (Stevens et al., 1995) found CSA to be significantly elevated among HIV-infected women. In Stevens et al.'s (1995) study, all of the women were prisoners, but the HIV-negative women represented a broader range of clinic patients, and their racial and ethnic makeup was different from that of HIV-infected women. In the other four studies, HIV-negative women were matched to the HIV-infected women on important variables. In the study of Wyatt et al. (2002), although the proportion of women who experienced CSA was higher among the HIV-infected women compared with the HIV-negative women (52% vs. 43% when collapsed across racial and ethnic groups), this difference was not statistically significant. In this case, the HIV-negative women were demographically and geographically matched to the HIV-infected women. In the two multicenter studies (Cohen et al., 2000; Vlahov et al., 1998), in which the HIV-negative women were matched to the HIV-infected women on HIV risk behavior (presumed mediators of any CSA–HIV link), the proportions of CSA among the HIV-negative and HIV-infected women were equally high (see Table 3.1). Moreover, in the fifth study (Hein et al., 1995), although the difference in proportions for HIV-infected and HIV-negative girls was not specifically tested, the proportion of HIV-negative female adolescents who had been sexually abused (28%) was nearly as high as that of HIV-infected female adolescents (32%). In this study, HIV-infected adolescents were matched to the HIV-negative adolescents on sexual initiation. (See also Miller & Paone, 1998, who did not report the proportion of female opiate users who had experienced CSA but indicated in text that there was no relation between prior sexual abuse and HIV status.) Taken together, the studies with an HIV-negative comparison group suggest that although CSA seems to be overrepresented among women with HIV infection, it is also highly prevalent among HIV-negative women who engage in HIV risk behaviors.

In sum, a history of CSA is not uncommon among women with HIV infection, affecting one third to one half of them. These proportions appear to be consistently higher than those that would be expected from estimates of CSA from national probability samples, which range from 8% to 27%

among representative samples. The validity of these findings is further supported by the fact that these high proportions were obtained in the two large, multicenter domestic cohort studies of HIV among women—the National Institutes of Health's Women's Interagency HIV Study (Cohen et al., 2000) and the Centers for Disease Control and Prevention's HIV Epidemiologic Research Study (Vlahov et al., 1998)—that include the samples most representative of the HIV/AIDS epidemic in the United States. Although it may seem inconsistent that in the larger cohort studies, CSA was highly prevalent among the HIV-negative women in the comparison groups, this appears to be due to the fact that the HIV-infected and HIV-negative women were matched on sexual and drug use risk behaviors. Specifically, CSA appears to be highly prevalent among women who engage in sexual and drug risk behaviors, suggesting the importance of these behaviors in understanding the factors that link CSA to HIV.

Prevalence of Child Sexual Abuse Among Women in HIV Risk Groups

Although only a limited number of studies reported the prevalence of CSA among women with HIV infection, the possible link between CSA and HIV can also be examined by considering the prevalence of CSA among women who are members of recognized HIV risk groups. Because an STD serves as a reliable proxy for unprotected sex, women with a current STD or currently attending an STD clinic are considered at high risk for HIV infection. Injection drug users and commercial sex workers (CSWs) are also at high risk for HIV.

Child Sexual Abuse and Sexually Transmitted Disease

Five studies reported the prevalence of CSA among women who had a current STD (Champion, Shain, Piper, & Perdue, 2001; Sikstrom, Hellberg, Nilsson, Brihmer, & Mardh, 1996; Vermund, Alexander-Rodriquez, Macleod, & Kelley, 1990) or who were patients of STD or sexual health clinics (Petrak, Byrne, & Baker, 2000; Thompson, Potter, Sanderson, & Maibach, 1997). With one exception (Thompson et al., 1997), the prevalence of CSA was quite high, though the proportions varied predictably according to definition and the methods used for ascertaining CSA. Proportions of more than 45% were obtained in studies in which CSA was self-reported in response to a question about a broad array of sexual experiences throughout childhood and adolescence (i.e., "any unwanted sexual experience before the age of 18," 45.2%; Petrak et al., 2000) or not specifically defined in the study (47%; Sikstrom et al., 1996). A lower, but nevertheless large proportion of CSA survivors (32%) was reported by each of two studies that used narrower definitions for ascertaining or defining the acts constituting CSA (i.e., documentation in chart review of child or adolescent rape, incest, or molestation; Vermund et al., 1990) or that used self-report in response to the questions "Have you ever had a really bad experience like sexual abuse or rape?" and then "Was your first experience of anal or vaginal sex willing or forced?" (Champion et al., 2001). Only Thompson et al. (1997), who defined CSA as a forced act of sex (i.e., "ever forced to have sex against your will before the age of 18?") reported a prevalence (16.7%) that was not above the national average. Moreover, in both of the studies that included comparison groups without an STD (Sikstrom et al., 1996; Vermund et al., 1990), CSA occurred significantly more often in the histories of currently STD-infected women than in those of women who were not STD-infected.

Data obtained from studies of the lifetime history of STD (see Table 3.2) are consistent with those obtained from studies of current STD clinic patients. In 6 of 7 studies of women with and women without a history of sexual abuse during childhood (Browning & Laumann, 1997) or during childhood or adolescence (Fergusson, Horwood, & Lynskey, 1997; Greenberg et al., 1999; Hillis, Anda, Felitti, Nordenberg, & Marchbanks, 2000; Kenney, Reinholtz, & Angelini, 1998; Wingood & DiClemente, 1997), the women who had been sexually abused as children or adolescents reported more STDs. Similar results were obtained in 3 studies using composite measures of abuse (physical, sexual, or emotional; Liebschutz et al., 2000; Petrak et al., 2000; Plichta & Abraham, 1996). In 6 of the 10 studies shown in Table 3.2 (Browning & Laumann, 1997; Fergusson et al., 1997; Greenberg et al., 1999; Hillis et al., 2000; Petrak et al., 2000; Plichta & Abraham, 1996), analyses suggested that the association between STDs and abuse (sexual and other forms) during childhood remained significant or marginally significant even after confounding variables such as age, age at sexual initiation, and family dysfunction were statistically controlled. Although investigators in only 1 study (Browning & Laumann, 1997) specifically noted that they ensured that none of the STDs assessed had resulted directly from the sexual abuse, it is not likely that direct transmission of STDs accounted for most of the STDs reported.

In sum, most of the findings in the STD literature are consistent with those in the HIV literature. That is, with only one exception, CSA appears to be highly prevalent among women with STDs, affecting at least one third of the currently infected or STD clinic population. Moreover, significantly more women who have experienced CSA have had an STD at some time. Although many studies suggest that this association is independent of other family characteristics that may co-occur with abuse, equivocal findings suggest the need for further evaluation.

Child Sexual Abuse and Commercial Sex Work

The relation between early abuse and commercial sex work (CSW) was of interest long before the emergence of the HIV epidemic, and theorists have speculated that abusive family environments play a critical role in the life experiences and choices of CSW. We found eight published studies that documented the prevalence of CSA in a (nonredundant) sample of female CSWs (Table 3.3). The prevalences reported from four of these studies were

TABLE 3.2

Sexually Transmitted Disease Outcomes Among Women With Abuse Histories

Study/year	Sample	CSA or abuse definition/measure	Adjusted for	Outcome for CSA compared with non-CSA
		Women With CSA Histories		
Browning and Laumann (1997)	1,749 National Health and Social Life Survey participants, ages 18–59	Physical sexual contact between prepubescent child and partner of age 14 and ≥ 4 years older	Age, race, class, family structure, age at menses	1.6 times more likely to have had at least 1 lifetime STD
Ferguson et al. (1997)	New Zealand; 520 from representative cohort, followed to age 18	Retrospective: involvement in noncontact/contact abuse, attempted/completed intercourse	Dysfunctional family characteristics	15–17 year-olds had 5.6 times greater likelihood of STDs. Remained marginally significant ($p < .10$) after adjustment.
Greenberg et al. (1999)	NYC[a], Baltimore, Seattle; 825 WINGS[b] participants at risk for HIV	Before age 18: made to do something sexual, touched in way that made uncomfortable, or persuasive or forced sexual contact by older person	Age, race	Significantly higher mean lifetime history of STDs
Hillis et al. (2000)	5,060 HMO[c] patients from ACES[d] study	Before age 18: fondled, forced into touching, attempted/completed intercourse by adult > 5 years older	Age, race	1.9 times as likely to have lifetime STD
Kenney et al. (1998)	Southwestern U.S.; 1,194, multi-ethnic women, ages 18–22	Before age 18: contact molestation, coercion, attempted rape/rape using a modified SES[e]	None	Higher proportion with STD (29% vs. 15%); significantly higher for those coerced or raped
Noell et al. (2001)	216 homeless adolescents	Prepubertal sexual contact with older person, or nonconsensual sex after puberty	None	CSA unrelated to STD during 6-month follow-up period for those with no STD at baseline (85% of sample)

continues

TABLE 3.2 (Continued)

Study/year	Sample	CSA or abuse definition/measure	Adjusted for	Outcome for CSA compared with non-CSA
Wingood and DiClemente (1997)	165 sexually active low-income African Americans	Before age 16: forced, unwanted sex with man	None	1.4 times as likely to have lifetime STD, 2.4 times as likely to have > 2 lifetime STDs
Women With any Type of Child Abuse History				
Liebschutz et al. (2000)	New England; 50 primary care patients	Physical or sexual abuse determined by interview or records review of injuries from rape or abuse	NA	4.3 times as likely to have STD history at study entry
Petrak et al. (2000)	UK[f]; 303 inner-city sexual health clinic patients	Before age 18: Unwanted sexual experience; analyses collapsed across abuse type (physical, emotional, or sexual)	No.[g] of sex partners, condom use, IDU[h], commercial sex work	More likely to have STD history and > 1 STD
Plichta and Abraham (1996)	US[i]; 1,599 from representative phone survey	Respondent's assessment of, as a child, physical or sexual abuse	Socio-demographic characteristics, access to care	Higher proportion ever diagnosed with STD (58.9% vs. 18.8%); CSA doubled/tripled odds of gynecology problems for married/single women

Note. CSA = child sexual abuse. [a]New York City. [b]Women in Group Support. [c]Health maintenance organizations. [d]Adverse Childhood Experiences. [e]Sexual Experiences Survey. [f]United Kingdom. [g]Number. [h]Injection drug use. [i]United States.

TABLE 3.3
Prevalence of Child Sexual Abuse Among Commercial Sex Workers

Study/year	Sample			Sample characteristics		
	Sex workers No. (% SA)	Comparison No. (% CSA)	Different by statistical test?	CSW	Non-CSW comparison	CSA definition/ measure
Bagley and Young (1987)	45 (73.3)	45 (28.9)	Yes	Alberta, Canada; former prostitutes	Representative and age-matched community sample	Before age 16; sexually abused by adult > 18 years of age
Earls and David (1990)	1. 50 (26) 2. 50 (38)	1. 50 (6) 2. 50 (12)	1. Yes 2. Not tested	Montreal; actively engaged prostitutes	Recruited from similar locales; age and SES[a]-matched	1. Sexual interaction with family member 2. Before age 14; consensual sexual experience with partner ≥ 5 years older
Potterat et al. (1998)	237 (32)	407 (13)	Yes	Current and former prostitutes, STD clinic and HIV sites	407 STD clinic patients	Before age 11; penile penetration
Ross et al. (1990)	20 (55)	1. 20 (65) 2. 20 (85)	1. Not tested 2. No	Manitoba, Canada; prostitutes	1. 20 exotic dancers 2. 20 MPD[d] patients (1 male)	Identified from DDIS[b] & DES[c]
Rubenstein (1990)	32 (NR[e])	32 (NR)	Yes; CSWs had more age-inappropriate sexual experiences	LA[f]; women charged with soliciting	Matched for age, birth order, income, SES, marital status, no.[g] of children, education, history of therapy	ESEQ[h]; sex between ages 5–10

continues

TABLE 3.3 (Continued)

Study/year	Sample			Sample characteristics		
	Sex workers No. (% CSA)	Comparison No. (% CSA)	Different by statistical test?	CSW	Non-CSW comparison	CSA definition/ measure
James and Meyerding (1977)	136 (52)	NA	NA	Jailed prostitutes; 66 were addicts	NA	Before 1st sexual intercourse: person > 10 years older attempted sexual play or intercourse
Silbert and Pines (1982)	200 (60)	NA	NA	San Francisco; juvenile and adult current and former CSWs	NA	Before age 16: forced sexual activity
Vanwesenbeeck et al. (1995)	92 (15.2 by relatives; 8.8 by others)	NA	NA	Netherlands; prostitutes	NA	Before age 16; sexual abuse
El-Bassel et al. (2001)	106 (29.2)	NA	NA	NY; 106 street-based sex workers	NA	Before age 18; sexual abuse

Note. [a]Socioeconomic status. [b]Dissociative Disorders Interview Schedule. [c]Dissociative Experiences Scale. [d]Multiple personality disorder. [e]Not reported. [f]Los Angeles. [g]Number. [h]Early Sexual Experiences Questionnaire.

exceptionally high—more than 50% (Bagley & Young, 1987; James & Meyerding, 1977; Ross, Anderson, Heber, & Norton, 1990; Silbert & Pines, 1982). The prevalences reported from the other four were average to moderately high: one quarter to one third of women reported CSA (Earls & David, 1990; El-Bassel, Witte, Wada, Gilbert, & Wallace, 2001; Potterat, Rothenberg, Muth, Darrow, & Phillips-Plummer, 1998; Vanwesenbeeck, DeGraff, van Zessen, Straver, & Visser, 1995).

The five studies of female CSWs that included a matched comparison group (Bagley & Young, 1987; Earls & David, 1990; Potterat et al., 1998; Ross et al., 1990; Rubenstein, 1990) provide more consistent support for a link between CSA and commercial sex work. In four of these (Bagley & Young, 1987; Earls & David, 1990; Potterat et al., 1998; Rubenstein, 1990), CSA was significantly more common among CSWs than among other women. Indeed, only Ross et al. (1990)—whose comparison groups comprised exotic dancers and strippers (many of whom may barter sex but not self-identify as CSWs) and patients with multiple personality disorder (a disorder associated with early abuse; American Psychiatric Association, 1994)—did not find CSA to be more common among CSWs.

A second way to examine the relation between CSA and commercial sex work is by directly assessing the strength of this association in a specified sample. We found 11 studies of women that examined and reported the association between CSA and behaviors related to commercial sex work (see Table 3.4). Most of these studies were conducted in populations known to be at risk for CSA or survival sex, such as the homeless, drug users, or jail detainees. Unlike the case control studies in which the sample comprised women who engaged in sex work for their livelihood, many of these studies identified the bartering of sex at some point in time, including the trading of sex for drugs or shelter, as the outcome measure. As such, they document the association between CSA and engagement in risk behaviors, rather than prevalence of CSA among members of a specific high-risk group.

Of these 11 studies, only 1 used a case control design. Widom and Kuhns (1996) studied 76 women who had experienced CSA (located through cases processed in county courts when the girls were less than 11 years of age) and a comparison group of women who had not been abused or neglected (located through birth certificates and elementary school records). The groups were matched for age, sex, race, and family social class. At 20-year follow-up, the women who had experienced CSA were 2.5 times more likely than those not sexually abused to have "ever been paid for having sex with someone" (10.5% for those who had experienced CSA vs. 2.9% for those who had not). (Analyses controlled for demographics and welfare status as a child.) Although not exclusive to sexual abuse (a similarly high risk was associated with child physical abuse), the association could not be explained by running away, which, when statistically controlled, reduced but did not eliminate the association.

TABLE 3.4
Bartering Sex Among Women With Child Sexual Abuse Histories

Study/year	Sample	CSA definition or measure	Bartering measure	Adjusted for	Outcome for CSA compared with non-CSA
Widom and Kuhns (1996)	Metropolitan Midwest; 76 women with substantiated CSA cases; 244 controls matched for age, race, and birth hospital	Before age 11; court case processed with charges such as sexual assault, fondling, incest	Ever paid for having sex	Demographics, welfare as a child	2.54 times as likely to have been paid for sex
Simons and Whitbeck (1991)	40 adolescent runaways and 90 homeless adults	Before age 18; verbal request for sexual acts, fondling, or attempted sexual contact by relative or foster parent, or for adolescents, was reason for leaving home	Since runaway/homeless, ever sold sexual favors	None	1.23/1.3 times greater odds for adolescents/adults ($r_{csa, sex work}$ = .33 adolescents, .26 adults, p < .05)
Goodman and Fallott (1998)	99 mentally ill women from hospitals and shelters	Unwanted sexual experiences during childhood, ranging from forcible contact to rape	Report of prostitution by case manager (available for 70% of sample)	None	6.4 times as likely to have prostituted
Boyer and Fine (1992)	WA[a]; 535 pregnant adolescents	History of molestation, attempted rape, or rape by detailed questionnaire	Traded sex for money, shelter, or drugs/alcohol	None	Significantly more likely to have traded sex for money (11% vs. 1%), shelter (14% vs. 2%), and drugs (14% vs. 1%)
McClanahan et al. (1999)	1,142 jail detainees	Before age 16; unwanted sexual experiences	Solicited money for sex or routinely (> once/week) or episodically prostituted	None	Significantly more likely to have ever (44.2% vs. 28.5%) and routinely (34.6% vs. 20.6%) prostituted

Study	Sample	Abuse measure	Outcome measure	Controls	Findings
Mullings et al. (2000)	500 newly admitted prisoners	Sexual maltreatment, sexual abuse, or rape while growing up	Traded sex for drugs or money; prostituted > 30 days prior to incarceration	None	Significantly more likely to have traded sex for money/drugs and to have prostituted
Medrano et al. (1999)	179 illicit drug users in treatment	Childhood Trauma Questionnaire	Ever traded sex for drugs or money; also measured frequency	None	No difference in likelihood of having traded sex for drugs or money
Parillo et al. (2001)	1,490 female sex partners of IDUs[b] from WHEEL[c] study	Sexual abuse during childhood or adolescence involving anal, oral, and/or vaginal penetration	Ever traded sex for money or drugs	Adult rape, recent hard drug use, recent sex with IDU	Greater risk of trading sex (2.3 times greater if abused as child, 1.7 if abused as adolescent, 3.4 if abused as child and as an adolescent)
Zierler et al. (1991)	83 women with or at risk for HIV infection	Forced sex or rape as a child or adolescent	Current or prior work as a prostitute	None	2.8 times more likely to have worked as a prostitute (20.7% vs. 7.4%)
Cohen et al. (2000)	1,645 women with or at risk for HIV infection	Before age 18; pressured or forced to have sexual contact	Traded sex for money, drugs, or shelter	None	2.6 times more likely to have traded sex
Runtz and Briere (1986)	278 college undergraduates	Before age 15; sexual contact with person ≥ 5 years older	Provided sex for money during adolescence	None	No difference

Note. [a]Washington state. [b]Intravenous drug users. [c]Women Helping to Empower and Enhance Lives.

Of the 10 remaining studies, only 2 (Medrano, Desmond, Zule, & Hatch, 1999; Runtz & Briere, 1986) did not find a significant association. According to the 6 studies that reported an effect size statistic (Cohen et al., 2000; Goodman & Fallot, 1998; Parillo, Freeman, Collier, & Young, 2001; Simons & Whitbeck, 1991; Widom & Kuhns, 1996; Zierler et al., 1991), the odds that women who had experienced CSA had engaged in commercial sex work or bartered sex ranged from 1.3 to 6.4. According to 4 of these studies, the women who had been sexually abused as children were 2.5 times more likely than those not sexually abused to engage in commercial sex work or the bartering of sex as an adult.

Taken together, these findings suggest that CSA or its concomitants predispose women to commercial sex work or sexual bartering. Among the high-risk populations studied, women who have experienced CSA are more likely to engage in sexual bartering, and CSWs are more likely than other women with similar characteristics to have experienced CSA. Although prevalence estimates of CSA among CSWs differ across studies, the findings of most studies suggest that one third to one half of female CSWs were sexually abused as children.

Child Sexual Abuse and Injection Drug Use

Although many studies have addressed the relation between CSA and substance use (broadly defined), few studies of female injection drug users exist. We found only one published study (Mullings, Marquart, & Diamond, 2001) that reported the prevalence of CSA among a sample of female injection drug users. Among 122 female prisoners who injected drugs, Mullings et al. (2001) found that 33% had experienced sexual maltreatment, abuse, or rape while growing up, significantly higher than the 24% of 328 female prisoners who did not inject drugs and who had experienced CSA. Prevalence rates of 48% to 54% have been reported for samples of former injectors (Neaigus et al., 2001) and opiate users (90% of whom had a history of injection drug use; Miller & Paone, 1998), but these studies used lifetime measures of sexual (Miller & Paone, 1998) or multiple forms (Neaigus et al., 2001) of abuse. However, similar to the proportion reported by Mullings et al. (2001), 30% of women in the study of Miller and Paone (1998) reported that their first sexual contact occurred through abuse.

In addition, we found eight published studies that did not recruit injection drug users but nevertheless examined the association between CSA and injection drug use in a particular population, often one at risk for substance use (see Table 3.5). In only two of the eight studies was there a significant association between CSA and injection drug use or needle-sharing behaviors. Mullings, Marquart, and Brewer (2000; presumably the same sample as in Mullings et al., 2001) found that after controlling for age, race and ethnicity, education, and marginal living conditions, significantly more of the CSA victims (56.2%) had a history of injection drug use than did women who had not experienced CSA (44.1%). Kirkham and Lobb (1998) reported that among 110 HIV-infected women, significantly more of those with a history of CSA reported injection drug use as the risk behavior that led to their HIV infection (86.4% vs. 30.2% of those who had not experienced CSA). In one additional study (Thompson et al., 1997), the relation between CSA and injection drug use history approached statistical significance ($p = .07$). Specifically, more of the STD clinic patients with a history of CSA reported having ever injected drugs (14%) than did those without a history of CSA (4%). Four studies of women who were either HIV-infected or engaged in high-risk sexual or drug-use behavior (Cohen et al., 2000; Greenberg et al., 1999; Medrano et al., 1999; Zierler et al., 1991) and one study of White high school students (Lodico & DiClemente, 1994) found no significant association between CSA and needle sharing, injection frequency, or recent or lifetime injection drug use.

At present, the literature on women who inject drugs is too limited for us to draw conclusions about the prevalence of CSA in this population. The published studies do suggest that as many as one third of female injection drug users may have experienced CSA, somewhat higher than the national average. Moreover, unlike the women in studies of the relationship between CSA and STD or commercial sex work, women who have experienced CSA do not appear to be at increased risk specifically for injection drug use. The absence of such an association may relate to the strong link between CSA and general substance use (see chap. 8, this volume). That is, CSA may increase the risk for substance abuse but may be causally unrelated to the specific choice of drug or method of use.

CONCLUSION

Clinical reports and HIV risk-behavior studies have suggested that CSA may predispose women to risk behavior and subsequent infection with HIV. However, to our knowledge, ours is the first systematic review to examine the extent to which CSA and HIV infection co-occur. In addition, many reviews of adult risk behavior among people who have experienced CSA have grouped together the studies of men and women, sexual abuse and other forms of abuse (physical, emotional), or abuse occurring during childhood and adulthood. Because CSA may affect girls and boys differently, and because the demographics of men and women differ in the HIV/AIDS epidemic in the United States, we limited our review to studies of women. Moreover, although sexual abuse often co-occurs with physical and emotional abuse of children (as well as other family disruptions), whenever possible, we limited our studies to those that addressed sexual abuse specifically. Although not all studies were designed to allow the differential effects of sexual abuse

TABLE 3.5
Association Between Child Sexual Abuse and Injection Drug Use (IDU)

Study/year	Sample	CSA definition or measure	Outcome for CSA compared with non-CSA
Medrano et al. (1999)	181 illicit drug-using women, ≥ age 18	Childhood Trauma Questionnaire	No difference in injection frequencies or needle-sharing behaviors during past month
Kirkham and Lobb (1998)	Canada; 110 HIV-infected women	Sexual abuse as a child	Significantly more likely to identify IDU as HIV transmission mode (86.4% vs. 30.2%)
Greenberg et al. (1999)	825 WINGS[a] participants, at risk for HIV	Before age 18; forced sexual contact with an older person	No difference in rates of IDU during past month (13% vs. 11%)
Lodico and DiClemente (1994)	2,582 9th and 12th grade White females	Being fondled or forced to touch someone else	Relative risk for ever injecting drugs (2.8) or needle-sharing (15.1) was not significant
Cohen et al. (2000)	1,645 urban women at risk for HIV (1,288 HIVP[b], 357 HIVN[c])	Before age 18; fondling or attempted/forced intercourse	Likelihood of recent IDU (OR[d] = 1.2) was not significant
Mullings et al. (2000)	500 female prisoners	Sexual treatment, sexual abuse, and/or rape while growing up	Significantly more likely to have ever injected drugs (56.2% vs. 44.1%)
Zierler et al. (1991)	83 women at risk for HIV	Rape or forced sex during childhood and/or adolescence	No difference in lifetime IDU (28% vs. 24%)
Thompson et al. (1997)	83 women attending STD clinic	Before age 18; forced sex	Nonsigninificant tendency toward more lifetime IDU (14% vs. 4%)

Note. [a]Women in Group Support. [b]HIV-positive. [c]HIV-negative. [d]Odds ratio.

to be separated from those of other forms of abuse, we considered this selectivity necessary to estimate the prevalence of sexual abuse history among women with or at risk for HIV infection.

The studies we reviewed do suggest that CSA is overrepresented among women with HIV, true of at least one third to one half of HIV-infected women. It also appears to be overrepresented among women in certain groups considered at high risk for HIV. Studies of CSA among CSWs have produced numbers similar to those from studies of women with HIV infection. That is, most indicate that at least one third, and perhaps as many as one half, of women engaged in commercial sex work have experienced CSA. Moreover, significantly more women who have experienced CSA compared with those who have not, have bartered sex for money, drugs, or shelter. CSA also appears to be overrepresented among women with STDs, although the literature is less consistent here. One third of women treated for an STD may have experienced CSA, and CSA is more common in the histories of women who have ever had an STD than among women who have not.

Currently, however, studies do not provide evidence for an association between CSA and injection drug use. This may be due, in part, to the limited number of studies that have addressed this issue (we found only one that clearly presented the prevalence of CSA among female injection drug users). However, most of the studies that examined history of injection drug use among women with and women without a history of CSA did not find an association. Although more studies are needed, this lack of association may suggest that CSA is either unrelated to injection drug use or unrelated to women's choice of drug or method of use. With respect to the relation between CSA and HIV infection, the lack of association may also suggest that any psychosocial or life-course sequelae of CSA that predispose women to HIV infection do so through sexual rather than needle transmission.

What, if any, implications do these findings have for HIV prevention? CSA has been associated with psychological and behavioral sequelae that could be associated with the risk of acquiring an STD, including HIV. But the path from early sexual abuse to an STD in adulthood is likely a long and complex one. Research has not yet established and tested a causal model that would account for the mediating or moderating mechanisms that likely play a role in this outcome. Development and testing of an articulated model clearly represents a research need, particularly in light of recent findings (Greenberg, 2001) suggesting that standard communication and condom skills-building interventions are less effective for women with a history of sexual abuse. Nevertheless, much is currently known about the effects of sexual abuse on basic psychological processes (see, e.g., chaps 5, 6, 7, & 10, this volume). Better understanding of these effects, particularly among HIV prevention researchers, may provide important suggestions for how and where prevention messages are delivered. Integrating this knowledge into the development of HIV prevention interventions tailored to the needs of woman who have experienced CSA should ultimately help to decrease their risk of acquiring HIV infection.

REFERENCES

American Psychiatric Association. (1994). *Diagnostic and statistical manual of mental disorders* (4th ed.). Washington, DC: Author.

Bagley, C., & Young, L. (1987). Juvenile prostitution and child sexual abuse: A controlled study. *Canadian Journal of Community Mental Health, 6,* 5–26.

Bedimo, A. L., Kissinger, P., & Bessinger, R. (1997). History of sexual abuse among HIV-infected women. *International Journal of STD and AIDS, 8,* 332–335.

Boyer, D., & Fine, D. (1992). Sexual abuse as a factor in adolescent pregnancy and child maltreatment. *Family Planning Perspectives, 24,* 4–11.

Browning, C. R., & Laumann, E. O. (1997). Sexual contact between children and adults: A life course perspective. *American Sociological Review, 62,* 540–560.

Centers for Disease Control and Prevention. (2001a). *A glance at the HIV epidemic* [Fact sheet]. Atlanta, GA: Author. Retrieved March 13, 2002, from http://www.cdc.gov/nchstp/od/news/At-a-Glance.pdf

Centers for Disease Control and Prevention. (2001b). *HIV/AIDS among US women: Minority and young women at continuing risk* [Fact sheet]. Atlanta, GA: Author. Retrieved March 13, 2002, from http://www.cdc.gov/hiv/pubs/facts/women.htm

Centers for Disease Control and Prevention. (2001c). *HIV/AIDS Surveillance Report, 12*(2), 1–44. Retrieved March 13, 2002, from http://www.cdc.gov/hiv/stats/hasr1202.htm

Champion, J. D., Shain, R. N., Piper, J., & Perdue, S. T. (2001). Sexual abuse and sexual risk behaviors of minority women with sexually transmitted diseases. *Western Journal of Nursing Research, 23,* 241–254.

Cohen, M., Deamant, C., Barkan, S., Richardson, J., Young, M., Holman, S., et al. (2000). Domestic violence and childhood sexual abuse in HIV-infected women and women at risk for HIV. *American Journal of Public Health, 90,* 560–565.

Earls, C. M., & David, H. (1990). Early family and sexual experiences of male and female prostitutes. *Canada's Mental Health, 38,* 7–11.

El-Bassel, N., Witte, S. S., Wada, T., Gilbert, L., & Wallace, J. (2001). Correlates of partner violence among female street-based sex workers: Substance abuse, history of childhood abuse, and HIV risks. *AIDS Patient Care and STDs, 15,* 41–51.

Elliott, D. M., & Briere, J. (1992). Sexual abuse trauma among professional women: Validating the Trauma Symptom Checklist–40 (TSC-40). *Child Abuse and Neglect, 16,* 391–398.

Fergusson, D. M., Horwood, L. J., & Lynskey, M. T. (1997). Childhood sexual abuse, adolescent sexual behaviors and sexual revictimization. *Child Abuse and Neglect, 21,* 789–803.

Fergusson, D. M., & Mullen, P. E. (1999). The prevalence of sexual abuse during childhood. In D. M. Fergusson & P. E. Mullen (Eds.), *Childhood sexual abuse: An evidence-based perspective* (pp. 13–33). Thousand Oaks, CA: Sage.

Finkelhor, D., Hotaling, G., Lewis, I. A., & Smith, C. (1990). Sexual abuse in a national survey of adult men and women: Prevalence, characteristics, and risk factors. *Child Abuse and Neglect, 14,* 19–28.

Gielen, A. C., McDonnell, K. A., Wu, A. W., O'Campo, P., & Faden, R. (2001). Quality of life among women living with HIV: The importance violence, social support, and self-care behaviors. *Social Science and Medicine, 52,* 315–322.

Goodman, L. A., & Fallot, R. D. (1998). HIV risk-behavior in poor urban women with serious mental disorders: Association with childhood physical and sexual abuse. *American Journal of Orthopsychiatry, 68,* 73–83.

Greenberg, J., Hennessy, M., Lifshay, J., Kahn-Krieger, S., Bartelli, D., Downer, A., et al. (1999). Childhood sexual abuse and its relationship to high-risk behavior in women volunteering for an HIV and STD prevention intervention. *AIDS and Behavior, 3,* 149–156.

Greenberg, J. B. (2001). Childhood sexual abuse and sexually transmitted diseases in adults: A review of and implications for STD/HIV programmes. *International Journal of STD and AIDS, 12,* 777–783.

Hader, S. L., Smith, D. K., Moore, J. S., & Holmberg, S. D. (2001). HIV infection in women in the United States: Status at the millennium. *Journal of the American Medical Association, 285,* 1186–1192.

Hein, K., Dell, R., Futterman, D., Rotheram-Borus, M. J., & Shaffer, N. (1995). Comparison of HIV+ and HIV– adolescents: Risk factors and psychosocial determinants. *Pediatrics, 95,* 96–104.

Hillis, S. D., Anda, R. F., Felitti, V. J., Nordenberg, D., & Marchbanks, P. A. (2000). Adverse childhood experiences and sexually transmitted diseases in men and women: A retrospective study. *Pediatrics, 106,* e11.

James, J., & Meyerding, J. (1977). Early sexual experience as a factor in prostitution. *Archives of Sexual Behavior, 7,* 31–42.

Kenney, J. W. R., Reinholtz, C. M., & Angelini, P. J. B. (1998). Sexual abuse, sex before age 16, and high-risk behaviors of young females with sexually transmitted diseases. *Journal of Obstetric, Gynecologic, and Neonatal Nursing, 27,* 54–63.

Kilpatrick, D. G., Acierno, R., Saunders, B., Resnick, H. S., Best, C. L., & Schnurr, P. P. (2000). Risk factors for adolescent substance abuse and dependence: Data from a national sample. *Journal of Consulting and Clinical Psychology, 68,* 19–30.

Kimerling, R., Armistead, L., & Forehand, R. (1999). Victimization experiences and HIV infection in women: Associations with serostatus, psychological symptoms, and health status. *Journal of Traumatic Stress, 12,* 41–58.

Kirkham, C. M., & Lobb, D. J. (1998). The British Columbia Positive Women's Survey: A detailed profile of 110 HIV-infected women. *Canadian Medical Association Journal, 158,* 317–323.

Liebschutz, J. M., Feinman, G., Sullivan, L., Stein, M., & Samet, J. (2000). Physical and sexual abuse in women infected with the human immunodeficiency virus:

Increased illness and health care utilization. *Archives of Internal Medicine, 160,* 1659–1664.

Lodico, M. A., & DiClemente, R. J. (1994). The association between childhood sexual abuse and prevalence of HIV-related risk behaviors. *Clinical Pediatrics, 33,* 498–502.

Lynch, D. A., Kranz, S., Russell, J. M., Hornberger, L. L., & VanNess, C. J. (2000). HIV infection: A retrospective analysis of adolescent high-risk behaviors. *Journal of Pediatric Health Care, 14,* 20–25.

Lyon, M. E., Richmond, D., & D'Angelo, L. J. (1995). Is sexual abuse in childhood or adolescence a predisposing factor for HIV infection during adolescence? *Pediatric AIDS and HIV Infection, 6,* 271–275.

McClanahan, S. F., McClelland, G. M., Abram, K. M., & Teplin, L.A. (1999). Pathways into prostitution among female jail detainees and their implications for mental health services. *Psychiatric Services, 50,* 1606–1613.

McMahon, P. M., & Puett, R. C. (1999). Child sexual abuse as a public health issue: Recommendations of an expert panel. *Sexual Abuse: A Journal of Research and Treatment, 11,* 257–266.

Medrano, M. A., Desmond, D. P., Zule, W. A., & Hatch, J. P. (1999). Histories of childhood trauma and the effects on risky HIV behaviors in a sample of women drug users. *American Journal of Drug and Alcohol Abuse, 25,* 593–606.

Miller, M., & Paone, D. (1998). Social network characteristics as mediators in the relationship between sexual abuse and HIV risk. *Social Science and Medicine, 47,* 765–777.

Molnar, B. E., Buka, S. L., & Kessler, R. C. (2001). Child sexual abuse and subsequent psychopathology: Results from the National Comorbidity Survey. *American Journal of Public Health, 91,* 753–760.

Moore, K., Nord, C., & Peterson, J. (1989). Nonvoluntary sexual activity among adolescents. *Family Planning Perspectives, 21,* 110–114.

Mullings, J. L., Marquart, J. W., & Brewer, V.E. (2000). Assessing the relationship between child sexual abuse and marginal living conditions on HIV/AIDS-related risk behavior among women prisoners. *Child Abuse and Neglect, 24,* 677–688.

Mullings, J. L., Marquart, J. W., & Diamond, P. M. (2001). Cumulative continuity and injection drug use among women: A test of the downward spiral framework. *Deviant Behavior, 22,* 211–238.

Neaigus, A., Miller, M., Friedman, S. R., Hagen, D. L., Sifaneck, S. J., Ildefonso, G., et al. (2001). Potential risk factors for the transition to injecting among non-injecting heroin users: A comparison of former injectors and never injectors. *Addiction, 96,* 847–860.

Neal, J. J., Fleming, P. L., Green, T. A., & Ward, J. W. (1997). Trends in heterosexually acquired AIDS in the United States, 1988 through 1995. *Journal of Acquired Immune Deficiency Syndromes, 14,* 465–474.

NIMH Multisite HIV Prevention Trial. (2001). A test of factors mediating the relationship between unwanted sexual activity during childhood and risky sexual practices among women enrolled in the NIMH Multisite HIV Prevention Trial. *Women and Health, 33*, 163–179.

Noell, J., Rohde, P., Seeley, J., & Ochs, L. (2001). Childhood sexual abuse, adolescent sexual coercion and sexually transmitted infection acquisition among homeless female adolescents. *Child Abuse and Neglect, 25*, 137–148.

Parillo, K. M., Freeman, R. C., Collier, K., & Young, P. (2001). Association between early sexual abuse and adult HIV-risky sexual behaviors among community-recruited women. *Child Abuse and Neglect, 25*, 335–346.

Petrak, J., Byrne, A., & Baker, M. (2000). The association between abuse in childhood and STD/HIV risk behaviours in female genitourinary (GU) clinic attendees. *Journal of Sexually Transmitted Infections, 76*, 457–461.

Plichta, S. B., & Abraham, C. (1996). Violence and gynecological health in women <50 years old. *American Journal of Obstetrics and Gynecology, 174*, 903–907.

Potterat, J. J., Rothenberg, R. B., Muth, S. Q., Darrow, W. W., & Phillips-Plummer, L. (1998). Pathways to prostitution: The chronology of sexual and drug abuse milestones. *Journal of Sex Research, 35*, 333–340.

Ross, C. A., Anderson, G., Heber, S., & Norton, G. R. (1990). Dissociation and abuse among multiple-personality patients, prostitutes, and exotic dancers. *Hospital and Community Psychiatry, 41*, 328–330.

Rubenstein, R. (1990). Antecedents of prostitution: Flawed attachments and early sexual experiences. In K. Pottharst (Ed.), *Research explorations in adult attachment* (pp. 269–299). New York: Peter Lang.

Runtz, M., & Briere, J. (1986). Adolescent "acting out" and childhood history of sexual abuse. *Journal of Interpersonal Violence, 1*, 326–334.

Sedlak, A. J., & Broadhurst, D. D. (1996). *Executive summary of the third national incidence study of child abuse and neglect.* Retrieved March 13, 2002, from http://www.calib.com/nccanch/pubs/statinfo/nis3.cfm

Sikstrom, B., Hellberg, D., Nilsson, S., Brihmer, C., & Mardh, P. A. (1996). Sexual risk behavior in women with cervical human papillomavirus infection. *Archives of Sexual Behavior, 25*, 361–372.

Silbert, M. H., & Pines, A. M. (1982). Entrance into prostitution. *Youth and Society, 13*, 471–500.

Simoni, J. M., & Ng, M. T. (2000). Trauma, coping, and depression among women with HIV/AIDS in New York City. *AIDS Care, 12*, 567–580.

Simons, R. L., & Whitbeck, L. B. (1991). Sexual abuse as a precursor to prostitution and victimization among adolescent and adult homeless women. *Journal of Family Issues, 12*, 361–379.

Stevens, J. A., Zierler, S., Cram, V., Dean, D., Mayer, K. H., & DeGroot, A. S. (1995). Risks for HIV infection in incarcerated women. *Journal of Women's Health, 4*, 569–577.

Thompson, N. J., Potter, J. S., Sanderson, C. A., & Maibach, E. W. (1997). The relationship of sexual abuse and HIV risk behaviors among heterosexual adult female STD patients. *Child Abuse and Neglect, 21*, 149–156.

Vanwesenbeeck, I., DeGraff, R., van Zessen, G., Straver, C. J., & Visser, J. H. (1995). Professional HIV risk taking, levels of victimization, and well-being in female prostitutes in the Netherlands. *Archives of Sexual Behavior, 24,* 503–515.

Vermund, S. H., Alexander-Rodriquez, T., Macleod, S., & Kelley, K. (1990). History of sexual abuse in incarcerated adolescents with gonorrhea or syphilis. *Journal of Adolescent Health Care, 11,* 449–452.

Vlahov, D., Weintge, D., Moore, J., Flynn, C., Schuman, P., Schoenbaum, E., & Zierler, S. (1998). Violence among women with or at risk for HIV infection. *AIDS and Behavior, 2,* 53–60.

Widom, C. S., & Kuhns, J. B. (1996). Childhood victimization and subsequent risk for promiscuity, prostitution, and teenage pregnancy. *American Journal of Public Health, 86,* 1607–1612.

Wilsnack, S. C., Vogeltanz, N. D., Klassen, A. D., & Harris, T. R. (1997). Childhood sexual abuse and women's substance abuse: National survey findings. *Journal of Studies on Alcohol, 58,* 264–271.

Wingood, G. M., & DiClemente, R. J. (1997). Child sexual abuse, HIV sexual risk, and gender relations of African-American women. *American Journal of Preventive Medicine, 13,* 380–384.

Wyatt, G. E., Myers, H. F., Williams, J. K., Kitchen, C. R., Loeb. T., Carmona, J. V., et al. (2002). Does a history of trauma contribute to HIV risk for women of color? Implications for prevention policy. *American Journal of Public Health, 92,* 660–665.

Wyatt, G. E., Loeb, T. B., Solis, B., & Carmona, J. V. (1999). The prevalence and circumstances of child sexual abuse: Changes across a decade. *Child Abuse and Neglect, 23,* 45–60.

Zierler, S., Feingold, L., Laufer, D., Velentgas, P., Kantrowitz-Gordon, L., & Mayer, K. (1991). Adult survivors of childhood sexual abuse and subsequent risk of HIV infection. *American Journal of Public Health, 81,* 572–575.

4

SEXUAL ABUSE OF BOYS: SHORT- AND LONG-TERM ASSOCIATIONS AND IMPLICATIONS FOR HIV PREVENTION

DAVID W. PURCELL, ROBERT M. MALOW, CURTIS DOLEZAL, AND ALEX CARBALLO-DIÉGUEZ

The aim of this chapter is to explore the complex associations between the sexual abuse of boys and adult functioning in a variety of domains, including sexual behavior. Public concerns about sexual threats to children, particularly girls, have deep historical roots, but until about 20 years ago, the effects of child sexual abuse (CSA) received little research attention (Haugaard, 2000). Most research has focused on women (Haugaard, 2000), and studies that have included men have either lacked methodological rigor (Holmes & Slap, 1998) or failed to analyze for gender effects (e.g., Kamsner & McCabe, 2000). This pattern has continued despite the growing evidence that gender seems to moderate the effect of CSA (Molnar, Buka, & Kessler, 2001; Rind, Tromovitch, & Bauserman, 1998). More recently, focus has

This chapter was authored or coauthored by an employee of the United States government as part of official duty and is considered to be in the public domain. Any views expressed herein do not necessarily represent the views of the United States government.

Robert M. Malow's contribution was supported in part by grants from the National Institute on Drug Abuse and from the National Institute on Alcohol Abuse and Alcoholism.

shifted from individual psychopathology and intervention to a complementary, population-based epidemiologic orientation, especially in attempts to understand the contribution of CSA to morbidity risks with heavy public health burdens.

Most reviews of the effects of CSA on males have noted serious methodological problems but have concluded that the effects of CSA on diverse emotional and social domains are pervasive and long-lasting (e.g., Holmes & Slap, 1998; Mendel, 1995). In their review of 166 studies of sexual abuse of boys, Holmes and Slap attempted to summarize the data by using meta-analysis, but they concluded that the procedure was not feasible because most studies were cross-sectional, used nonprobability samples and widely varying definitions of abuse, and differed in methods of assessing sexual abuse histories. Although accumulating evidence suggests that CSA of boys is not rare and that it may produce clinical symptoms of trauma affecting cognitive, emotional, interpersonal, and sexual domains, another line of research has focused on clarifying the role that perception may play in how trauma is manifested in boys (Rind et al., 1998).

Researchers with this latter focus recently completed three reviews (Bauserman & Rind, 1997; Rind & Tromovitch, 1997; Rind et al., 1998) and concluded that the association between CSA of boys and adult adjustment is small in nonclinical or more representative samples and that many more men compared with women reported neutral or positive responses to early sexual experiences. On the basis of these reviews, Rind and his colleagues argued that CSA is not as damaging as is assumed in the research and clinical literature. Outrage over these conclusions led to scientific attack (Dallam et al., 2001; Ondersma et al., 2001) and condemnation by the U.S. Congress (see Rind, Bauserman, & Tromovitch, 2000). Meanwhile, Rind and his colleagues have vigorously defended their conclusions (Rind, Tromovitch, & Bauserman, 2001). This conflict highlights the fact that researchers looking at the same data can draw very different conclusions about the effects of CSA on men. Discussion among researchers and policy makers, as well as more research studies, might help to clarify and resolve these issues. For our purposes, the work by Rind and his colleagues is a reminder that perception of harm may be important in determining adult functioning. However, as we explore later, the absence of feeling harmed by early sexual activity, even if it is consensual, does not necessarily mean that the event was harmless to the individual or to the public health goal of reducing HIV risk behavior.

DEFINING CHILD SEXUAL ABUSE AND DETERMINING PREVALENCE

Recent reviews have underscored the lack of consensus on how to define CSA (Haugaard, 2000; Holmes & Slap, 1998; Rind & Tromovitch,

1997; Rind et al., 1998; Romano & De Luca, 2001), which makes it diffi-cult to compare and generalize the findings of studies. CSA definitions usually involve, to varying degrees, a focus on (a) the ages of the youth and abuser, (b) the behaviors of both, including the presence of force or coer-cion (often defined as *rape*), and (c) the perception of the boy that he was abused, either at the time or later. Although these components are multi-dimensional, researchers and the law usually dichotomize experiences into "abuse" or "no abuse" (Haugaard, 2000). In addition, when asking partici-pants about their experiences, researchers often require a forced choice (e.g., "were you abused as a child?") rather than collecting data on the various aspects of the experiences. Estimates of the long-term effects of CSA decrease as the definition of abuse is broadened to include noncontact (Collings, 1995).

Estimating CSA prevalence among boys is problematic because cases are likely to be underreported (Boney-McCoy & Finkelhor, 1995; Feiring, Taska, & Lewis, 1999) as a result of stigma regarding same-sex behavior and a socialization of boys that emphasizes interpersonal autonomy. Holmes and Slap (1998) reported that the prevalence rates of CSA among boys varied dramatically from 4% to 76%, although in the larger studies with more rep-resentative samples, rates ranged from 4% to 16%. The prevalence rates in a given sample decrease by about half when physical touch was a criterion (Holmes & Slap, 1998; West, 1998). Gorey and Leslie (1997) found that half of the variability in prevalence estimates was due to differences in the definition of abuse and in response rates (a lower response rate was associ-ated with higher prevalence).

By excluding noncontact abuse from the CSA definition, Gorey and Leslie (1997) estimated prevalence in the general male population at 5% to 8%. Similarly, in another population-based study, 6.8% of men reported con-tact CSA (Bensley, Van Eenwyk, & Simmons, 2000). Generally, more gay or bisexual men (men who have sex with men [MSM]) report CSA than do heterosexual men: The rates for MSM (20% to 39%) are comparable with those for women (Bartholow et al., 1994; Doll et al., 1992; Finkelhor, 1994; Jinich et al., 1998; Lenderking et al., 1997; Paul, Catania, Pollack, & Stall, 2001). Although most of these studies have used convenience samples, Paul et al. (2001) used a more representative sample of MSM and found 20.6% prevalence of coercive CSA with physical contact. Thus, the rate of CSA for MSM is approximately three times that of the general male population (see also Duncan, 1990), and this difference may even be larger because the over-all rate of CSA includes MSM. Given that, in general, more men of color experience CSA than do White men (Holmes & Slap, 1998), the preva-lence for gay men of color may be particularly high (Carballo-Diéguez & Dolezal, 1995; Doll et al., 1992). Given the differences in prevalence, MSM and men of color are subgroups requiring particular attention and treatment resources (Relf, 2001).

One of the challenges to making links between a childhood experience such as CSA and adult functioning is the passage of time and the number of experiences that precede and follow abuse (Haugaard, 2000). A pervasive pattern of violent abuse is likely to have greater immediate and long-term effects than an isolated incident, but even severe and pervasive CSA is probably insufficient to fully explain adult functioning. The most common research design used to determine the "effects" of CSA has been cross-sectional surveys about childhood experiences and adult adjustment—designs that cannot establish effects but only correlates between simultaneously reported childhood and adulthood functioning. Errors in recall about childhood and method variance are particularly likely in these studies (Feiring et al., 1999) and may confound CSA with general family environment (Rind et al., 1998). It is necessary to conduct longitudinal research to separate the effects of CSA from difficulties that precede it or continue after it (Saywitz, Mannarino, Berliner, & Cohen, 2000).

Research has suggested a few general principles regarding the consequences of CSA for boys and girls. The key principle, which is surprising given the broad range of definitions used for CSA, is that the effects are highly variable and that no single symptom or syndrome characterizes sexually abused children (Oddone Paolucci, Genuis, & Violato, 2001; Saywitz et al., 2000). Two important general findings flow from this principle. First, regarding immediate effects, some children show no effects of CSA, whereas others show severe psychological distress (Feiring et al., 1999). Second, for long-term effects, CSA is a risk factor for adult distress and psychopathology, although not all adults who have been abused develop abuse-related problems (Saywitz et al., 2000). Thus, the long-term effects of CSA should be thought of as a potential vulnerability to a negative outcome, not destiny. The goals for researchers are to understand vulnerability and resiliency among those who experienced CSA and other childhood stressors so that society can prevent or successfully treat the individual and community effects of these problems.

We developed a model in an effort to understand the complex associations between CSA and adult functioning in boys (see Figure 4.1). The model we propose should be viewed heuristically rather than as a complete and validated model for predicting behavior. Antecedents to CSA include family and individual factors that make it more likely that a boy will experience CSA. It is beyond the scope of this chapter to cover all of the antecedents to CSA, and many are the same for boys and girls. Because of its specific relevance for boys, the only individual factor we examine here is the relationship between CSA and gender-related behavior or sexual orientation. During or after CSA, these family and individual factors also are potential

Figure 4.1. A model of the links between child sexual abuse and HIV risk behavior for males. Although the model is organized temporally, it is not intended to suggest that events earlier in time caused later events.

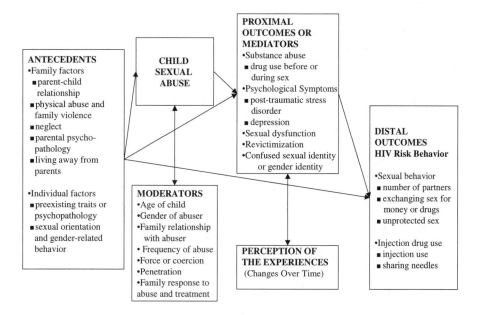

mediators or moderators of outcomes. The model also highlights proximal outcomes of CSA such as substance use and psychological symptoms, as well as distal outcomes, focusing specifically on those related to HIV risk behavior.

SEXUAL ORIENTATION, GENDER-RELATED BEHAVIOR, AND CHILD SEXUAL ABUSE OF BOYS

MSM are more likely to have been abused than heterosexual men, and MSM are particularly likely to have been abused by men (Paul et al., 2001). Gender role confusion or same-sex attractions may precede abuse, be affected by abuse, or both. Longitudinal studies have reliably related gender-nonconforming behavior in boys to being gay or bisexual in adulthood (without examining or accounting for abuse; Bailey & Zucker, 1995). However, no longitudinal studies have examined the relationship between CSA and the development of gender role and sexual orientation. Male youths who recognize their same-sex attractions or who are gender nonconforming may seek partners at a young age and initiate sexual behavior that is labeled CSA (Carballo-Diéguez & Dolezal, 1995). Male youths may also place themselves in situations in which they are more likely to be unexpectedly abused. In a recent study of gay men, 20% of the men reported a sexual relationship with a man during adolescence, but very few of the men reported believing that these experiences had a role in creating their same-sex interest, instead reporting feeling that the same-sex interest already existed (Rind, 2001). Clearly, some early sexual relationships, regardless of sexual orientation, are voluntary or initiated by the youths as part of exploring emerging sexual feelings, even though these experiences may be illegal and exploitive (Carballo-Diéguez & Dolezal, 1995; Dolezal & Carballo-Diéguez, 2002). Because we know little about the development of sexual orientation in the absence of abuse, it is not surprising that the relative contributions of personality characteristics and abuse experiences to sexual orientation are unknown.

CHARACTERIZING CHILD SEXUAL ABUSE AND MODERATORS AFFECTING OUTCOMES

It is important for researchers to carefully characterize CSA among boys to be able to develop a better understanding of contextual factors or moderators that may affect childhood and adulthood correlates of CSA.

Characteristics of Abused Males

When Holmes and Slap (1998) reviewed the literature on the CSA of boys, in studies using larger samples they found some common characteristics among those who were abused. First, the mean and median age at abuse was about 10 years. In studies of substantiated cases of abuse, boys were slightly younger than girls (Romano & De Luca, 2001). Research findings are inconsistent about whether the age of abuse is related to worse outcomes, probably due to differences in CSA definitions and outcomes. A few smaller studies found that non-White males were more likely to be abused than White males (Holmes & Slap, 1998).

Characteristics of Abusers

Regarding the gender of the abusers of boys, most (53% to 94%) were male, and about half of the female abusers were teenage babysitters (Holmes & Slap, 1998). The proportion of female abusers is highest in reports of adolescents and young adults and then decreases among adults, suggesting that as men age, they may not report the experiences as abuse but now consider them normative. Men who were abused only by women have been found to have the best adult functioning (Mendel, 1995). Regarding age of the abuser, Romano and De Luca (2001) found that the age difference between male victims and abusers was less than for female victims as boys appeared more likely to be abused by same-age peers or older adolescents. However, in a recent study with a more representative sample, the average age difference between abusers and gay men who were abused as children was 16 years (Paul et al., 2001). It is unclear whether greater age differences are associated with greater psychological trauma.

Significantly more boys are abused by nonfamily members than are girls (Gold, Elhai, Lucenko, Swingle, & Hughes, 1998; Romano & De Luca, 2001). Holmes and Slap (1998) found that although most of the abusers (54% to 89%) were not family members, less than half (21% to 40%) were unknown to the boy. A closer relationship with the abuser may be related to greater distress and worse psychological functioning in adulthood (Romano & De Luca, 2001). The fact that abusers are less likely to be family members and thus less likely to inflict "betrayal trauma" (Freyd, 1996) may mean that CSA could be less traumatic or less likely to be repressed by boys than by girls.

Contextual Factors Affecting the Outcomes of Child Sexual Abuse

Various factors such as duration or frequency of abuse, use of force, the sexual behavior involved in the experience, and family response may affect outcomes.

Duration and Frequency

The duration of abuse for boys is shorter than for girls (Bensley et al., 2000), possibly because duration is related to whether the abuser is a family member. From 46% to 73% of the incidents of abuse of boys were single occurrences (Holmes & Slap, 1998). However, for 17% to 53% of boys, abuse was chronic, ranging from months to years. Research on frequency of abuse, which is correlated with duration ($r = .66$; Paul et al., 2001), has consistently found that increased frequency of abuse is associated with more negative outcomes during adulthood (Romano & De Luca, 2001). Paul et al. (2001) found that, among measures of severity, frequency of abuse was the most powerful correlate of adult outcomes.

Use of Force or Coercion

Romano and De Luca (2001) concluded that physical force is more often used on boys than on girls, although in most studies, physical force was used in less than 25% of abusive acts (Holmes & Slap, 1998). Force and coercion were used more often if the boy was older and if the abuser was a man. In more than 90% of cases in which the abuser was female, persuasion rather than force or threats was used. Those who experienced force or coercion consistently reported greater distress (Kendall-Tackett, Williams, & Finkelhor, 1993; Romano & De Luca, 2001).

Type of Sexual Behavior

Regarding the types of sexually abusive acts, fondling (of child or adult) was the most commonly reported act (55% to 91%), whereas exhibitionism was the least reported act (as low as 6%), with anal penetration and oral-genital contact falling somewhere in between (Holmes & Slap, 1998). In one study, when anal penetration of boys was compared with anal or vaginal penetration of girls, frequencies did not differ (Gold et al., 1998). According to Holmes and Slap's review, the prevalence of anal penetration was moderated by age of the boy: Anal penetration was reported for less than 10% of boys abused before age 2 and 71% of boys abused between ages 9 and 11. Generally, CSA involving more invasive acts, physical contact, or defined as more severe by mental health professionals has been associated with worse outcomes (Bryant & Range, 1997; Collings, 1995; Kendall-Tackett et al., 1993; Mendel, 1995).

Family Response and Help-Seeking Behavior

For all boys, disclosure to, or discovery by, family members is a potentially important moderator. For example, communicating acceptance and not blaming the child can potentially decrease or minimize the harm from CSA. Among Latinos, relatives who wanted to save the family honor by preventing further disclosure often silenced boys who had disclosed to a family member (Carballo-Diéguez & Dolezal, 1995). Feeling self-blame may be related to ongoing developmental effects in the form of enduring negative self-attributes (Feiring et al., 1999), whereas addressing the experience more positively may minimize future effects by decreasing self-blame. Boys may be more likely to blame themselves if (a) the abuser or family members blame them; (b) they became aroused by the experiences or received side benefits, favors, or special treatment; (c) they believe they should have been able to protect themselves; or (d) they believe the societal myth that men should always be ready for sex, regardless of the circumstances (Mendel, 1995; Romano & De Luca, 2001). In addition, treatment for CSA and related effects will moderate the relationship between CSA and both proximal and distal outcomes.

Perceptions of Those Who Were Abused

People's perception of CSA and their memory of it can change with time. Important cognitive processing differences affect perception and memory depending on whether the CSA was a sudden, unexpected, isolated act such as a stranger rape; an ongoing voluntary sexual relationship between an older man and a teenager; or ongoing incest by a relative. Despite their changeability, perceptions should be discussed because they seem to be important to the outcomes of CSA. In our model (see Figure 4.1), we considered perception of the experience separately because it is not clearly in the causal chain as either a moderator or a mediator.

Perhaps surprisingly, not all men portray their experience of CSA as unequivocally negative (Carballo-Diéguez & Dolezal, 1995; Dolezal &

Carballo-Diéguez, 2002; West, 1998). This is at least partly due to the historically broad definitions used for CSA. In various studies, the participants who reported negative reactions to CSA ranged from 15% to 68%: The more negative reactions were related to the use of force or penetration, greater age difference between the two persons, and a male perpetrator (Holmes & Slap, 1998). Men who did not report negative reactions were evenly divided between those who reported a positive reaction and those who reported a neutral reaction, and more than 90% of those who had reacted positively remembered the experience as physically pleasurable. Positive responses to CSA also were related to being older than 12, longer duration, and a female abuser (Holmes & Slap, 1998). In a study using a restrictive definition of CSA (coercion and contact) and in which the men reported high levels of penetrative sex and physical force, 66% of the men said that the abuse was moderately or extremely upsetting at the time, and 48% still found the experience upsetting (Paul et al., 2001). This pattern suggests that current perceptions may underestimate the immediate effects of the abuse.

Positive and neutral perceptions go against the belief that CSA is traumatic and negative (Rind et al., 1998). It has been suggested that positive or neutral reactions may be due to defensive reactions (e.g., denial) that act as a coping mechanism or may reflect the belief that men should be able to protect themselves. Boys are socialized differently from girls from a very early age and are taught to talk less about emotions and feelings than girls are (Fivush, Brotman, Buckner, & Goodman, 2000). Thus, some boys may have difficulty expressing how CSA experiences made them feel or may feel pressure to minimize the experience rather than admit weakness. Conversely, positive reactions to early sexual experiences may also become more negative through involvement in self-help groups, reading books on CSA, or therapy.

Some support for the denial theory comes from a study of almost 2,000 gay men (Jinich et al., 1998). When the researchers looked at coercion by age, 44% of the men who had been abused when they were 13 to 15 years old reported no coercion, and 26% of those abused before age 13 reported no coercion. This points to how perceptions of abuse, by themselves, can be problematic. For those men abused before age 13, the mean age of first sexual contact was 8 years, and the abusers had a mean age 23. Even if, as adults, the men do not perceive the experience as coercive, they may have perceived it that way initially but their perceptions may become more favorable over time. In any case, this reportedly noncoercive sexual behavior between boys (average age of 8) and men (average age of 23) is, at the very least, inappropriate and may have been harmful. It would be useful to conduct a qualitative study among men who were abused at such a young age so that we can better understand their perceptions of the event, how it might have changed over time, and how it may have affected their later sexual behavior.

Positive or neutral reactions to CSA may accurately reflect individual perceptions. However, analysis of sexual behavior among groups of abused men may reveal differences that are not perceived individually. For example, in a study of Latino gay men who did and did not experience CSA before age 13, risky sexual behavior was highest among unwilling participants, at a medium level among willing participants, and at lowest levels among those who had not had sexual experience before age 13 (Carballo-Diéguez & Dolezal, 1995). Thus, participants who perceived their early sexual experiences as voluntary were still potentially affected by the experience in that they exhibited higher levels of sexual risk behavior than did men who had not been abused. Similarly, Bartholow and his colleagues (Bartholow et al., 1994) found differences in the timing of developmental sexual milestones among gay men depending on whether they were abused and whether those who had been abused perceived their first sexual experience as abusive. The earliest sexual milestones were reported by abused men who reported that their first sexual experience was not abusive, followed by men whose first sexual experience was abusive, and the latest milestones were reported by men who had never been abused. The milestones for this last group were more in line with those for heterosexual male adolescents.

Clearly, the perceptions of men who report early sexual activities are important for elucidating how these events are understood and how they affect future behavior. Adults who perceive CSA as voluntary may have fewer psychological symptoms and feel uninjured, but the effects may still be evident at a group level when examining sexual behavior and milestones.

PROXIMAL AND DISTAL OUTCOMES OF CHILD SEXUAL ABUSE

Because of our interest in HIV transmission, our model is organized by *proximal* outcomes or mediators such as psychopathology, substance abuse, and revictimization, and *distal* outcomes, in this case HIV risk behavior (see Figure 4.1). In the model, the proximal outcomes are hypothesized to mediate the relationship between CSA and the distal outcomes.

Proximal Outcomes During Childhood

Research with boys who have been sexually abused is limited because most of this research relies on cases that have been reported to the police or mental health system. In addition, in longitudinal research, abused boys may receive intervening treatment, which affects long-term outcomes. During childhood, the effects of abuse seem to be twofold: (a) localized effects (common, short-lived symptoms such as avoidance and fearfulness) and (b) developmental effects (more generalized and pervasive effects that interfere with important development tasks such as emotional regulation; Finkelhor, 1995). Large age differences in cognitive, interpersonal, and emotional domains make it important to understand the correlates of CSA among children from a developmental perspective (Celano, 1992). Unfortunately, the research to date with male youths does not allow such fine-grained distinctions.

Kendall-Tackett and her colleagues (Kendall-Tackett et al., 1993) reviewed 45 studies (most were cross-sectional) on the immediate effects of CSA on boys and girls and found that for almost every outcome assessed, children who were sexually abused exhibited more symptoms (e.g., fears and nightmares; posttraumatic stress disorder [PTSD]; lower self-esteem; internalizing problems such as depression, self-blame, and guilt; externalizing problems such as aggression, sexually inappropriate behavior, and self-harm) than those who were not abused. However, one third of the youths exhibited no symptoms, and about two thirds showed recovery during the first 1 to 2 years after the abuse. Boney-McCoy and Finkelhor (1996), who used a longitudinal, prospective design in a study of a national sample of children ages 10 to 16, found that sexual victimization between Time 1 (T1) and Time 2 (T2) was related to depression and PTSD-related symptoms in boys at T2 (an average of 15 months after T1). Although psychological symptoms and the parent–child relationship at T1 were covariates of the relationship between CSA and symptoms at T2, their inclusion did not eliminate the relationship, providing evidence that CSA plays a causal role in symptoms.

Regarding gender differences, some researchers have concluded that sexual abuse and related outcomes are different for boys and girls (e.g., Chandy, Blum, & Resnick, 1996; Feiring et al., 1999); others have concluded that there are few differences (e.g., Dallam et al., 2001; Romano & De Luca, 2001). There is even conflicting evidence for whether boys exhibit more externalizing problems and girls more internalizing problems (Chandy et al., 1996; Feiring et al., 1999; Romano & De Luca, 2001), although this is a generalized sex difference that has been observed in clinical samples of children, regardless of abuse status (American Psychiatric Association, 1994). One relatively established difference is that boys who report CSA also report early or current use of a variety of substances, including alcohol, marijuana, cocaine, as well as intravenous drug use and multidrug use (Chandy et al., 1996; Holmes & Slap, 1998), and substance use may be an important mediator of sexual risk (Leigh & Stall, 1993). All the symptoms and syndromes associated with CSA have the potential to lead to long-term negative outcomes, especially in the absence of appropriate intervention.

Proximal Outcomes During Adulthood

Men who have experienced CSA are at increased risk for substance abuse and psychopathology such as PTSD, depression, suicide attempts, anxiety disorders, borderline and antisocial personality disorders, paranoia, dissociation, somatization, bulimia, anger, aggressive behavior, poor self-esteem, self-blame, interpersonal problems such as lack of assertiveness, poor school performance, and legal trouble (Dhaliwal, Gauzas, Antonowicz, & Ross, 1996; DiIorio, Hartwell, & Hansen, for the NIMH HIV Prevention Trial Group, 2002; Holmes & Slap, 1998; Johnson, Cohen, Brown, Smailes, & Bernstein, 1999; Whiffen, Thompson, & Aube, 2000; Widom, 1999; Widom, Weiler, & Cottler, 1999). Evidence from a recent population-based sample suggests that lifetime rates of psychopathology are greater among women who were physically or sexually abused than among men who experienced CSA (MacMillan et al., 2001). CSA also has been linked to substance use before or during sex (Lodico & DiClemente, 1994; Paul et al., 2001). However, because CSA is embedded in developmental and family processes, it is unclear whether potential mediators such as family environment explain the outcomes or whether CSA is the crucial link to negative outcomes (Emery & Laumann-Billings, 1998; Saywitz et al., 2000).

Rosen and Martin (1996) found that physical or emotional abuse and sexual abuse were independently related to psychological symptoms among male soldiers in the U.S. Army. Molnar et al. (2001), who studied a nationally representative sample, found that CSA was independently related to PTSD and three different substance use disorders in men, even when controlling for family adversity. The most significant family adversity in this study was parental psychopathology, particularly among mothers. CSA was related to adult psychopathology for the men who reported no family adversity and for men who reported five or more family adversities, suggesting that regardless of family background and adversities, CSA was significantly related to adult psychopathology. One study directly compared the psychological symptoms of men and women entering an outpatient treatment program for CSA (Gold, Lucenko, Elhai, Swingle, & Sellers, 1999). Although there were no differences in raw scores, when the scores were examined using gender-specific norms, men exhibited significantly more anxiety, depression, interpersonal sensitivity, and phobic anxiety than women. However, the data from men seeking treatment for CSA may not be generalizable.

Psychological symptoms and syndromes are important proximate outcomes because they may mediate the relationship between CSA and sexual risk. Although depression has often been studied, one review found that negative affective states were only weakly related to risky sexual behavior (Crepaz & Marks, 2001). Another study found that depression did not mediate the relationship between CSA and sexual risk behavior among gay men (Paul et al., 2001). Other likely mediators besides psychiatric syndromes are substance abuse as well as interpersonal problems that may not be reflected in a psychiatric diagnosis but are important in situations that require assertiveness and sexual negotiation skills (Whiffen et al., 2000).

Researchers have proposed specific mechanisms to explain the association between CSA and substance abuse, including the hypotheses that substances provide (a) emotional or psychological escape from the abusive environment or from symptoms related to these experiences; (b) self-medication to gain control over negative experiences; (c) self-enhancement to help the person improve self-esteem, reduce isolation and loneliness, and connect with a peer group; and (d) expression of self-destructive feelings due to low self-esteem and self-blame (Holmes & Slap, 1998; Widom et al., 1999). Research support for any of these specific mechanisms for sexually abused men is lacking because cross-sectional studies predominate.

Widom and her colleagues (Widom et al., 1999) took the important step of comparing prospective and retrospective data from the same sample regarding the relationship among CSA, physical abuse, and neglect and adult substance abuse. The sample included 676 youths with documented cases of trauma or abuse and 520 matched youths who had not been abused and followed them into adulthood. It is interesting that not all participants with documented cases of abuse during childhood reported abuse when asked about their abuse history as adults. Other research also has found a low concordance between documented cases of child abuse and adult recall of abuse (e.g., Johnson et al., 1999). Not surprisingly, retrospective findings for the sample were most similar to the findings of cross-sectional studies: Significantly more of the men who reported child abuse or neglect met lifetime and current diagnoses of substance use or dependence. However, prospective data showed no differences in lifetimes rates of substance abuse or dependence, possibly because the rates of substance abuse in both groups were much higher than in population-based samples.

When prospective data and retrospective recall of abuse were crossed in a 2 × 2 table, rates of current substance abuse diagnoses were as follows, from highest to lowest: (a) men with documented cases of abuse and self-reported abuse; (b) men with self-reported abuse, but no documented abuse; (c) men with documented abuse, but no self-reported abuse; and (d) men with no indication of abuse (Widom et al., 1999). For the men whose abuse had been documented but who as adults did not report child abuse, it is unclear whether their low level of substance abuse represents resiliency, denial, or memory problems. These data highlight the importance of the perception and memory of abuse that is carried into adulthood in understanding the array of correlates of CSA.

Another proximal outcome that may be relevant for sexually abused men is revictimization. The literature on women shows that CSA is related to later sexual abuse and that revictimization is related to sexual risk behavior in consensual relationships, but the literature on men is more equivocal. In Widom's (1999) longitudinal sample, regardless of type of abuse, significantly more abused participants were raped than were matched controls. Similarly, Kalichman et al. (2001), who conducted a cross-sectional study of gay and bisexual men, found that revictimization, but not CSA, was related to risky sexual behavior. In contrast, another recent cross-sectional study with more rigorous sampling and assessment methods found that adult revictimization was not a predictor of risky sexual behavior among gay men (Paul et al., 2001).

The final proximal outcomes or mediators in the model are sexual functioning, gender identity, and sexual identity. According to cross-sectional studies, more of the men who have been sexually abused report problems with controlling sexual feelings, sexual dysfunction, and sexually coercive and aggressive behavior (especially with other men; Holmes & Slap, 1998; Romano & De Luca, 2001). There is some evidence that CSA may be related to later sexual scripts among MSM: Significantly more of the men who reported CSA engaged in sexual scripts that focus on dominant and submissive roles (Paul et al., 2001). Holmes and Slap (1998) concluded that more sexual dysfunction and sexually coercive behavior is observed among men who were abused chronically and men abused at a younger age. However, most of the studies on which they based their conclusion were conducted with gay and bisexual men or nonrepresentative or clinical samples (Raj, Silverman, & Amaro, 2000).

Regarding increases in sexuality-related problems and dysfunction among abused men, two recent cross-sectional studies with nonpsychiatric, primarily heterosexual samples found no evidence of such a relationship. In the first study, 359 heterosexual men who sought treatment at a clinic for sexual dysfunction were asked about CSA, and CSA was not related to current sexual dysfunction (Sarwar, Crawford, & Durlak, 1997). This study had a built-in gender control because the same analyses had been conducted with the men's wives, and CSA was significantly related to sexual problems for the wives (Sarwar & Durlak, 1996). Similarly, Kinzl, Mangweth, Traweger, and Biebl (1996) examined CSA and sexual dysfunction among 301 male college students in Austria and found that adverse family environment was related to all sexual dysfunctions but that CSA was not. In a similar study with women, Kinzl and his colleagues found that both family atmosphere and CSA contributed to sexual problems (Kinzl, Traweger, & Biebl, 1995). Given that less than 10% of the men in each sample were abused and that the extent of abuse was not assessed, these studies are limited by their small sample size and assessment methods. Also, it may be that men have a harder time admitting sexual dysfunction than women do.

Sexually abused males sometimes have concerns about the effect of CSA on their gender role and sexual orientation, as well as fears of intimacy both with men and women (Holmes & Slap, 1998; Romano & De Luca, 2001). Sexual orientation and gender identity can be particularly confusing for men who experienced arousal during the abuse. Some abused men may avoid friendship with other men or may engage in antigay activities in an attempt to reassert their masculinity or to manage fears that they are gay or that their femininity contributed to their abuse (Bartholow et al., 1994; Carballo-Diéguez & Dolezal, 1995; Lisak, 1994). Heterosexual and gay men who had been abused have been found to be more homophobic (some heterosexual men doubt their sexuality, and some gay men are repulsed by various same-sex behaviors; Bartholow et al., 1994; Dhaliwal et al., 1996). Struggles with gender identity and sexual orientation may be related both to proximal and distal outcomes in our model.

Distal Outcomes, HIV Risk Behavior

Finally, the model focuses on the potential distal effects of CSA, specifically, risky sexual behavior and intravenous drug use. Cross-sectional studies of sexually abused men show elevated levels of hypersexuality and high-risk sexual behavior, including prostitution, unprotected sex, and having many partners (Bartholow et al., 1994; Bensley et al., 2000; Carballo-Diéguez & Dolezal, 1995; DiIorio et al., 2002; Jinich et al., 1998; Lenderking et al., 1997; Lodico & DiClemente, 1994; Morrill, Kasten, Urato, & Larson, 2001; O'Leary, Purcell, Remien, & Gomez, 2003; Paul et al., 2001). Higher rates of sexually transmitted diseases, including HIV, as well as higher rates of partner pregnancy, are biological markers of elevated sexual risk among men with a history of CSA (Anda et al., 2001; Jinich et al., 1998; Lodico & DiClemente, 1994). As one example, in a population-based sample, more of the gay men who reported CSA were HIV-seropositive (24% vs. 14%; Paul et al., 2001). The amount of sexual risk men engage depends on characteristics of the abuse (Carballo-Diéguez & Dolezal, 1995). Greater frequency of abuse also was related to higher rates of risk behavior (Paul et al., 2001), and greater coercion during the CSA was associated with greater levels of sexual risk and HIV infection (Jinich et al., 1998).

Paul et al. (2001) examined CSA and adult sexual risk behavior among gay and bisexual men and tried to address many of the weaknesses of earlier research by (a) carefully defining CSA, (b) trying to account for other contextual and family variables, and (c) using a more representative sample by recruiting through random-digit dialing. Overall, CSA was associated with risky sexual behavior, and the relationship was mediated by engaging in one-night stands, frequent drug use during sex, and recent experience with an abusive partner (Paul et al., 2001). Surprisingly, depression and adult victimization were not significant mediators. Adverse family events and severity of CSA interacted: (a) With no adverse family event, CSA was related to risky sexual behavior; (b) with a moderate level of adverse family events, only men who reported more than six sexually abusive incidents reported increased risky behavior; and (c) with a high level of adverse family events, the severity of CSA had no differential effect on risk, suggesting a ceiling on the joint effect of these two potential influences on risky sexual behavior. Jinich et al. (1998) also explored the relationships between CSA and risky sexual behavior among almost 2,000 gay men: 28% of the men met their definition of having been abused, and when they added the requirement of subjective coercion, the proportion dropped to 19%. Significantly more of the men who had been abused reported that they had engaged in risky sexual behavior during the past 30 days and reported risky behavior with a casual partner during the past year.

Two recent studies focused on heterosexual men to determine whether sexual risk behavior was also elevated in this group. In a study of over 4,000 male and female high school students in Massachusetts, 9.3% of sexually experienced boys reported CSA ("sexual contact against your will"; Raj et al., 2000). Three times as many boys who experienced CSA reported (a) multiple sex partners (lifetime and during the past 3 months) and (b) engaging in sex that resulted in pregnancy, compared with boys who had not been abused, even after controlling for delinquent and aggressive behaviors, substance use, depressive symptoms, and sexual orientation. Boys who reported CSA were at higher risk than girls who reported CSA for having multiple sex partners and having sex that resulted in a pregnancy. In a similar representative, statewide survey of 3,473 people in Washington state, CSA was associated with an eight-fold increase in HIV risk behavior for men (Bensley et al., 2000). Physical abuse was related to a threefold increase in HIV risk behavior and to a similar increase in heavy drinking. Although only 19% of the men reported any type of abuse, this group accounted for 50% of the HIV risk behavior.

In contrast to most cross-sectional data, in Widom and Kuhns's (1996) matched, prospective sample, CSA, physical abuse, and family neglect of boys were not associated with later promiscuity, prostitution, or involvement in a teenager's pregnancy. Widom and Kuhns noted that because their sample was drawn from official records and represented families with a lower socio-economic status and less education, it was not representative. These boys also may reflect the ceiling effect found in the study by Paul and his colleagues (Paul et al., 2001) in that they had experienced many adverse events in their lives, so CSA may have been a less important single determinant of risky sexual behavior.

Injection drug use is related to HIV risk directly (sharing needles) or indirectly (through exchanging sex for drugs or vice versa). Data from two studies indicate that CSA is related to injection drug use. Among a sample of students in Grades 9–12 in Minnesota, Lodico and DiClemente (1994) found that nine times as many male students who had been abused also injected drugs compared with those who had not been abused. Similarly, Holmes (1997) found that more men with a history of CSA reported injection drug use and were younger when they began to inject. Clearly, CSA is related to distal outcomes such as injection drug use and risky sexual behaviors that place men at risk of acquiring or transmitting HIV.

IMPLICATIONS FOR RESEARCH, TREATMENT, AND HIV PREVENTION PROGRAMS

Understanding and breaking the links between CSA and psychopathology, substance abuse, revictimization, and HIV risk behaviors require more research. It is clear that the empirical models of abuse based on data gathered from girls and women cannot be simply applied to boys and men. Future studies should focus on addressing the methodological issues that have hampered most of the research with males. For example, clearly defining CSA is important, as is assessing multiple aspects of the experience. More careful studies of the various aspects of CSA can help determine what is related to poor outcomes and help define a more valid construct that does not mix such a wide variety of experiences. Better control for potential confounding variables, using larger and more representative samples, and using longitudinal prospective designs, are improvements in some recent studies.

It also is important to provide early and ongoing treatment to sexually abused boys, as treatment may be an important mediator between CSA and adult functioning. Most studies find that less than a third of abused boys have disclosed (during childhood or adulthood) abuse to medical care providers or other treatment professionals (Holmes & Slap, 1998). Reasons for not disclosing include wanting to forget, not wanting to be perceived as feminine or a victim, wanting to protect the abuser, and fearing others' reactions to the disclosure. Family members may also pressure boys to be silent about their abuse to protect family honor (Carballo-Diéguez & Dolezal, 1995). When male college students were presented with sexual abuse vignettes, they attributed significantly less responsibility to abusers when the victim was a boy rather than a girl (Broussard & Wagner, 1988). Even in cases of abuse discovered during childhood, only about half of the victims were referred to mental health treatment (Holmes & Slap, 1998). Working with families is also important, because some parents and family members deny that boys can be the victims of CSA. Families should be encouraged to improve channels of communication with young boys so that the boys can trust that they will be heard if they disclose an abusive act (Carballo-Diéguez & Dolezal, 1995).

Among men and women who experienced physical, sexual, or emotional abuse during childhood, those with a helpful mental health provider demonstrated higher self-esteem and better family functioning (Palmer, Brown, Rae-Grant, & Loughlin, 2001). Clinicians must be sure to ask about abuse and offer treatment when appropriate: Research indicates that male patients are rarely questioned about sexual abuse and that many professionals have little knowledge or training in treating men who have been sexually abused (Lab, Feigenbaum, & De Silva, 2000). In addition, male clinicians should receive specific training because they are less likely to believe allegations of abuse, regardless of the sex of the victim (Jackson & Nuttall, 1993).

HIV prevention programs also should focus on men who have been abused, whether or not the men perceive the early sexual experiences as coercive. Although many abused men suffer negative consequences, many others do not report personal harm, even though more of them report risky sexual behavior. To address the public health effect on the HIV epidemic, it is important to better understand the pathways between CSA and risky sexual behavior and how events that are perceived in adulthood as nontraumatic or coercive may affect behavior. Although research is exploring the links between CSA and risk behavior, work can be done to identify relevant intervention strategies to help abused men reduce their sexual risk (Paul et al., 2001). By pulling together research, clinical, and prevention resources, we can better understand CSA and risky sexual behavior and help both the individual and the public to reduce the spread of HIV.

REFERENCES

American Psychiatric Association. (1994). *Diagnostic and statistical manual of mental disorders* (4th ed.). Washington, DC: Author.

Anda, R. F., Felitti, V. J., Chapman, D. P., Croft, J. B., Williamson, D. F., Santelli, J., et al. (2001). Abused boys, battered mothers, and male involvement in teen pregnancy. *Pediatrics, 107*, E19.

Bailey, J. M., & Zucker, K. J. (1995). Childhood sex-typed behavior and sexual orientation: A conceptual analysis and quantitative review. *Developmental Psychology, 31*, 43–55.

Bartholow, B., Doll, L., Joy, D., Douglas, J., Bolan, G., Harrison, J., et al. (1994). Emotional, behavioral, and HIV risks associated with sexual abuse among adult homosexual and bisexual men. *Child Abuse and Neglect, 18*, 747–761.

Bauserman, R., & Rind, B. (1997). Psychological correlates of male child and adolescent sexual experiences with adults: A review of the nonclinical literature. *Archives of Sexual Behavior, 26*, 105–141.

Bensley, L. S., Van Eenwyk, J., & Simmons, K. W. (2000). Self-reported childhood sexual and physical abuse and adult HIV-risk behaviors and heavy drinking. *American Journal of Preventive Medicine, 18*, 151–158.

Boney-McCoy, S., & Finkelhor, D. (1995). Psychological sequelae of violent victimization in a national youth sample. *Journal of Consulting and Clinical Psychology, 63*, 726–736.

Boney-McCoy, S., & Finkelhor, D. (1996). Is youth victimization related to trauma symptoms and depression after controlling for prior symptoms and family relationships? A longitudinal, prospective study. *Journal of Consulting and Clinical Psychology, 64*, 1406–1416.

Broussard, S. D., & Wagner, W. G. (1988). Child sexual abuse: Who is to blame? *Child Abuse and Neglect, 12*, 563–569.

Bryant, S. L., & Range, L. M. (1997). Type and severity of child abuse and college students' lifetime suicidality. *Child Abuse and Neglect, 21*, 1169–1176.

Carballo-Diéguez, A., & Dolezal, C. (1995). Association between history of childhood sexual abuse and adult HIV-risk sexual behavior in Puerto Rican men who have sex with men. *Child Abuse and Neglect, 19*, 595–605.

Celano, M. (1992). A developmental model of victims' internal attributions of responsibility for sexual abuse. *Journal of Interpersonal Violence, 7,* 57–69.

Chandy, J. M., Blum, R. W., & Resnick, M. D. (1996). Gender-specific outcomes for sexually abused adolescents. *Child Abuse and Neglect, 20,* 1219–1231.

Collings, S. J. (1995). The long-term effects of contact and noncontact forms of child sexual abuse in a sample of university men. *Child Abuse and Neglect, 19,* 1–6.

Crepaz, N., & Marks, G. (2001). Are negative affective states associated with HIV sexual risk behaviors? A meta-analytic review. *Health Psychology, 20,* 291–299.

Dallam, S. J., Gleaves, D. H., Cepeda-Benito, A., Silberg, J. L., Kraemer, H. C., & Spiegel, D. (2001). The effects of child sexual abuse: Comment on Rind, Tromovitch, and Bauserman (1998). *Psychological Bulletin, 127,* 715–733.

Dhaliwal, G. K., Gauzas, L., Antonowicz, D. H., & Ross, R. R. (1996). Adult male survivors of childhood sexual abuse: Prevalence, sexual abuse characteristics, and long-term effects. *Clinical Psychology Review, 16,* 619–639.

DiIorio, C., Hartwell, T., & Hansen, N., for the NIMH HIV Prevention Trial Group. (2002). Childhood sexual abuse and risk behaviors among men at high risk for HIV infection. *American Journal of Public Health, 92,* 214–219.

Dolezal, C., & Carballo-Diéguez, A. (2002). Childhood sexual experiences and the perception of abuse among Latino men who have sex with men. *Journal of Sex Research, 39,* 165–173.

Doll, L., Joy, D., Bartholow, B., Harrison, J., Bolan, G., Douglas, J., et al. (1992). Self-reported childhood and adolescent sexual abuse among adult homosexual and bisexual men. *Child Abuse and Neglect, 16,* 855–864.

Duncan, D. F. (1990). Prevalence of sexual assault victimization among heterosexual and gay/lesbian university students. *Psychological Reports, 66,* 65–66.

Emery, R. E., & Laumann-Billings, L. (1998). An overview of the nature, causes, and consequences of abusive family relationships: Toward differentiating maltreatment and violence. *American Psychologist, 53,* 121–135.

Feiring, C., Taska, L., & Lewis, M. (1999). Age and gender differences in children's and adolescents' adaptation to sexual abuse. *Child Abuse and Neglect, 23,* 115–128.

Finkelhor, D. (1994). Current information on the scope and nature of child sexual abuse. *The Future of Children, 4*(2), 31–53.

Finkelhor, D. (1995). The victimization of children: A developmental perspective. *American Journal of Orthopsychiatry, 65,* 177–193.

Fivush, R., Brotman, M. A., Buckner, J. P., & Goodman, S. H. (2000). Gender differences in parent–child emotion narratives. *Sex Roles, 42,* 233–253.

Freyd, J. J. (1996). *Betrayal trauma: The logic of forgetting child abuse.* Cambridge, MA: Harvard University Press.

Gold, S. N., Elhai, J. D., Lucenko, B. A., Swingle, J. M., & Hughes, D. M. (1998). Abuse characteristics among childhood sexual abuse survivors in therapy: A gender comparison. *Child Abuse and Neglect, 23,* 1005–1012.

Gold, S. N., Lucenko, B. A., Elhia, J. D., Swingle, J. M., & Sellers, A. H. (1999). A comparison of psychological/psychiatric symptomatology of women and men sexually abused as children. *Child Abuse and Neglect, 22,* 683–692.

Gorey, K. M., & Leslie, D. R. (1997). The prevalence of child sexual abuse: Integrative review adjustment for potential response and measurement biases. *Child Abuse and Neglect, 21,* 391–398.

Haugaard, J. (2000). The challenge of defining child sexual abuse. *American Psychologist, 55,* 1036–1039.

Holmes, W. C. (1997). Association between a history of childhood sexual abuse and subsequent, adolescent psychoactive substance use disorder in a sample of HIV seropositive men. *Journal of Adolescent Health, 20,* 414–419.

Holmes, W. C., & Slap, G. B. (1998). Sexual abuse of boys: Definition, prevalence, correlates, sequelae, and management. *Journal of the American Medical Association, 280,* 1855–1862.

Jackson, H., & Nuttall, R. (1993). Clinician responses to sexual abuse allegations. *Child Abuse and Neglect, 17,* 127–143.

Jinich, S., Paul, J., Stall, R., Acree, M., Kegeles, S., Hoff, C., et al. (1998). Childhood sexual abuse and HIV risk-taking behavior among gay and bisexual men. *AIDS and Behavior, 2,* 41–51.

Johnson, J. G., Cohen, P., Brown, J., Smailes, E. M., & Bernstein, D. P. (1999). Childhood maltreatment increases risk for personality disorders during early adulthood. *Archives of General Psychiatry, 56,* 600–606.

Kalichman, S., Benotsch, E., Rompa, D., Gore-Felton, C., Austin, J., Luke, W., et al. (2001). Unwanted sexual experiences and sexual risks in gay and bisexual men: Associations among revictimization, substance use, and psychiatric symptoms. *Journal of Sex Research, 38,* 1–9.

Kendall-Tackett, K. A., Williams, L. M., & Finkelhor, D. (1993). Impact of sexual abuse on children: A review and synthesis of recent empirical studies. *Psychological Bulletin, 113,* 57–62.

Kinzl, J. F., Mangweth, B., Traweger, C., & Biebl, W. (1996). Sexual dysfunction in males: Significance of adverse childhood experiences. *Child Abuse and Neglect, 20,* 759–766.

Kinzl, J. F., Traweger, C., & Biebl, W. (1995). Sexual dysfunctions: Relationship to childhood sexual abuse and early family experiences in a nonclinical sample. *Child Abuse and Neglect, 19,* 785–792.

Lab, D. D., Feigenbaum, J. D., & De Silva, P. (2000). Mental health professionals' attitudes and practices towards male childhood sexual abuse. *Child Abuse and Neglect, 24,* 391–409.

Leigh, B. C., & Stall, R. S. (1993). Substance use and risky sexual behavior for exposure to HIV. *American Psychologist, 48,* 1035–1045.

Lenderking, W. R., Wold, C., Mayer, K. H., Goldstein, R., Losina, E., & Seage, G. R. (1997). Childhood sexual abuse among homosexual men: Prevalence and association with unsafe sex. *Journal of General Internal Medicine, 12,* 250–253.

Lisak, D. (1994). The psychological impact of sexual abuse: Content analysis of interviews with male survivors. *Journal of Traumatic Stress, 7*, 525–548.

Lodico, M. A., & DiClemente, R. J. (1994). The association between childhood sexual abuse and prevalence of HIV-related risk behaviors. *Clinical Pediatrics, 33*, 498–502.

MacMillan, H. L., Fleming, J. E., Streiner, D. L., Lin, L., Boyle, M. H., Jamieson, E., et al. (2001). Childhood abuse and lifetime psychopathology in a community sample. *American Journal of Psychiatry, 158*, 1878–1883.

Mendel, M. P. (1995). *The male survivor: The impact of sexual abuse*. Thousand Oaks, CA: Sage.

Molnar, B. E., Buka, S. L., & Kessler, R. C. (2001). Child sexual abuse and subsequent psychopathology: Results from the national comorbidity survey. *American Journal of Public Health, 91*, 753–760.

Morrill, A. C., Kasten, L., Urato, M., & Larson, M. J. (2001). Abuse, addiction, and depression as pathways to sexual risk in women and men with a history of substance abuse, *Journal of Substance Abuse, 13*, 169–184.

Oddone Paolucci, E., Genuis, M. L., & Violato, C. (2001). A meta-analysis of the published research on the effects of child sexual abuse. *Journal of Psychology, 135*, 17–36.

O'Leary, A., Purcell, D., Remien, R. H., & Gomez, C. (2003). Childhood sexual abuse and sexual transmission risk behavior among HIV-seropositive men who have sex with men. *AIDS Care, 15*, 17–26.

Ondersma, S. J., Chaffin, M., Berliner, L., Cordon, I., Goodman, G. S., & Barnett, D. (2001). Sex with children is abuse: Comment on Rind, Tromovitch, and Bauserman (1998). *Psychological Bulletin, 127*, 707–714.

Palmer, S. E., Brown, R. A., Rae-Grant, N. I., & Loughlin, M. J. (2001). Survivors of childhood abuse: Their reported experience with professional help. *Social Work, 46*, 136–145.

Paul, J. P., Catania, J., Pollack, L., & Stall, R. (2001). Understanding childhood sexual abuse as a predictor of sexual risk-taking among men who have sex with men: The Urban Men's Health Study. *Child Abuse and Neglect, 25*, 557–584.

Raj, A., Silverman, J. G., & Amaro, H. (2000). The relationship between sexual abuse and sexual risk among high school students: Findings from the 1997 Massachusetts Youth Risk Behavior Survey. *Maternal and Child Health Journal, 4*, 125–134.

Relf, M. V. (2001). Childhood sexual abuse in men who have sex with men: The current state of the science. *Journal of the Association of Nurses in AIDS Care, 12*, 20–29.

Rind, B., Bauserman, R., & Tromovitch, P. (2000). Science versus orthodoxy: Anatomy of the congressional condemnation of a scientific article and reflections on remedies for future ideological attacks. *Applied and Preventive Psychology, 9*, 211–226.

Rind, B., & Tromovitch, P. (1997). A meta-analytic review of findings from national samples on psychological correlates of child sexual abuse. *Journal of Sex Research, 34*, 237–255.

Rind, B., Tromovitch, P., & Bauserman, R. (1998). A meta-analytic examination of assumed properties of child sexual abuse using college samples. *Psychological Bulletin, 124*, 22–53.

Rind, B., Tromovitch, P., & Bauserman, R. (2001). The validity and appropriateness of methods, analyses, and conclusions in Rind et al. (1998): A rebuttal of victimological critique from Ondersma et al. (2001) and Dallam et al. (2001). *Psychological Bulletin, 127*, 734–758.

Romano, E., & De Luca, R. V. (2001). Male sexual abuse: A review of effects, abuse characteristics, and links with later psychological functioning. *Aggression and Violent Behavior, 6*, 55–78.

Sarwar, D. B., Crawford, I., & Durlak, J. A. (1997). The relationship between childhood sexual abuse and adult male sexual dysfunction. *Child Abuse and Neglect, 21*, 649–655.

Sarwar, D. B., & Durlak, J. A. (1996). Childhood sexual abuse as a predictor of adult female dysfunction: A study of couples seeking sex therapy. *Child Abuse and Neglect, 20*, 963–972.

Saywitz, K. J., Mannarino, A. P., Berliner, L., & Cohen, J. A. (2000). Treatment for sexually abused children and adolescents. *American Psychologist, 55*, 1040–1049.

West, D. J. (1998). Boys and sexual abuse: An English opinion. *Archives of Sexual Behavior, 27*, 539–559.

Whiffen, V. E., Thompson, J. M., & Aube, J. A. (2000). Mediators of the link between childhood sexual abuse and adult depressive symptoms. *Journal of Interpersonal Violence, 15*, 1100–1120.

Widom, C. S. (1999). Posttraumatic stress disorder in abused and neglected children grown up. *American Journal of Psychiatry, 156*, 1223–1239.

Widom, C. S., & Kuhns, J. B. (1996). Childhood victimization and subsequent risk for promiscuity, prostitution, and teenage pregnancy: A prospective study. *American Journal of Public Health, 86*, 1607–1612.

Widom, C. S., Weiler, B. L., & Cottler, L. B. (1999). Childhood victimization and drug abuse: A comparison of prospective and retrospective findings. *Journal of Consulting and Clinical Psychology, 67*, 867–880.

III

THEORETICAL BASES FOR ADULT RISK AND REVICTIMIZATION: COGNITIVE, SOCIAL, AND BEHAVIORAL MEDIATORS

5

COGNITIVE AND ATTITUDINAL PATHS FROM CHILDHOOD TRAUMA TO ADULT HIV RISK

KATHRYN QUINA, PATRICIA J. MOROKOFF,
LISA L. HARLOW, AND EILEEN L. ZURBRIGGEN

In the search for links between childhood trauma and adult HIV risk, two conclusions seem clear from the data: First, there is a connection, and second, it is not a simple, direct link (Whitmire, Harlow, Quina, & Morokoff, 1999). Little is known about the nature of the pathways between these two life points, hence this volume. This chapter examines ways in which initial reactions to traumatic childhood experiences might become translated over time to increased HIV-risky sexual behavior in adult women.

Although a few studies have demonstrated an association between child sexual abuse (CSA) and HIV risk among adult men (Bartholow et al., 1994) and adolescents (Lodico & DiClemente, 1994), most of the work on CSA and on the nature of the connections has focused on women. Studies have identified cognitive and attitudinal predictors in gay (Aspinwall, Kemeny, Taylor, Schneider, & Dudley, 1991) and heterosexual (Sheeran, Abraham, & Orbell, 1999) men's sexual risk-related choices. Noar and Morokoff (2002)

The authors thank Seth Noar for his assistance in the preparation of this chapter.

found that college men with a traditional masculine ideology held more negative attitudes toward condom use, and those negative attitudes translated into less readiness to use condoms. We look forward to extensions of the work that follows to issues for men.

Figure 5.1 lays out a mediational model[1] for the CSA–HIV risk connection, beginning with the child abuse event and its traumagenic effects. If left unabated, the adult may develop cognitions and beliefs about herself; her behavioral responses to these may lead to HIV risky behaviors. Although cognitions and attitudes do not act alone in this path, they may be among the HIV risk predictors most amenable to interventions with at-risk women (Exner, Seal, & Ehrhardt, 1997; St. Lawrence et al., 1998). This chapter is not an exhaustive review of the literature, nor a well-tested model. Rather, we offer a framework both for assessing the current research in the field and for encouraging future research on these or similar connections.

CHILDHOOD TRAUMA EVENTS AND THEIR IMPACTS

There are a number of well-documented impacts of trauma, particularly CSA (see reviews by Briere & Runtz, 1993; Finkelhor & Hashima, 2001; Quina & Carlson, 1989). Finkelhor and Browne (1985) outlined traumagenic dynamics that result from abuse (or from the events surrounding the abuse, such as responses of others to disclosure of the abuse). These dynamics can become incorporated into the child's self-concept and affect her worldview and her interactions with her world. Adapting this model to our focus on cognitive and attitudinal outcomes, we have focused on the following: stigmatization (the child is abused because she is bad or deserved it) and betrayal of trust; powerlessness (there is no way to prevent the assaults); and sexualization (men dominate sexual options). Across these dynamics, there is a pervasive effect of fear. Sexual abuse often creates terror in children, even when it does not involve physical violence. When attempts to take control of safety fail, for example, when the child is physically beaten for fighting back or telling another adult, the child's reality may become a far-reaching fear of violence as an adult.

These effects are more dramatic when the abuse takes place within the family, in which it is likely to start earlier and go on for an extended period of

---

[1]Mediation occurs when one identifies a variable that intervenes between an independent variable (IV) and a dependent variable (DV), such that there is a strong relationship between the IV and the mediator and a strong relationship between the mediator and the DV (Collins, Graham, & Flaherty, 1998). Any direct relationship between the IV and the DV should diminish or drop when the mediator is included in analyses. For example, Whitmire et al. (1999) found that adult sexual victimization was a significant mediator between the IV of CSA and the DV of unprotected sex in a longitudinal sample of women at risk for HIV. In contrast, a moderator variable interacts with the IV to change the nature of the relationship to the DV (Baron & Kenny, 1986). Although it is possible that some of these variables may be moderator variables, the mediational approach seems more appropriate at this preliminary stage.

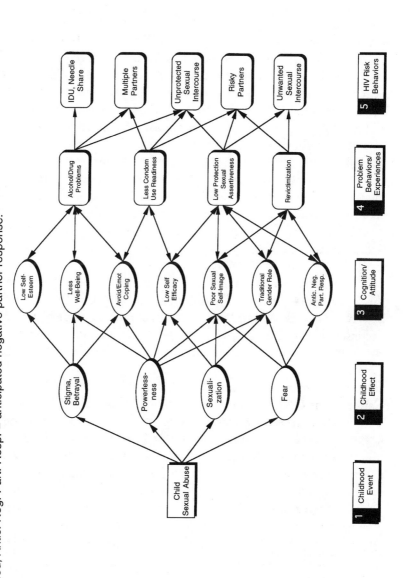

Figure 5.1. Proposed model of the path from child sexual abuse to adult HIV risk. The arrows between columns 3 and 4 are double-headed to indicate that cognitions and attitudes interact with behaviors and experiences; for example, low self-esteem may cause alcohol- and drug-related problems, or it may be the reverse, or they may continually enhance each other. IDU = injection drug use; Avoid/Emot = avoidant/emotion focused; Antic. Neg. Part. Resp. = anticipated negative partner response.

time, and to involve a direct betrayal of trust (Freyd, 1996; Wyatt, Newcomb, & Riederle, 1993). Furthermore, we found that women who experienced penetrative sexual abuse showed more heterosexual HIV risk than women with nonpenetrative sexual abuse experiences, regardless of relationship to the abusers or number of incidents (Whitmire et al., 1999).

COGNITIVE AND ATTITUDINAL SEQUELAE IN ADULT SURVIVORS

Seven constructs have consistent support in the research literature both as an outcome of CSA and as a predictor of HIV risky behavior: poor self-esteem, lack of psychosocial well-being, avoidant coping strategies, low self-efficacy, belief in traditional gender roles, poor psychosexual functioning, and anticipated negative partner response. It is likely that there is overlap among them, they co-occur (e.g., Nyamathi, Stein, & Swanson, 2000; Quina, Harlow, Morokoff, Burkholder, & Deiter, 2000), and there are others. However, this structure will permit a systematic review of the literature supporting their importance as variables in the HIV risk equation. Each of these is addressed in turn.

Self-Esteem

A number of researchers have identified lowered self-esteem as one of the sequelae of CSA (e.g., Finkelhor, 1990; Vanwesenbeeck, de Graaf, van Zessen, Straver, & Visser, 1995). Among community women in New Zealand, those reporting more than 10 episodes of childhood abuse also had significantly lower self-esteem (Romans, Martin, Anderson, O'Shea, & Mullen, 1995).

Self-esteem has also been associated with HIV risk. Among Black and Caribbean college women, Braithwaite and Thomas (2001) found that self-esteem was negatively correlated with sexual risk taking. Among minority women who were homeless and in drug recovery, Nyamathi (1991) found that those women with higher self-esteem and a stronger sense of coherence reported significantly fewer HIV risky behaviors. Somlai et al. (2000) found similar results for inner-city women attending a health clinic. In their cluster analysis of community-based women, Harlow et al. (1998) found self-esteem was significantly lower for the women who were in the two highest HIV risk level clusters; these two groups of women also had experienced the most child and adult victimization.

Psychosocial Well-Being

Characterized in the literature as purpose and meaning in life, hopefulness, and low demoralization, psychological well-being has been found to be lower among women with CSA histories in samples of Black and White adults (Whitmire et al., 1999; Wyatt, 1988, 1991), middle-class college students (Johnsen & Harlow, 1996), women in methadone maintenance (El-Bassel, Simoni, Cooper, Gilbert, & Schilling, 2001), and women in prison (Morrow, Mitchell, Quina, & Hevey, 1999). Extremely poor psychological functioning has been linked with more severe forms of sexual abuse. In a large survey of 9,000 adults, Felitti et al. (1998) found a significant relationship between depression and suicidality and the number of different types of child abuse. Wyatt (1988) found that well-being was lower in adult survivors whose abuse involved more severe body intrusion and a longer duration of incidents.

In a number of studies, poorer psychological well-being predicts HIV risk for adult women, particularly among the most at-risk women. Somlai et al. (2000) found that inner-city women at highest risk for HIV expressed more personal fatalism, less optimism concerning the future, and greater life dissatisfaction than peers at the lowest levels of risk. Among Black women, Orr, Celentano, Santelli, and Burwell (1994) found that HIV risky behaviors were more frequent among women who were depressed. Among women in serodiscordant couples, Kennedy et al. (1993) found that condom use was less likely among women who were psychologically distressed. Harlow et al. (1998) observed that the women engaging in the most HIV risky sexual behaviors scored lower on purpose and meaning in life and higher on hopelessness measures, and they were more likely to have experienced severe forms of CSA. Morrill, Ickovics, Golubchikov, Beren, and Rodin (1996) found that women who were initially higher in optimism for the future were four times as likely to initiate safer sex following training than women with lower optimism.

Ehrhardt, Yingling, Zawadzski, and Martinez-Ramirez (1992) suggested that overwhelming life circumstances reduced cognitive decision-making skills: In focus groups with various ethnic groups, they found that women who were demoralized were not able to determine whether they were at risk for infection. Consistent with this view, Harlow, Newcomb, and Bentler (1986) found that purpose and meaning in life was associated with a range of maladaptive behaviors, including alcohol and drug use and suicidality.

Passive and Avoidant Coping

CSA increases reliance on avoidant strategies: either more directly, as the child may choose to not engage in protective or fighting stances because of the futility of those strategies in past experiences; or less directly, as she tries to avoid her pain and fear through drug and alcohol use, dissociation (mentally "splitting" from the immediate situation, going to "another place" in one's mind; see chap. 6, this volume), or denial (not recognizing or minimizing the genuine risk of a situation). Deblinger, McLeer, Atkins, Ralphe, and Foa (1989) found greater avoidant and dissociative symptoms among adults reporting CSA. Among women in prison, Morrow et al. (1999) found that a history of CSA was positively correlated with avoidant coping and negatively correlated with active problem solving. Several researchers have suggested that CSA survivors may consume alcohol and other drugs to avoid or "mask" painful memories, anxiety, stress, and low self-esteem (Miller, Downs, & Testa, 1993).

Coping strategies have also been linked to HIV risk-related behaviors. Nyamathi et al. (2000) found that drug use and low self-esteem were associated with emotion-focused coping such as eating, drinking, sleeping, being alone, or taking stress out on others. Emotion-focused coping, in turn, was associated with having a recent sexually transmitted infection. Problem-focused coping, consisting of such active strategies as becoming informed, thinking and talking about the issue, and making an action plan, was associated with less drug use, less risky behavior, and seeking an HIV test (hence becoming more aware of level of risk).

Arata (1999) found that adult rape survivors who had also been sexually abused as children were less likely to use active coping strategies in the face of a dangerous sexual situation. Zlotnick et al. (1994) suggested that responding to stress with dissociation may be an important link to HIV risk. Denial of risk may also be a coping strategy. Quina et al. (2000) found that women who had been sexually abused as children were less likely to ask their sexual partners for information that would help them assess their HIV risk, even though they reported greater suspicions that their partners had had a risk factor. In a related vein, Harlow et al. (1998) found that women with the highest levels of abuse reported less confidence that they knew their partners' HIV risk status.

Self-Efficacy

In the face of repeated overwhelming physical and emotional force, it is not surprising that some survivors doubt that they can protect themselves (Perez, Kennedy, & Fullilove, 1995). Bandura (1990) introduced self-efficacy—the conviction that a person can successfully execute behaviors required to produce a desired outcome—into the HIV risk equation. A childhood without apparent options may lead to a belief that one can never control outcomes, particularly true of options with respect to sexuality. Bandura suggested that the more confident a woman feels regarding her ability to use condoms to prevent diseases, the more likely she will be to insist on their use. Yet for a CSA survivor, the ability to contemplate successful outcomes, and the confidence that she can apply the strategies necessary to achieve them, may be difficult.

Wingood and DiClemente (1996) reviewed research on self-efficacy and HIV risk among women and found a number of studies that have shown that higher self-efficacy for birth control and condom use is associated with stronger intentions to engage consistently in their use. They concluded that women who reported they were less efficacious about their ability to insist on condom use or to avoid being infected with HIV, and women who reported lower confidence about their ability to control condom use, were more likely to engage in HIV-related sexual risk. Furthermore, from intervention studies designed to increase HIV prevention efforts, they concluded that programs increasing women's self-efficacy for using condoms and negotiating their use with sexual partners increased HIV prevention in women.

The relationship between self-efficacy for condom use and protection from HIV infection is fairly robust, observed with sexually active college students (Harlow, Quina, Morokoff, Rose, & Grimley, 1993), women with steady partners (Morrison, Gilmore, & Baker, 1995), Latinas (Gomez & Marin, 1996), and adult women living in the community (Harlow et al., 1998), although this last study found that women in minority groups reported lower levels of self-efficacy overall. In a random household survey of 1,600 unmarried Latino adults, Marin, Tschann, Gomez, and Gregorich (1998) also found that self-efficacy was related to condom use, for men and women, but further clarified the nature of this relationship. Women reported that condom use was most challenging when asking regular partners to use condoms. There were few demographic differences in self-efficacy, although less educated men and women reported more difficulties when partners were resistant and when asking steady partners to use condoms.

There are at least three studies describing self-efficacy as a mediating link between CSA and HIV risk. Brown, Kessel, Lourie, Ford, and Lipsitt (1997) found that among adolescent female psychiatric patients, 38% reported CSA, and self-efficacy for condom use was lower for them than for teens not reporting CSA. These data were particularly powerful in that 16% of the variance was uniquely accounted for by a history of CSA. In our cluster analysis of older community women, those in the least efficacious group were at highest risk for HIV and most likely to have experienced CSA (Harlow et al., 1998). Among clients at a sexually transmitted disease (STD) clinic, Thompson, Potter, Sanderson, and Maibach (1997) found that those who reported CSA also had lower expectations for partner-related condom use efficacy.

Gender Role Beliefs

CSA appears to enhance traditional gender roles for women in sexual situations, as passive and deferent to male partners' choices and pressures (Holland, Ramazanoglu, Scott, Sharpe, & Thomson, 1990) and as sexual objects (Davis & Petretic-Jackson, 2000; Tharinger, 1990). Jehu (1988) and Maltz and Holman (1987) both examined how sexual abuse enhances gender roles, reporting that adult women CSA survivors were more likely to view sexual relationships as something men expect and feel that they have no rights to assert otherwise. Zurbriggen, Quina, and Freyd (2001) found that college women and men who had experienced sexual abuse from a close family member tended to have more traditional attitudes toward women than nonabused students, although this relationship did not reach statistical significance.

Links between gender role adherence and HIV risk are less studied, but there are important connections identified. Amaro (1995), Gomez and Marin (1996), and Quina, Harlow, Morokoff, and Saxon (1997) viewed traditional feminine gender norms of passivity and submission to men as risk predictors in and of themselves. Bowleg, Belgrave, and Reisen (2000) found that gender roles and more direct power strategies were significant predictors of sexual self-efficacy around HIV risk reduction. Clay, Noar, Zimmerman, and Stewart (2002) and Zurbriggen et al. (2001) found that women with less traditional attitudes on the Attitudes Toward Women Scale had higher condom assertiveness, and the latter study found condom assertiveness was associated with safer sex practices.

Sexual Self-Image

Perhaps the most pervasive result of early sexual objectification of a child is a sense of one's sexual self, which lacks purpose and meaning (except to please the male partner), in which one has little power over sexuality or its uses, and in which the woman (as the child) defers to male domination. This adaptation to abuse may also be reinforced by abusers. Finkelhor and Browne (1985) suggested that whereas abuse teaches the child she is powerless to resist another's sexual suggestions or advances, compliance with sexual advances is rewarded if it results in acceptance and approval from the more powerful male abuser. Briere and Runtz (1993) suggested that abused children learn that intimacy only occurs in sexual contacts.

CSA is also related to number of adult sexual partners and HIV risk levels of those partners. In a survey of 9,000 adults, Felitti et al. (1998) found a strong relationship between the number of categories of exposure to CSA and adult levels of promiscuity and number of STDs. Wyatt et al. (1993) found that women who had been sexually abused as children reported more sexual partners, a finding echoed by Thompson et al. (1997) among clients at an STD clinic. Our data supported this observation: Although frequency of sexual intercourse was comparable across groups, community women who reported sexual penetration as a child had more different partners, and these partners were reported to have a higher level of risk (Whitmire et al., 1999).

Fewer studies have actually looked at the links between psychosexual attitudes and HIV risk. Using a new measure of purpose and meaning in sexual life, based on more general measures of well-being, Harlow et al. (1998) found strong associations between poorer psychosexual attitudes and greater

HIV risk. Quina et al. (2000) observed that women with poorer psycho-sexual attitudes had more sexual partners with more known indicators of sexual risk. In the Netherlands, Vanwesenbeeck et al. (1995) observed that even among commercial sex workers, those who had been sexually abused as children could be characterized as more likely to take risks that suggested a lack of a sense of power over their own sexual encounters.

Anticipated Negative Partner Response

The terror experienced during childhood traumas does not easily go away. It can become an adult fear of men, or a fear of male anger, which the woman will try to avoid whenever possible—and one good strategy is to avoid angering her partner. The co-occurrence of different types of trauma can be statistically dramatic. Quina et al. (2000) found high intercorrelations among CSA, adult relationship violence, and anticipation of negative responses to requests for condom use from men.

There is ample evidence that having a violent partner is associated with greater acceptance of risky behaviors with that partner (e.g., Molina & Basinait-Smith, 1998; Wingood & DiClemente, 1997). Experiences with a violent partner do not have to be direct, however. Anticipating a negative partner response also affects HIV risk reduction strategies. Quina et al. (2000) found that anticipated negative partner response was greater among women who reported more known partner HIV-related risk factors; in addition, that anticipation was associated with less refusal assertiveness, poorer psycho-social attitudes, and lower self-efficacy. Harlow et al.'s (1998) highest partner risk group had experienced more of each type of interpersonally negative event assessed, including anticipated negative partner response.

RISK-RELATED BEHAVIORS AND EXPERIENCES

Another set of behavioral and experiential factors appear to transform cognitions and attitudes into HIV risky sexual practices. Alcohol and drug use are perhaps the most obvious, as these substances increase vulnerability in a number of emotional and behavioral ways (e.g., El-Bassel, Gilbert, Rajah, Foleno, & Frye, 2000; Miller et al., 1993; Testa, Livingston, & Collins, 2000). Willingness to adopt condom use, discussed here as readiness to use condoms, is a specific statement of the individual of her intentions to put cognitions and attitudes into action, and is highly related to actual condom use (Evers, 1999; Lauby et al., 1998; Redding & Rossi, 1999). Sexual assertiveness is the self-reported ability of a woman to refuse unwanted sex, insist on condom use by her partner, and discuss with her partner his HIV risk potential. Sexual revictimization as an adult has been shown to link closely to HIV risk (Goodman & Fallot, 1998; Letourneaux, Resnick, Kilpatrick, Saunders, & Best, 1996; Whitmire et al., 1999). As with the other lists presented in this chapter, the selection of these four behavioral and experiential factors is preliminary, based on the evidence available, but by no means to be considered exhaustive or nonoverlapping. Because substance use problems and revictimization are covered extensively in other chapters in this volume, and the transtheoretical model is discussed extensively in other sources (Harlow et al., 1999; Prochaska, Norcross, & DiClemente, 1994), we focus the present discussion on sexual assertiveness.

Our research group conceptualized and developed a psychometrically sound Sexual Assertiveness Scale (SAS), which takes a rights-based approach to women's sexual choices to initiate wanted sexual activity, refuse unwanted (and not forced) sexual activity, and insist on condoms to prevent infections or pregnancy (Morokoff et al., 1997). Johnsen and Harlow (1996) found that college women who reported CSA scored significantly lower on the SAS subscales for refusal and condom and birth control assertiveness, even though they were also less sure of their partner's HIV risk status. Zurbriggen et al. (2001) observed lower SAS scores among women and men who had been sexually abused as children. Harlow et al.'s (1998) most at-risk cluster showed lower SAS scores for condom use and higher levels of prior sexual abuse.

Of particular interest is assertiveness for condom use, which is negatively correlated with unprotected vaginal sex (Harlow et al., 1998; Morokoff et al., 1997). Wingood and DiClemente (1998) found that Black women who had not used a condom in the past 3 months were less likely to be sexually assertive. Zamboni, Crawford, and Williams (2000) found sexual assertiveness was the strongest predictor of condom use among women college students.

Communication assertiveness—the ability to communicate a desire for safe sex—has been positively related to condom use (Catania et al., 1992; Quina et al., 2000). In a study of Black and Latina clients of methadone clinics, condom use was related to women's attitudes toward the negotiation of safer sex with a partner and their comfort with communication skills with that partner (Schilling, El-Bassel, Gilbert, & Schinke, 1991). Deiter (1994) introduced communication subscales to the SAS, for requesting information about a partner's sexual history and asserting one's sexual preferences. Using these scales, Lang (1998) found that sexual communication assertiveness was one of the strongest predictors of HIV risky behavior in adolescent women but not men, suggesting that responses on this variable are strongly gender based. Quina et al. (2000) concluded that communication of HIV risk information was used by some as an HIV risk reduction strategy, although not always effectively.

TOWARD A MODEL: CAVEATS

There are important caveats to address before building more formal models with these and other constructs. First, any review of potential mediators requires us to consider the contexts in which risk occurs. First and foremost must be the sociocultural considerations of gender, ethnicity, sexuality, class, and power (Connell, McKevitt, & Low, 2001; Goldstein & Manlowe, 1997; Pequengnat & Stover, 1999; Wingood & DiClemente, 2000). Prediction models for White middle-class gay men will be different from prediction models for heterosexual Black women living in poverty, even though both groups are among the most vulnerable to HIV infection (Amaro, 1995; Wyatt, 1988, 1991, 1994). Understanding risk to a woman who survives through sex work, who has little education and inadequate skills to earn a living otherwise, a woman who is drug- or alcohol-dependent, or a woman in a violent relationship is different from understanding risk for a well-educated, financially secure college student (El-Bassel et al., 2000; Kalichman, Williams, Cherry, Belcher, & Nachimson, 1998; Kline, Kline, & Oken, 1992; Muller & Boyle, 1996; Shayne & Kaplan, 1991). Defining and measuring risky behavior in a neighborhood where HIV infection rates are high becomes a different task than defining and measuring risk on a college campus, where estimates of seroprevalence are low; indeed, differences may be observed among similar women in settings in which the local seroprevalence rates vary (Wood, Tortu, Rhodes, & Deren, 1998). Thus this chapter is undertaken with the caution that cognitive and attitudinal predictors can only be viewed within the specific context of a person's life.

In a related vein, there are significant structural factors that may enhance or diminish the CSA–HIV link. The most at-risk women are located in a constellation of poverty, drugs, racism, marginal living conditions including homelessness, and violence from partners (Mullings, Marquart, & Brewer, 2000; O'Leary & Martins, 2000; Quina et al., 2000). The Multifaceted Model of HIV Risk (Harlow et al., 1993) posited that HIV risky sexual behavior was complex, with behavioral, interpersonal, cognitive and attitudinal, and gender or cultural predictors working together to enhance or diminish risky behavior. Indeed, most studies of HIV risk find multiple predictors, overlap among variables, and involve complex interrelationships (e.g., Rotheram-Borus, Mahler, Koopman, & Langabeer, 1996). It would be far too naïve to presume that cognitions or beliefs could outweigh all other forces.

Furthermore, any model must be respectful of the ways in which power, particularly interpersonal power, shapes the influence of any predictor or mediator for each individual (Quina et al., 1997; Wingood & DiClemente, 2000). Lack of power may undermine any efforts of an individual to choose or initiate protective strategies. For example, Kline et al. (1992) found a link between low levels of condom use and women's lack of power in relationships; indeed, although some women reported condom use with secondary partners, who had little power over them, condoms were not likely to be used with their main partners, with whom presumably they had less power. The more dependent a woman is on the monetary contributions of her partner—and thus the "security" of the relationship—the more she may be subjected to her partner's (often violent) sexual and other demands (Shayne & Kaplan,

1991). Power is a greater issue in relationships in which violence has been used to enforce the power differential. In focus groups, we found that young mothers with violent partners were explicit about the tradeoffs they made in their relationships: They would demand safety and support for their children, but they understood that to succeed in achieving that goal they would not make sexual demands such as condom use (Quina et al., 1999).

A final caveat recognizes that these are not predetermined outcomes; at any point in time good interventions or experiences—a teacher who believes in the child, a helpful emotional partner—can help the child or the adult feel good about herself, cope well, and develop a healthy sexual life. By the same token, further negative experiences, in particular further violence and abuse, can magnify the potential for negative outcomes, as suggested by Whitmire et al. (1999).

In spite of these caveats, we believe researchers can proceed in the testing of proposed models across groups of adult women and careful generalizations of results. Although studies comparing ethnically different samples of women have found differences in levels of risk-related behaviors (e.g., Harlow et al., 1998) and condom use (e.g., Gomez & Marin, 1996), these studies have found no significant differences in the pattern of predictors. Furthermore, in the absence of large-scale societal change, cognitions and attitudes hold some promise for individual change in those women whose living conditions permit (Sutton, McVey, & Glanz, 1999). Interesting new research by Noar, Morokoff, and Redding (2001) and Noar (2002) has found that young men's condom use decisions are responsive to women's attitudes and behavioral messages. Indeed, developing the belief that it is possible to have control over her own life might enable a woman to enact the structural changes that would allow her to use risk-reduction strategies.

CONCLUSION

This framework, and the literature review that accompanies it, are not exhaustive, nor are they ideal. We developed the framework to help researchers, including ourselves, to begin to examine those constructs in more depth, with conceptual and empirical support from the literature. Although the links we suggest are informed by existing data, we must underscore that for the most part, the mediated relationships we outline are hypothetical, and we urge readers to consider further research to pursue this important line of discovery. More importantly, we hope that this approach can inform cognitive and attitudinally based interventions, to reduce the harm of HIV risk-related behaviors.

REFERENCES

Amaro, H. (1995). Love, sex, and power: Considering women's realities in HIV prevention. *American Psychologist, 50,* 437–447.

Arata, C. (1999). Coping with rape: The roles of prior sexual abuse and attributions of blame. *Journal of Interpersonal Violence, 14,* 62–78.

Aspinwall, L. G., Kemeny, M. E., Taylor, S. E., Schneider, S. G., & Dudley, J. P. (1991). Psychosocial predictors of gay men's AIDS risk-reduction behavior. *Health Psychology, 10,* 432–444.

Bandura, A. (1990). Perceived self-efficacy in the exercise of control over AIDS infection. *Evaluation and Program Planning, 13,* 9–17.

Baron, R. M., & Kenny, D. A. (1986). The moderator–mediator variable distinction in social psychological research: Conceptual, strategic, and statistical considerations. *Journal of Personality and Social Psychology, 51,* 1173–1182.

Bartholow, B. N., Doll, L. S., Joy, D., Douglas, J. M., Bolan, G., Harrison, J. S., et al. (1994). Emotional, behavioral, and HIV risks associated with sexual abuse among adult homosexual and bisexual men. *Child Abuse and Neglect, 18,* 747–761.

Bowleg, L., Belgrave, F. Z., & Reisen, C. A. (2000). Gender roles, power strategies, and precautionary sexual self-efficacy: Implications for Black and Latina women's HIV/AIDS protective behaviors. *Sex Roles, 42,* 613–638.

Braithwaite, K., & Thomas, V. G. (2001). HIV/AIDS knowledge, attitudes, and risk-behaviors among African-American and Caribbean college women. *International Journal for the Advancement of Counselling, 23,* 115–129.

Briere, J., & Runtz, M. (1993). Childhood sexual abuse: Long-term sequelae and implications for psychological assessment. *Journal of Interpersonal Violence, 8,* 312–330.

Brown, L. K., Kessel, S. M., Lourie, K. J., Ford, H. H., & Lipsitt, L. P. (1997). Influence of sexual abuse on HIV-related attitudes and behaviors in adolescent psychiatric inpatients. *Journal of the American Academy of Child and Adolescent Psychiatry, 36,* 316–322.

Catania, J. A., Coates, T. J., Kegeles, S., Thompson Fullilove, M., Peterson, J., Marin, B., et al. (1992). Condom use in multi-ethnic neighborhoods of San Francisco: The population-based AMEN (AIDS in Multi-Ethnic Neighborhoods) study. *American Journal of Public Health, 82,* 284–287.

Clay, C., Noar, S. M., Zimmerman, R. S., & Stewart, G. (2002, August). *The influence of gender roles on safer sexual behaviors.* Poster presented at the 110th Annual Convention of the American Psychological Association, Chicago, IL.

Collins, L. M., Graham, J. W., & Flaherty, B. P. (1998). An alternative framework for defining mediation. *Multivariate Behavioral Research, 33,* 295–312.

Connell, P., McKevitt, C., & Low, N. (2001). Sexually transmitted infections among Black young people in south-east London: Results of a rapid ethnographic assessment. *Culture, Health and Sexuality, 3,* 311–327.

Davis, J. L., & Petretic-Jackson, P. A. (2000). The impact of child sexual abuse on adult interpersonal functioning: A review and synthesis of the empirical literature. *Aggression and Violent Behavior, 5,* 291–328.

Deblinger, E., McLeer, S. V., Atkins, M. S., Ralphe, D., & Foa, E. B. (1989). Posttraumatic stress in sexually abused, physically abused, and nonabused children. *Child Abuse and Neglect, 13,* 403–408.

Deiter, P. J. (1994). Sexual assertiveness training for college women: An intervention study. *Dissertation Abstracts International: Section B, 55*(9-B), 4116.

Ehrhardt, A. A., Yingling, S., Zawadzki, R., & Martinez-Ramirez, M. (1992). Prevention of heterosexual transmission of HIV: Barriers for women. *Journal of Psychology and Human Sexuality, 5,* 37–67.

El-Bassel, N., Gilbert, L., Rajah, V., Foleno, A., & Frye, V. (2000). Fear and violence: Raising the HIV stakes. *AIDS Education and Prevention, 12,* 154–170.

El-Bassel, N., Simoni, J. M., Cooper, D. K., Gilbert, L., & Schilling, R. F. (2001). Sex trading and psychological distress among women on methadone. *Psychology of Addictive Behaviors, 15,* 177–184.

Evers, K. E. (1999). Quantitative methods for assessing change: Application to condom use. *Dissertation Abstracts International: Section B, 59*(8-B), 4448.

Exner, T. M., Seal, D. W., & Ehrhardt, A. A. (1997). A review of HIV interventions for at-risk women. *AIDS and Behavior, 1,* 93–124.

Felitti, V. J., Anda, R. F., Nordenberg, D., Williamson, D. F., Spitz, A. M., Edwards, V., et al. (1998). Relationship of childhood abuse and household dysfunction to many of the leading causes of death in adults: The Adverse Childhood Experiences (ACE) study. *American Journal of Preventive Medicine, 14,* 245–258.

Finkelhor, D. (1990). Early and long-term effects of child sexual abuse: An update. *Professional Psychology: Research and Practice, 21,* 325–330.

Finkelhor, D., & Browne, A. (1985). The traumatic impact of child sexual abuse: A conceptualization. *American Journal of Orthopsychiatry, 55,* 530–541.

Finkelhor, D., & Hashima, P. Y. (2001). The victimization of children and youth: A comprehensive overview. In S. O. White (Ed.), *Handbook of youth and justice* (pp. 49–78). New York: Kluwer Academic/Plenum.

Freyd, J. J. (1996). *Betrayal trauma: The logic of forgetting childhood abuse.* Cambridge, MA: Harvard University Press.

Goldstein, N., & Manlowe, J. (Eds.). (1997). *The gender politics of HIV/AIDS in women.* New York: New York University Press.

Gomez, C. A., & Marin, B. V. (1996). Gender, culture, and power: Barriers to HIV-prevention strategies for women. *Journal of Sex Research, 33,* 355–362.

Goodman, L. A., & Fallot, R. D. (1998). HIV risk-behavior in poor urban women with serious mental disorders: Association with childhood physical and sexual abuse. *American Journal of Orthopsychiatry, 68,* 73–83.

Harlow, L. L., Newcomb, M. D., & Bentler, P. M. (1986). Depression, self-derogation, substance use, and suicide ideation: Lack of purpose in life as a mediational factor. *Journal of Clinical Psychology, 42,* 5–21.

Harlow, L. L., Prochaska, J. O., Redding, C. A., Rossi, J. R., Velicer, W. F., Snow, M. G., et al. (1999). Stages of condom use in a high-risk sample. *Psychology and Health, 14,* 143–157.

Harlow, L. L., Quina, K., Morokoff, P. J., Rose, J. S., & Grimley, D. M. (1993). HIV risk in women: A multifaceted model. *Journal of Applied Biobehavioral Research, 1,* 3–38.

Harlow, L. L., Rose, J. S., Morokoff, P. J., Quina, K., Mayer, K., Mitchell, K., & Schnoll, R. (1998). Women HIV sexual risk takers: Related behaviors, issues and attitudes. *Women's Health: Research on Gender, Behavior, and Policy, 4,* 407–439.

Holland, J., Ramazanoglu, C., Scott, S., Sharpe, S., & Thomson, R. (1990). Sex, gender and power: Young women's sexuality in the shadow of AIDS. *Sociology of Health and Illness, 12,* 336–350.

Jehu, D. (1988). *Beyond sexual abuse: Therapy with women who were childhood victims.* New York: Wiley.

Johnsen, L. W., & Harlow, L. L. (1996). Childhood sexual abuse linked with adult substance use, victimization, and AIDS-risk. *AIDS Education and Prevention, 8,* 44–57.

Kalichman, S. C., Williams, E. A., Cherry, C., Belcher, L., & Nachimson, D. (1998). Sexual coercion, domestic violence, and negotiating condom use among low-income African American women. *Journal of Women's Health, 7,* 371–378.

Kennedy, C. A., Skurnick, J., Wan, J. Y., Quattrone, G., Sheffet, A., Quinones, M., et al. (1993). Psychological distress, drug and alcohol use as correlates of condom use in HIV-serodiscordant heterosexual couples. *AIDS, 7,* 1493–1499.

Kline, A., Kline, E., & Oken, E. (1992). Minority women and sexual choice in the age of AIDS. *Social Science and Medicine, 34,* 447–457.

Lang, M. A. (1998). A quantitative and qualitative assessment of adolescent HIV-risk predictors. *Dissertation Abstracts International, 58*(8-B), 4491.

Lauby, J. L., Semaan, S., Cohen, A., Leviton, L., Gielen, A., Pulley, L., et al. (1998). Self-efficacy, decisional balance and stages of change for condom use among women at risk for HIV infection. *Health Education Research, 13,* 343–356.

Letourneaux, E. J., Resnick, H. S., Kilpatrick, D. G., Saunders, B. E., & Best, C. L. (1996). Comorbidity of sexual problems and posttraumatic stress disorder in female crime victims. *Behavior Therapy, 27,* 321–336.

Lodico, M. A., & DiClemente, R. J. (1994). The association between childhood sexual abuse and prevalence of HIV-related risk behaviors. *Clinical Pediatrics, 33,* 498–502.

Maltz, W., & Holman, B. (1987). *Incest and sexuality: A guide to understanding and healing.* Lexington, MA: Lexington Books.

Marin, B. V., Tschann, J. M., Gomez, C. A., & Gregorich, S. (1998). Self-efficacy to use condoms in unmarried Latino adults. *American Journal of Community Psychology, 26,* 53–71.

Miller, B. A., Downs, W. R., & Testa, M. (1993). Interrelationships between victimization experiences and women's alcohol use. *Journal of Studies on Alcohol, 11,* 109–117.

Molina, L. D., & Basinait-Smith, C. (1998). Revisiting the intersection between domestic abuse and HIV risk. *American Journal of Public Health, 88,* 1267–1268.

Morokoff, P. J., Quina, K., Harlow, L. L., Whitmire, L., Grimley, D. M., Gibson, P. R., & Burkholder, G. J. (1997). Sexual Assertiveness Scale (SAS) for women:

Development and validation. *Journal of Personality and Social Psychology, 73,* 790–804.

Morrill, A. C., Ickovics, J. R., Golubchikov, V. V., Beren, S. E., & Rodin, J. (1996). Safer sex: Social and psychological predictors of behavioral maintenance and change among heterosexual women. *Journal of Consulting and Clinical Psychology, 64,* 819–828.

Morrison, D. M., Gilmore, M. R., & Baker, S. A. (1995). Determinants of condom use among high-risk heterosexual adults: A test of the theory of reasoned action. *Journal of Applied Social Psychology, 25,* 651–676.

Morrow, J. A., Mitchell, K. J., Quina, K., & Hevey, C. E. (1999, March). *Coping with stress among women offenders: The impact of parental/adult substance use and exposure to domestic violence.* Poster presented at the annual meeting of the Academy of Criminal Justice Sciences, Orlando, FL.

Muller, R. B., & Boyle, J. S. (1996). "You don't ask for trouble": Women who do sex and drugs. *Family and Community Health, 19*(3), 35–48.

Mullings, J. L., Marquart, J. W., & Brewer, V. E. (2000). Assessing the relationship between child sexual abuse and marginal living conditions on HIV/AIDS-related risk behavior among women prisoners. *Child Abuse and Neglect, 24,* 677–688.

Noar, S. M. (2002, Summer). Eyes wide shut or open? What are we learning about men, masculinity, and safer sex? *SPSMM Bulletin,* 7–9.

Noar, S. M., & Morokoff, P. J. (2002). The relationship between masculinity ideology, condom attitudes, and condom use stage of change: A structural equation modeling approach. *International Journal of Men's Health, 1,* 43–58.

Noar, S. M., Morokoff, P. J., & Redding, C. A. (2001). An examination of transtheoretical predictors of condom use in late-adolescent heterosexual men. *Journal of Applied Biobehavioral Research, 6,* 1–26.

Nyamathi, A. M. (1991). Relationship of resources to emotional distress, somatic complaints, and high-risk behaviors in drug recovery and homeless minority women. *Research in Nursing and Health, 14,* 269–277.

Nyamathi, A. M., Stein, J. A., & Swanson, J. M. (2000). Personal, cognitive, behavioral, and demographic predictors of HIV testing and STDs in homeless women. *Journal of Behavioral Medicine, 23,* 123–147.

O'Leary, A., & Martins, P. (2000). Structural factors affecting women's HIV risk: A life-course example. *AIDS, 14,* 568–572.

Orr, S. T., Celentano, D. D., Santelli, J., & Burwell, L. (1994). Depressive symptoms and risk factors for HIV acquisitions among Black women attending urban health centers in Baltimore. *AIDS Education and Prevention, 6,* 230–236.

Pequengnat, W., & Stover, E. (1999). Considering women's contextual and cultural issues in HIV/STD prevention research. *Cultural Diversity and Ethnic Minority Psychology, 5,* 287–291.

Perez, B., Kennedy, G., & Fullilove, M. (1995). Childhood sexual abuse and AIDS: Issues and interventions. In A. O'Leary & L. Jemmott (Eds.), *Women at risk: Issues in the primary prevention of AIDS* (pp. 38–101). New York: Plenum Press.

Prochaska, J. O., Norcross, J. C., & DiClemente, C. C. (1994). *Changing for good*. New York: William Morrow.

Quina, K., & Carlson, N. (1989). *Rape, incest, and sexual harassment: A guide to helping survivors*. New York: Praeger.

Quina, K., Harlow, L. L., Morokoff, P. J., Burkholder, G., & Deiter, P. J. (2000). Sexual communication in relationships: When words speak louder than actions. *Sex Roles: A Journal of Research, 42*, 523–549.

Quina, K., Harlow, L. L., Morokoff, P. J., & Saxon, S. (1997). Interpersonal power and women's HIV risk. In N. Goldstein & J. Manlowe (Eds.), *Gender and the politics of HIV* (pp. 188–206). New York: New York University Press.

Quina, K., Morokoff, P. J., Harlow, L. L., Dieter, P. J., Lang, M. A., & Rose, J. S. (1999). Focusing on participants: Feminist process model for survey modification. *Psychology of Women Quarterly, 23*, 459–483.

Redding, C. A., & Rossi, J. S. (1999). Testing a model of situational self-efficacy for safer sex among college students: Stage of change and gender-based differences. *Psychology and Health, 14*, 467–486.

Romans, S. E., Martin, J. L., Anderson, J. C., O'Shea, M. L., & Mullen, P. E. (1995). Factors that mediate between child sexual abuse and adult psychological outcome. *Psychological Medicine, 25*, 127–142.

Rotheram-Borus, M. J., Mahler, K. A., Koopman, C., & Langabeer, K. (1996). Sexual abuse history and associated multiple risk behavior in adolescent runaways. *American Journal of Orthopsychiatry, 66*, 390–400.

Schilling, R. F., El-Bassel, N., Gilbert, L., & Schinke, S. P. (1991). Correlates of drug use, sexual behavior, and attitudes toward safer sex among African-American and Hispanic women in methadone maintenance. *Journal of Drug Issues, 21*, 685–698.

Shayne, V. T., & Kaplan, B. J. (1991). Double victims: Poor women and AIDS. *Women and Health, 17*, 21–37.

Sheeran, P., Abraham, C., & Orbell, S. (1999). Psychosocial correlates of heterosexual condom use: A meta-analysis. *Psychological Bulletin, 125*, 90–132.

Somlai, A. M., Kelly, J. A., Heckman, T. G., Hackl, K., Runge, L., & Wright, C. (2000). Life optimism, substance use, and AIDS-specific attitudes associated with HIV risk behavior among disadvantaged innercity women. *Journal of Women's Health and Gender-Based Medicine, 9*, 1101–1111.

St. Lawrence, J. S., Eldridge, G. D., Reitman, D., Little, C. E., Shelby, M. C., & Brasfield, T. L. (1998). Factors influencing condom use among African American women: Implications for risk reduction interventions. *American Journal of Community Psychology, 26*, 7–27.

Sutton, S., McVey, D., & Glanz, A. (1999). A comparative test of the theory of reasoned action and the theory of planned behavior in the prediction of condom use intentions in a national sample of English young people. *Health Psychology, 18*, 72–81.

Testa, M., Livingston, J. A., & Collins, R. L. (2000). The role of women's alcohol consumption in evaluation of vulnerability to sexual aggression. *Experimental and Clinical Psychopharmacology, 8*, 185–191.

Tharinger, D. (1990). Impact of child sexual abuse on developing sexuality. *Professional Psychology: Research and Practice, 21*, 331–337.

Thompson, N. J., Potter, J. S., Sanderson, C. A., & Maibach, E. W. (1997). The relationship of sexual abuse and HIV risk behaviors among heterosexual adult female STD patients. *Child Abuse and Neglect, 21*, 149–156.

Vanwesenbeeck, I., de Graaf, R., van Zessen, G., Straver, C., & Visser, J. H. (1995). Professional HIV risk taking, levels of victimization, and well-being in female prostitutes in the Netherlands. *Archives of Sexual Behavior, 24*, 503–515.

Whitmire, L. E., Harlow, L. L., Quina, K., & Morokoff, P. J. (1999). *Childhood trauma and HIV: Women at risk.* New York: Taylor & Francis.

Wingood, G. M., & DiClemente, R. J. (1996). HIV sexual risk reduction interventions for women: A review. *American Journal of Preventive Medicine, 21*, 209–217.

Wingood, G. M., & DiClemente, R. J. (1997). The effects of an abusive primary partner on the condom use and sexual negotiation practices of African-American women. *American Journal of Public Health, 87*, 1016–1018.

Wingood, G. M., & DiClemente, R. J. (1998). Partner influences and gender-related factors associated with noncondom use among young adult African-American women. *American Journal of Community Psychology, 26*, 29–53.

Wingood, G. M., & DiClemente, R. J. (2000). Application of the theory of gender and power to examine HIV-related exposures, risk factors, and effective interventions for women. *Health Education and Behavior, 27*, 539–565.

Wood, M. M., Tortu, S., Rhodes, F., & Deren, S. (1998). Differences in condom behaviors and beliefs among female drug users recruited from two cities. *Women and Health, 27*, 137–160.

Wyatt, G. E. (1988). The relationship between child sexual abuse and adolescent sexual functioning in Afro-American and White American women. *Annals of the New York Academy of Sciences, 528*, 111–122.

Wyatt, G. E. (1991). Examining ethnicity versus race in AIDS related sex research. *Social Science and Medicine, 33*, 37–45.

Wyatt, G. E. (1994). The sociocultural relevance of sex research: Challenges for the 1990s and beyond. *American Psychologist, 49*, 748–754.

Wyatt, G. E., Newcomb, M. D., & Riederle, M. H. (1993). *Sexual abuse and consensual sex: Women's developmental patterns and outcomes.* Newbury Park, CA: Sage.

Zamboni, B. D., Crawford, I., & Williams, P. G. (2000). Examining communication and assertiveness as predictors of condom use: Implications for HIV prevention. *AIDS Education and Prevention, 12*, 492–504.

Zlotnick, C., Begin, A., Shea, M. T., Pearlstein, T., Simpson, E., & Costello, E. (1994). The relationship between characteristics of sexual abuse and dissociative experiences. *Comprehensive Psychiatry, 35*, 465–470.

Zurbriggen, E. L., Quina, K., & Freyd, J. J. (2001, August). *Sexual assertiveness, condom use, and attitudes toward women: Gender differences and similarities.* Paper presented at the 109th Annual Convention of the American Psychological Association, San Francisco, CA.

6

THE LINK BETWEEN CHILD SEXUAL ABUSE AND RISKY SEXUAL BEHAVIOR: THE ROLE OF DISSOCIATIVE TENDENCIES, INFORMATION-PROCESSING EFFECTS, AND CONSENSUAL SEX DECISION MECHANISMS

EILEEN L. ZURBRIGGEN AND JENNIFER J. FREYD

Previous research has demonstrated a connection between child sexual abuse (CSA) victimization and engaging in high-risk sexual behaviors as an adult (Allers, Benjack, White, & Rousey, 1993; Browne & Finkelhor, 1986; Fergusson, Horwood, & Lynskey, 1997; Knutson, 1995; Thompson, Potter, Sanderson, & Maibach, 1997; Urquiza & Capra, 1990). These behaviors include sexual compulsivity, indiscriminate or impulsive sex, a high number of sexual partners, substance abuse, prostitution, and a low incidence of condom use. Although some researchers have investigated possible psychological mediator variables such as condom use self-efficacy (Thompson et al., 1997), sex guilt (Walser & Kern, 1996), self-esteem (Low, Jones, MacLeod, Power, & Duggan, 2000), sexual assertiveness (Morokoff et al., 1997), and gender rigidity (Lisak, Hopper, & Song, 1996), much work remains to be done. In this chapter, we describe a set of cognitive mechanisms that may be important mediators of the relationship between abuse experiences and sexually risky behavior.

We come to this research from slightly different directions, but we share a belief in the importance of studying and understanding the cognitive processes that result from and underlie sexual abuse and aggression. Freyd has spent the last 10 years theorizing about and investigating the relationship between traumatic experience, especially CSA, and unawareness of that experience. The goal of this program of research has been to understand the reasons and mechanisms whereby people who are abused may remain unaware of that abuse or may not be able to recall the abuse for long periods of time. Freyd has approached the question of unawareness of abuse from a cognitive science perspective, and much of her empirical work in this area has involved laboratory investigations of cognitive mechanisms involved in dissociation. In the process of these years of theorizing and researching the relationship between dissociation and trauma, she has also considered particular consequences to sexual awareness and decision making, many of which may be relevant to the observed link between CSA and sexually risky behavior.

Zurbriggen has a long-standing interest in the relationship between cognition and personality and in the ways in which cognitive mechanisms might underlie or relate to individual differences in motivation, attitudes, and beliefs. In particular, she has studied unconscious psychological links between the concepts of *power* and *sex*, and shown that people with strong power–sex links are more likely to report acting in a sexually aggressive manner in dating relationships (Zurbriggen, 2000). She also has academic training and industry experience as a computer scientist and has helped develop computational models that accurately predict speeded performance for complex cognitive tasks (Glass et al., 2000; Meyer et al., 1995; Schumacher et al., 1999). These computational models were constructed using a production rule architecture—a set of "If-Then" rules that are hypothesized to describe and explain behavior. This sort of computational modeling may also prove useful in understanding the link between CSA and adult sexual behavior.

Our shared focus, then, is on cognitive science approaches to understanding the psychology of sexual abuse and aggression. Our theorizing takes an information-processing perspective and is concerned with cognitive structures, processes, and mechanisms. In this chapter, we first describe some of our ongoing work investigating cognitive mechanisms in the area of trauma, dissociation, and memory, and we then speculate about the implication for sexually risky behavior. Note that there are many theoretically plausible links between CSA and sexually risky behavior, ranging from third-variable explanations to a variety of mediating factors between the experience of abuse and subsequent behavior (some cognitive, others noncognitive). We believe that there are multiple explanations for this relationship; however, in this chapter, we consider just one set of plausible links, those based on information-processing theory. Although these links are unlikely to explain the entire observed relationship between CSA and sexually risky behavior, we believe that they are important links, and ones that have been understudied to date.

DISSOCIATION AND BETRAYAL TRAUMA THEORY

Dissociation

Individuals differ in the extent to which they report experiences of dissociation. Although most adults report only mild dissociative experiences, such as briefly losing awareness while reading or driving, some adults report more extreme dissociative experiences, such as finding items that they must have purchased but with no memory or awareness of having actually done so. Dissociative experiences such as temporarily losing track of one's identity, location, or place in time are marked by a lack of integration of consciousness, attention, and memory. It is therefore likely that basic cognitive mechanisms of memory and attention are implicated in the phenomenon of dissociation.

The word *dissociation* is often used in connection with diagnosable disorders of thinking or behavior. For example, Bernstein and Putnam (1986) defined dissociation as "a lack of normal integration of thoughts, feelings, and experiences into the stream of consciousness and memory" (p. 727). The *Diagnostic and Statistical Manual of Mental Disorders* (4th ed., *DSM–IV*; American Psychiatric Association, 1994) recognizes five distinct dissociative disorders. Common to all five is "the disruption in the usually integrated functions of consciousness, memory, identity, or perception of the environment." (American Psychiatric Association, 1994, p. 477). In addition, dissociation is now recognized by the *DSM–IV* as contributing to posttraumatic stress disorder (PTSD).

Dissociation has consistently been linked to a history of traumatic victimization. Janet (1889) was one of the early theorists and researchers to observe this relationship and develop an account for the connection. This observed relationship between dissociative disorders and trauma has now been documented in a large number of empirical studies, using a variety of measurement instruments (e.g., Chu & Dill, 1990; DiTomasso & Routh, 1993; Miller, McCluskey-Fawcett, & Irving, 1993; Sanders & Giolas, 1991; van der Kolk, Perry, & Herman, 1991). Importantly, this trauma–dissociation relationship has been found in studies with corroborated trauma samples, such as Putnam and Trickett's (1997) study of sexually abused girls.

Betrayal Trauma Theory

Many have suggested that dissociation is a defense against the psychological and emotional pain that results from traumatic experiences (e.g., Freud,

1913; Goleman, 1985; Green, 1992; Greenson, 1967). In contrast, Freyd (1994, 1996, 2002) has proposed that dissociation and related memory failures result from some kinds of traumatic experiences, not for the purpose of avoiding pain, but to allow the trauma victim to maintain a necessary system of attachment.

More specifically, consider what happens when a child, charged by life with the duty to become attached to (and elicit attachment from) his or her caregiver, is betrayed by that very person. We are frequently sensitive to cheating and betrayal when we know we have the choice to avoid the cheater or betrayer (Cosmides & Tooby, 1992). This exquisite sensitivity to betrayal usually motivates us to withdraw from the person who betrayed us. However, when the betrayer is someone we depend on for physical and emotional survival, the very mechanisms that are normally protective become, themselves, a problem. An infant or a child who responds to cheating in the "normal" way would pull back from that relationship, become less lovable, and become less likely to inspire the nurturing he or she requires for survival. Child abuse by a caregiver or trusted authority is especially likely to produce a social conflict for the victim. If a child processes the betrayal in the normal way, he or she will be motivated to stop interacting with the betrayer. To preserve the attachment, then, the child needs to *not* know about the abuse.

Betrayal trauma theory (Freyd, 1994, 1996) predicts varying frequencies of amnesia for different sorts of traumatic events depending on the presence or absence of factors related to social betrayal, as well as depending on the presence or absence of factors related to the cognitive feasibility of amnesia. More specifically, betrayal trauma theory posits that traumatic events can be broadly distinguished into two separate dimensions, one being the terror- or fear-inducing aspects of a situation and the other being social betrayal (see Figure 6.1). Symptoms of traumatic response are theorized to depend on the extent to which these dimensions are present in the traumatic episode. Immediately life-threatening events that produce great biological fear are hypothesized to lead to hyperarousal and anxiety, whereas events that include social betrayal are hypothesized to lead to numbing, amnesia, and dissociation. Because many traumatic events are highly loaded on both dimensions, many people will display both kinds of symptoms. In addition, though, we argue that those individuals who have experienced high degrees of social betrayal traumas may tend to create a particular *cognitive environment* that is marked by high levels of divided attention (as in multitasking) as opposed to selective or focused attention.

BETRAYAL TRAUMA THEORY, COGNITIVE MECHANISMS, AND DISSOCIATIVE TENDENCIES: LABORATORY STUDIES

To test the predictions of betrayal trauma theory, Freyd and her colleagues at the University of Oregon have been conducting a number of re-

Figure 6.1. A two-dimensional model of trauma. Copyright © 1996 by Jennifer J. Freyd. Reprinted with permission.

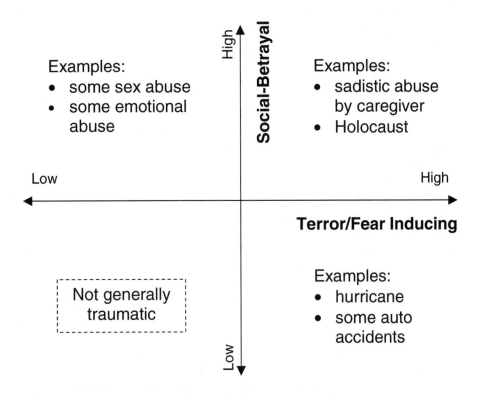

search projects investigating aspects of trauma, information processing, and betrayal trauma theory. One research direction evaluates predictions regarding the frequency of amnesia as a function of different features of trauma. Another research direction involves assessing the association of trauma, dissociative experiences, and performance on standard cognitive tasks. Results from both of these lines of research are summarized below.

Betrayal and Memory Impairment: Betrayal Trauma Inventory Studies

One of the key insights of betrayal trauma theory (Freyd, 1994, 1996) is that victims of abuse may remain unaware of the abuse, not to reduce suffering, but rather to maintain an attachment with a figure vital to survival, development, and thriving. The nature of the relationship between the victim and perpetrator (e.g., whether or not the perpetrator is a caregiver, that is, someone who provides food, clothing, shelter, and other resources necessary for survival) is therefore hypothesized to be highly relevant to whether memory for a traumatic incident is impaired and forgetting occurs. Ideally, this hypothesis would be tested by gathering detailed information about the victim–perpetrator relationship and the degree of dependency. To date, however, few data sets have included this information. The closest proxy to high dependence in the relationship in most published studies appears to be whether the abuse was perpetrated by a relative. Freyd (1996) reanalyzed a number of data sets, including Feldman-Summers and Pope (1994), Williams (1994, 1995), and Cameron (1993), focusing on the relationship between amnesia and whether the abuse was incestuous. In most cases this analysis indicated that memories for incest are more likely to be lost and recovered than are memories for other forms of abuse.

To more precisely test the specific hypotheses of betrayal trauma theory, we have been collecting new data that assess the victim–caretaker relationship in a much more detailed way. These studies use the Betrayal Trauma Inventory (BTI), a measure that is currently under development in the Freyd laboratory. The BTI assesses physical, emotional, and sexual abuse in childhood and some adulthood traumas. It consists of many behaviorally defined events (e.g., "Before you were the age of 16, did someone hold your head under water or try to drown you?"). If a participant indicates that this event happened, he or she is asked to answer follow-up questions. There are many factors probed in the follow-up questions, including age of the victim, relationship between victim and perpetrator, severity of injuries, and the victim's memory for the event. One follow-up question assessed caretaker status of the perpetrator: "Was the person responsible for caring for you (for example, providing you with food or shelter)?"

In a recent study using the BTI (Freyd, DePrince, & Zurbriggen, 2001), we administered this questionnaire to 202 men and women enrolled in an introductory psychology course. Within the three types of abuse (sexual, physical, and emotional), averages were computed across items (i.e., across the specific behaviors such as holding under water or hitting with a belt) for the age at which the abuse began, the duration of the abuse, and the amount of memory impairment. Duration scores and memory impairment scores were calculated on the basis of responses to follow-up questions. For duration, participants were asked to indicate "Over how long a period did it happen?" for any event endorsed. To determine memory impairment, we asked participants about their "knowledge of the event." Participants received a 1 for each abuse item in which they indicated any memory impairment (i.e., they endorsed "I now remember basically what happened, but I didn't always" or "I now remember the details of what happened, but I didn't always") and a 0 for all other abuse items. Average memory impairment scores thus ranged from zero to one. Note that this method of assessing memory impairment is conservative in that it does not identify people with (current) complete memory impairment, that is, those victims who currently have no memories (either general or detailed) of being abused.

Within sexual and physical abuse, caretaker status of the perpetrator was significantly related to average memory impairment in the predicted direction, with higher levels of memory impairment associated with caretaker

Figure 6.2. Average memory impairment for caretaker and noncaretaker sexual, physical, and emotional abuse. From "Self-Reported Memory for Abuse Depends Upon Victim–Perpetrator Relationship," by J. J. Freyd, A. P. DePrince, and E. L. Zurbriggen, 2001, *Journal of Trauma and Dissociation, 2*, p. 12. Copyright © 2001 by the International Society for the Study of Dissociation. Reprinted with permission.

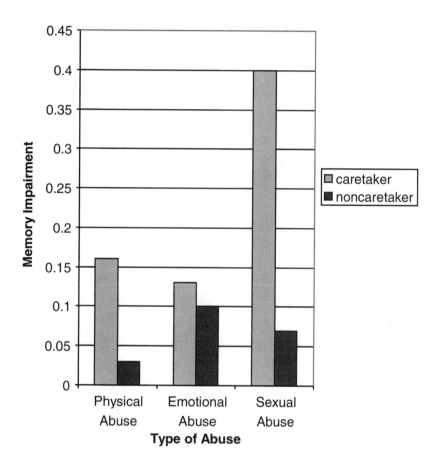

abuse (see Figure 6.2). To control for the possible effects of age at first abuse and duration of abuse on memory impairment, we conducted additional regression analyses. Even when the possible effects of age and duration of abuse were statistically controlled, however, the relationships between caretaker status and sexual and physical abuse were still significant. In other words, physical and sexual abuse perpetrated by caretakers was associated with greater memory impairment than physical and sexual abuse perpetrated by noncaretakers. This difference in memory impairment could not be accounted for by the fact that victimization by caretakers occurred at an earlier age and for a longer duration.

These results are consistent with the predictions made by betrayal trauma theory, which states that *knowledge isolation* (of which impaired memory is one example) is more likely to result from traumas that have a social betrayal component. Another type of knowledge isolation is the dissociation and withdrawal dimension of PTSD. In a recently completed study using a community sample of 75 individuals who self-reported one or more traumatic events, DePrince (2001) found that self-reported betrayal (associated with the trauma) predicted multiple measures of dissociation and PTSD withdrawal, but self-reported fear did not. We plan to conduct further studies concerning betrayal, fear, and knowledge isolation related to experiences of trauma.

Dissociation and Selective Attention: Stroop Studies

Another research direction involves the assessment of basic cognitive mechanisms related to attention for people with varying exposure to childhood trauma and with varying levels of dissociative tendencies. This basic research seeks to understand the repercussions of a dissociative style on specific cognitive tasks. We began by focusing on the basic function of selective attention: the ability to willfully select certain information while inhibiting the selection of other information simultaneously available. Human participants are generally impressive at selective attention, but it is not an all-or-none ability. Even though certain information is selected for focused processing, additional information may nonetheless intrude. We hypothesized that dissociative tendencies would be systematically related to selective attentional mechanisms.

The Stroop paradigm (Stroop, 1935), one of most widely used methodologies for studying selective attention, seemed to us a good starting place for exploring our hypothesis that participants varying in dissociative tendencies would show a difference in basic attentional processing. In the classic Stroop demonstration participants are asked to name the ink color of a list of words or strings of letters printed in different colors. In its simplest form in the experimental condition, the words are color names (e.g., *red* or *green*), and those words are incongruent with the ink colors (thus the word *red* is printed in green ink, and the word *green* is printed in blue ink). In a control condition the words are neutral terms (e.g., *table* or *tree*) or nonword stimuli such as strings of identical letters (e.g., *xxxxx*), and the ink colors are randomly assigned to the different words or strings of letters. Participants attempting to name the ink color take longer when the ink colors are paired with incongruent color words than when the ink colors are paired with neutral words, strings of letters, or congruent color terms. The fact that participants can name the ink colors and inhibit naming the words illustrates the power of selective attention. However, the fact that the meaning of the color words apparently interferes with ink-naming demonstrates the inability to completely exclude information that is not chosen for selection.

Note that our focus here is on the standard, rather than the emotional, Stroop task. The emotional Stroop task, in which participants view words that are emotionally charged for their particular fears (along with control words and control participants), has been widely used to study information processing in a variety of mental disorders. A number of studies with individuals who meet criteria for PTSD have shown biases toward threatening information in the emotional Stroop task (e.g., Foa, Feske, Murdock, Kozak, & McCarthy, 1991; McKenna & Sharma, 1995; McNally, Kaspi, Riemann, & Zeitlin, 1990). Although this literature increases understanding of biases in various forms of psychopathology, these studies do not examine the basic (non-emotional) Stroop effect that is well established in the cognitive literature (MacLeod, 1991). We used the standard Stroop task to better understand differences in basic attentional mechanisms (not dependent on emotional content) that might be important to dissociation and response to trauma.

In our first study on this topic (Freyd, Martorello, Alvarado, Hayes, & Christman, 1998), we found that women and men reporting high levels of dissociative experiences (as measured by the Dissociative Experiences Scale [DES]; Bernstein & Putnam, 1986) displayed a greater level of interference on the basic Stroop color-naming task. High-DES participants took longer to name the ink colors when the lists were conflicting color terms (e.g., naming the color *yellow* when the word *red* was printed in the ink color yellow) than did the low-DES participants. For all other categories but the conflicting color terms, reaction times for high dissociators were equivalent to or slightly faster than the reaction times of the low dissociators, indicating that the increased interference effect was not due to generalized slowing among the high-DES participants.

Although the first study showed a disadvantage for high dissociators in a particular task, we suspected that high dissociators must sometimes have an advantage. We considered under what conditions that might be and hypothesized that conditions of divided attention might advantage high dissociators just as low dissociators are apparently advantaged in a selective attention task. So we designed an experiment in which we looked for an interaction between performance in different attentional contexts as a function of dissociative tendencies.

In this second study (DePrince & Freyd, 1999), we sought to build on previous results (Freyd et al., 1998) by examining whether the relationship between dissociation and performance on the Stroop task would be different in a single-task (selective attention) as opposed to a multitask (divided attention) environment. In the divided attention condition, participants were asked to name the ink colors (as in the standard Stroop task) but at the same time were asked to memorize the words. We predicted an interaction between attentional context and DES score. For the selective attention condition, we expected to replicate the results of Freyd et al. (1998), with high dissociators showing impaired performance on the Stroop task. In contrast, we expected that low dissociators would show impaired performance in the divided attention condition.

We also wanted to investigate the relationship between dissociative tendencies and the emotional valence or "charge" of the words. Because we hypothesized that the function of dissociation is to keep emotionally threatening information from conscious awareness, we wanted to test whether high dissociators had particular difficulties recalling emotionally charged words. Because most people who are high dissociators have a history of traumatic experiences (see Freyd, 1996), the charged words that we used were ones associated with trauma (e.g., *assault, rape*).

In a replication of the results from Freyd et al. (1998), men and women reporting high levels of dissociative experiences (as measured by the DES) showed a greater level of interference on the basic (selective attention) Stroop color-naming task. However, high dissociators showed less interference when they were asked to divide their attention and accomplish two tasks at once. High dissociators also remembered fewer charged words than did low dissociators, a finding suggestive of the adaptive value of dissociation. Furthermore, we found (in line with other studies) that high dissociators reported significantly more trauma in their history.

Cognitive Environments

These results can best be understood by conceptualizing dissociation as a particular type of *cognitive environment*. This term is based in part on an analogy to modern computer software environments. These environments allow users to decide whether they want to have many "windows" and applications open to simultaneously handle a number of ongoing programs and tasks, or whether they prefer to have only a few windows and applications open, thus focusing fairly exclusively on a single task. A similar choice is available more generally as we work, play, and interact with others—we can choose to do many things at once or to focus more specifically on one person or task.

Because dissociation involves a lack of integration of thoughts, experiences, and emotions, it necessarily creates a cognitive environment in which many distinct windows are open at the same time, thus leading to a near-constant state of divided attention. People who habitually dissociate may therefore be most comfortable in environments that favor multitasking and divided control structures. Those who tend not to dissociate may be most comfortable in a more focused single-task environment. From this cognitive–environments perspective, high dissociators may find the selective attention task more challenging than the divided attention task. Thus high dissociators show greater Stroop interference than the low dissociators in the selective attention task as evidence of the difficulty. However, high dissociators may show less Stroop interference in the divided attention task because they are adept at engaging in dual tasks compared with low dissociators.

Much research remains to be completed before we can make statements about the causal link between attention and dissociation. At least one possibility that is consistent with the research to date is that in coping with trauma, individuals learn to multitask as a way of managing and controlling the flow of information. In particular, a cognitive environment based on dissociation and multitasking serves as a means of keeping threatening information (especially knowledge of social betrayal) out of conscious awareness. Such a cognitive environment can have both adaptive and maladaptive consequences, depending on the context and situation.

Clinical Implications

The therapeutic treatment goals and methods that are most appropriate for survivors of childhood abuse have much in common with the treatment goals and methods appropriate for trauma survivors more generally. Indeed, many of the therapeutic goals (e.g., the development of a healthy therapist–client relationship) are fundamental to the therapy process and are thus appropriate for all clients. However, betrayal trauma theory suggests that there are also specific concerns and goals that are either unique to or especially important for clients who were victimized by a caretaker (or whose traumatic victimization was in some other way an instance of a social betrayal).

According to betrayal trauma theory, survivors of childhood abuse by a caretaker have learned to cope with social conflicts they cannot escape by being disconnected internally. While abuse is ongoing, this mental disconnection (and the concomitant memory impairment) may be adaptive. However, disconnection and memory impairment regarding nonabusive relationships are likely to be problematic, as is a more general style of mental disconnection or dissociation. Because these problematic symptoms arose in the context of a close relationship, their treatment will require a focus on social relationships and the cognitive mechanisms that support such relationships.

One of the main treatment goals will therefore be the promotion of internal integration of disjointed and fragmentary sensory memories, as well as a deeper (and more veridical) connection to the external ("objective") world. This is an important goal for abuse victims more generally. However, it is especially important for victims whose abuse comprised a social betrayal, because they are more likely to suffer from disjointed and impaired memory. Note that this treatment goal need not be at odds with the treatment goals and methods for addressing other common symptoms of trauma (e.g., high levels of anxiety, fear, and hyperarousal). It can best be met, for example, within the context of a healthy therapist–client relationship, a relationship that is important for other treatment goals as well.

Another important goal for a therapist working with victims of caretaker childhood abuse is to provide support and assistance as the client works to develop close relationships with important others (e.g., friends, romantic partners, or family members). Again, this goal is not unique to victims of caretaker childhood trauma; close interpersonal relationships are important to everyone. However, victims of caretaker childhood abuse may be especially impaired in the development of such relationships because of the violent breach of trust that they experienced as a child. The development of healthy social relationships will of necessity entail the development of the client's active and appropriate use of trust and reality assessment mechanisms—exactly the mechanisms that are most likely to be damaged or underdeveloped. The clinician should therefore be prepared to encourage and assist the client, as well as to provide "reality checks" as needed and appropriate.

For clients who are survivors of caretaker childhood abuse, even more so than with other types of clients, the potential to heal internal disconnection is almost surely going to be most fully realized in the context of what was so broken in the first place: intimate and trusting relationships. It is thus absolutely crucial that the client be able to trust the therapist and that this trust not be betrayed. Betrayal trauma theory suggests that even small betrayals of trust (e.g., lying about the reason for canceling an appointment) could have large consequences for people whose internal and external disconnection were the direct result of childhood social betrayals.

While disconnection and dissociation can be truly problematic, high dissociators may have certain cognitive "deficits" and "strengths" depending on the task context. Clinicians might help high dissociators find appropriate contexts for their particular skills. When high dissociators make chaos in their lives, clinicians may be more helpful if they understand the cognitive and adaptive forces behind this chaos. Clinicians should remain alert to the possibility that, for some clients, certain dissociative responses may continue to have current adaptive value. They may also want to talk to their dissociative clients about the benefits and costs of dissociation (e.g., not being present during sex may help with anxiety but may be costly in terms of control over HIV risk).

Our results also suggest that the assessment of trauma history may be highly relevant to the diagnosis and treatment of other disorders. In particular, because we have shown that basic processes of attention are affected by dissociative tendencies, we recommend that clinicians who are working with clients with any kind of attention-based disorder (e.g., ADHD) always explore their clients' trauma history. The possible links between trauma and attention-based disorders like ADHD are speculative at this point, but we suspect that both of the following are likely to be true. First, it is possible that a substantial number of children diagnosed or medicated for purported ADHD have been misdiagnosed and are in fact showing dissociative and other posttraumatic reactions to childhood abuse or other traumatic experiences. Because of the misdiagnosis, these children are likely to be poorly understood by teachers and physicians. Second, children with underlying ADHD may have their symptoms significantly complicated by posttraumatic reactions, and the role that trauma plays in exacerbating or affecting the ADHD symptoms may be poorly understood by teachers and physicians.

If trauma is playing a role in children diagnosed with ADHD, it will be important to recognize and respond to the trauma, yet past research on ADHD in children has almost never included even an assessment of trauma history. In fact, in some cases (as with the National Institutes of Health Multimodal Treatment study for ADHD; Hinshaw et al., 1997), the recruitment procedures specifically excluded children who were experiencing abuse or neglect. As a result of this lack of research on ADHD in abused children, the authors of the recently published American Academy of Pediatrics Guidelines for diagnosing and treating ADHD (American Academy of Pediatrics, 2000) specifically state that the guidelines are not applicable to abused and neglected children.

Recent work in the Freyd laboratory was designed in part to fill this gap in the ADHD literature. Becker (2002) examined the relationship between trauma and abuse history, PTSD, and ADHD in community samples of preschool- and school-age (ages 8–11) children. She found reliable correlations between ADHD and PTSD symptoms for both groups of children. In addition, for the school-age children, boys and girls with a history of abuse had higher ADHD scores. These results underscore the need to screen all children suspected of an attention-based disorder for trauma and trauma symptoms.

DAMAGED COGNITIVE MECHANISMS: POSSIBLE MEDIATORS BETWEEN ABUSE EXPERIENCES AND SEXUALLY RISKY BEHAVIOR

In Figure 6.3 we present a partial list of cognitive mechanisms that may lead to specific HIV-relevant outcomes (including specific high-risk sexual behaviors). Because so little research on cognitive mediators has been conducted, many of the links in this figure are only speculative at this point. However, all of the hypothesized links are theoretically and conceptually plausible. We briefly discuss three hypothesized cognitive mechanisms and then focus in greater detail on the remaining two: a general dissociative style and consensual sex decision mechanisms (CSDMs)

Self-Esteem

One set of paths that already enjoys a fair amount of empirical support is the set of paths from abuse to lowered self-esteem and from self-esteem to behavioral outcomes. CSA is correlated with lowered self-esteem as an adult (Banyard, 1999; Romans, Martin, & Mullen, 1996). Higher levels of self-

Figure 6.3. Cognitive mechanisms that might mediate the path between childhood abuse experiences and risky sexual behavior. CSDMs = consensual sex decision mechanisms.

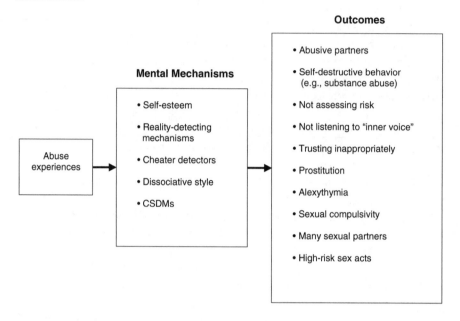

Mental Mechanisms

- Self-esteem
- Reality-detecting mechanisms
- Cheater detectors
- Dissociative style
- CSDMs

Abuse experiences

Outcomes

- Abusive partners
- Self-destructive behavior (e.g., substance abuse)
- Not assessing risk
- Not listening to "inner voice"
- Trusting inappropriately
- Prostitution
- Alexythymia
- Sexual compulsivity
- Many sexual partners
- High-risk sex acts

esteem are associated with less risky behavior under some circumstances, for example, between female sex workers and their clients (Fritz, 1998), among college students engaging in relatively unconventional sexual behavior (Hollar & Snizek, 1996), and among young women in casual sexual relationships (Seal, Minichiello, & Omodei, 1997). On the other hand, higher levels of self-esteem can also be associated with more risky behavior, for example, between female sex workers and their romantic partners (Fritz, 1998), among college students engaging in more conventional sexual behaviors (Hollar & Snizek, 1996), and among young women in more committed sexual relationships (Seal et al., 1997).

Reality-Detecting Mechanisms

Other paths have not been tested but make conceptual sense. For example, cognitive mechanisms that aid in the general assessment of reality are likely to be damaged by any long-term experience of CSA. This is because it is commonplace for perpetrators to lie and distort reality. While the child is being abused and is frightened and in pain, he or she is told "You like this." Afterward, the message may be "I did that because I love you" or "All daddies do that with their daughters." If the child tries to disclose the abuse, the response might be "You're lying" or "You must have imagined that" or "He would never do that; he loves you." The normal processes whereby a child learns to distinguish reality from fantasy are in danger of being sidetracked by these inaccurate (yet authoritatively delivered) statements. The end result may be an adult whose ability to assess reality is hampered. Valid intuitions may be brushed aside. For example, the fear that a potential sexual partner might be abusive is ignored. Risk may be assessed improperly (e.g., the high probability that an injecting partner is HIV-positive is not considered).

Cheater Detectors

Another set of cognitive mechanisms that is likely to be damaged (or not fully developed) in sexual abuse survivors is the set of particular cognitive mechanisms that are used to assess the trustworthiness of other people. Cosmides and Tooby (1992) discussed these *cheater detector* mechanisms and argued for the evolutionary adaptiveness of being able to recognize when other people are trying to take advantage of us. As described in the previous section, Freyd (1996) has argued that these mechanisms are exactly the mechanisms that need to be suppressed when a child is being abused by his or her caretaker. The automatic response to being cheated is either anger and confrontational behavior or to "leave the field" and avoid further contact with the cheater. Neither of these options is open to the dependent child, though, because of the need to maintain an attachment with the caregiver. One solution to the dilemma is to turn off the cheater-detector mechanisms. Should these mechanisms remain in a nonfunctioning state in adulthood, however, a host of negative outcomes are likely to ensue. These include remaining with an abusive partner, being unable to avoid exploitation (e.g., as a prostitute), and being at higher risk for date rape and sexual assault (because of the difficulty of accurately perceiving that someone is untrustworthy).

Dissociation, Divided Attention, and Sex

Victimization can lead to dissociation (DiTomasso & Routh, 1993; Putnam & Trickett, 1997; Sanders & Giolas, 1991). Like most behaviors, sexual behaviors can be performed in a highly dissociated state. In other words, someone can engage in sexual activity without attending to her or his own feelings of fear, pleasure, or safety. In addition to this inability to attend to aspects of one's own mental and emotional state, people with dissociative tendencies may also be unaware of external features of the event; for example, whether a condom is being used or even (in extreme cases) who they are with. Such dissociation would make it difficult for someone to make *any* decisions about sex, let alone good ones, because they are not mentally present.

Dissociation may also appear (although probably to a lesser degree) even when simply thinking or talking about sex, and even with a neutral third party. Thus, when safer sex practices or facts about sexually transmitted diseases (STDs) or AIDS are taught or even just discussed (e.g., in health classes, clinic settings, community agencies, or intervention programs), people who have been sexually victimized may have difficulty processing and encoding that information. Our data on lower memory scores for high-DES participants support this speculation. (Recall that the words high-DES participants had trouble remembering were those related to sex and to trauma, suggesting that they were "tuning out" when those words were presented.) This suggests that many abuse victims who are exposed to HIV/STD and pregnancy-prevention messages and who are taught risk prevention skills (e.g., condom use and negotiation) may not be fully present to process and store that information; thus, they will have difficulty using the information.

One obvious intervention for people with dissociative tendencies is to practice being present in sex—both when engaging in sexual activities and when merely talking about them. The former might best be accomplished with a supportive partner—someone who can gently remind the CSA survivor where she is and what is happening, who will ask about her emotional state. This could also be done alone, though; for example, by imagining consensual sex and then focusing on the feelings that come up. In either case, an intervention that starts small and builds gradually is advisable.

Note that helping someone to learn not to dissociate can also be done in nonerotic settings. For example, if any mention of sex causes someone to mentally disappear, then it would be useful to talk one-on-one with a counselor who knows about this tendency toward dissociation. Together, therapist and client could work toward having longer and longer discussions in which the client was mentally present.

Damaged Consensual Sex Decision Mechanisms

Freyd (1996) has proposed that under healthy conditions people develop consensual sex decision mechanisms, or CSDMs. Damage to one's sexual being, however, may cause a breakdown of the ability to freely consent to sexual activities with another person. Although there are probably many mental mechanisms involved in determining whether sex is consensual or not, for simplicity we label all of them as CSDMs.

CSDMs are the set of mental functions that, in the absence of external force, allow a person to make a choice about whether to engage in a sexual behavior (or continue to engage in it, once it has begun). Consensual sex is possible only when two necessary conditions are met, neither of which alone is sufficient: The situation must be free from all external force, even subtle force, and each participant must have a functioning set of CSDMs.

Damaged CSDMs may be thought of as inaccurate beliefs, unhealthy (unhelpful) cognitions about the self, a lack of access to one's internal affective state, and the presence of risk-seeking sexual decision rules. We are particularly interested in studying sexual decision rules that may be used by those who have been sexually victimized, and we are engaged in research to clarify the content and structure of these rules as well as their correlates. Currently, we conceptualize these rules as a collection of "if-then" statements, as in a computer programming language. *If* certain conditions are met, *then* certain outcomes will result. The *if* conditions can be situational (e.g., *if* a sexual partner says "I love you" . . .), affective (e.g., *if* I feel angry . . .), or cognitive (e.g., *if* I believe that premarital sex is immoral . . .). The *then* outcomes can also be affective or cognitive, or they can be behavioral (e.g., . . . *then* ask partner to use a condom). The process whereby these rules are executed is straightforward—if the conditions in the "if" portion of the decision rule are met, then the behaviors, affects, or cognitions in the "then" portion of the rule are enacted. An example of a simple decision rule might be:

if My sexual partner smiles at me . . . [situational input]

then Smile back. [behavior]

To give a better sense of how damaged or undeveloped CSDMs might lead to sexually risky behavior, we discuss some hypothetical examples. In particular, we consider three distinct scenarios: (a) the person in question does not want to be having sex at all (at least not with this particular partner), (b) the person wants to be doing something sexual but wants one or more things to be different (e.g., wants to be using a condom, or not having intercourse), and (c) the sexual activity is proceeding exactly as the person wants (even though it involves risky behavior).

Scenario 1: No Desire for Sexual Contact

Consider the case of a person who does not want to be sexual (at this moment or with this person), yet is doing so anyway. We can imagine a number of potentially helpful decision rules that are apparently damaged, not present, or not active. These include such rules as: "*If* I don't like what is happening sexually, *then* stop" or "*If* I don't feel safe, *then* don't continue with sex" or "*If* I don't trust my sexual partner, *then* don't engage in sexual behavior with him or her." One possibility is that these rules are simply not present. There is no cognitive connection between level of trust and choice of behavior, between assessment of affective state and decisions to continue or stop. Another possibility is that the rules are present in some form, but one or both of the two clauses (the *if* or the *then* clause) are damaged or cannot be accessed or executed. For example, the evaluation that is an inherent part of the *if* clause might not occur—I might not attempt to assess the trustworthiness of my partner or I might be unable (perhaps due to alexythymia) to evaluate my own affective state. In contrast, the evaluation portion of the rule may be operating in a satisfactory way, but the *then* clause is suboptimal. For example, a rule that said "*If* I don't like what is happening sexually, *then* dissociate" would have been a helpful and adaptive rule for a dependent child, but is likely to be unhelpful and dangerous for an adult, in that it would prevent him or her from ending an encounter that felt assaultive.

It is not difficult to imagine how decision rules such as the above, rules that would appear naturally during normal sexual development, might be damaged as a result of CSA. When a child is abused, he or she does not have the power to stop the sex act. The rules outlined above cannot be acted on, and thus cannot be incorporated as part of one's set of CSDMs. Instead, alternative rules (e.g., *if* it feels bad, *then* dissociate) are likely to develop.

Scenario 2: Desire for a Different Type of Sexual Contact

Now consider a second type of situation, one in which the person does want to be sexual, but there is something about the situation that he or she would like to change. For example, he might prefer to engage in mutual masturbation rather than anal sex, or she might want to have intercourse but with a condom rather than without one.

Here are some possibilities for beliefs, cognitions, and decision rules that might not be present: (a) My health is important; (b) I am important; (c) I deserve to be treated with respect; (d) I deserve to be listened to when I talk about what I want; (e) This person doesn't seem to care about me very much, but other people do; (f) *If* someone is treating me badly, *then* speak up about it; and (g) *If* someone continues to treat me badly even after I've asked them to stop, *then* stop spending time with them.

Again, it is not hard to imagine these kind of decision rules and cognitions being damaged or eliminated by an abuser and by the process of abuse. Because victimized children are not listened to and are not treated with respect, they internalize the idea that they are not deserving of respect. This is especially likely to happen when verbal abuse occurs (as it commonly does) and the child is explicitly told that he or she is unimportant, bad, and evil, that no one else cares about her, that he deserves to die. It is also easy to imagine the ways in which these types of cognitive constructs could lead to sexually risky behavior. If I believe that my health is unimportant, I am unlikely to take steps to protect it (e.g., I am less likely to screen partners carefully or to use condoms or other latex barriers on a regular basis). If I believe that I am not deserving of respect, it will be more difficult to break out of an abusive relationship, or to escape from an exploitative experience of prostitution.

Scenario 3: Sexual Contact Is Desired (Albeit Risky)

In this third scenario the sexual situation, while risky, is proceeding just as desired. One of the most important mental mechanisms contributing to such an experience might be dissociative style. If a general "tuning out" occurred whenever sex was discussed, the person might be woefully underinformed about AIDS and other STDs and may not understand the risk involved in the sexual behaviors he or she is engaged in. A second possibility is that the person might have some understanding of the risk involved but be using denial and rationalization to minimize the dissonance between his or her knowledge and behavior. The person may think, "just this once without a condom won't hurt" or "you can't get AIDS from heterosexual intercourse" or "the risk is really low" or "I only date 'nice' boys who don't have STDs" or "my boyfriend doesn't sleep with other women (or doesn't inject drugs)" or any number of other (inaccurate) cognitions. It makes sense that victims of sexual abuse would be especially likely to rely on denial as a defense mechanism. Denial (by the perpetrator and others) is a pervasive part of the experience of being abused, so denial is modeled as normative. Also, dissociation and repression are a form of denial, so to the extent that those defenses were used as coping strategies by the child, it makes sense that they would also be used by the adult.

A third possibility is that there might be an actual attraction to risk. Not all risk-seeking people are unconsciously suicidal, of course, but some are. Some percentage of people who were sexually victimized as children are likely to be depressed or even suicidal. More relevant for the focus on CSDMs are associations formed during victimization between sexual pleasure and risky behaviors. The victimization may contribute to an eroticization of risk and danger, or to an erotic association with particular context variables (e.g., an aggressive partner) that correlate with risk. This is in contrast to seeking risk merely for its own sake (perhaps as part of a self-destructive tendency), which could also be present in some adult survivors.

Conscious and Unconscious Consensual Sex Decision Mechanisms

We believe that some CSDMs are open to a person's conscious awareness (explicit cognitive mechanisms and decision rules) but that others might not be (implicit mechanisms and rules). Other researchers have investigated some explicit decision rules related to initiation and refusal of condom use (Morokoff et al., 1997). We are currently conducting research aimed at examining both implicit and explicit CSDMs and their relationship to child trauma and adult sexually risky behavior.

SUGGESTIONS FOR FURTHER RESEARCH

We have discussed a number of cognitive mechanisms that may be important mediators of the relationship between CSA and sexually risky behavior. To conclude this chapter, we describe a number of important research questions that remain and highlight some of our ongoing studies that attempt to address some of these questions.

Figure 6.3 summarizes many of the mediational pathways that we believe are the most deserving of immediate study, but it does so in a general way. That is, rather than drawing causal pathways from specific mental mechanisms to specific outcomes, we have left the picture more abstract. We do not believe, however, that every type of cognitive adaptation to abuse is equally likely to lead to every type of high-risk outcome. One research priority, then, is to attempt to link specific mental mediational mechanisms to specific behavioral outcomes.

To do that, one must describe and quantify the mental mechanisms in enough detail that they can be adequately assessed. Dissociative style and self-esteem can both be reliably measured using existing scales. Reality-detecting mechanisms, cheater detectors, and CSDMs, however, do not at this point have accepted and reliable methods of assessment. One of the major goals of our immediate research program is to find methods to assess both the conscious and unconscious components of these mental mechanisms. In particular, we are currently using several techniques from cognitive psychology to measure implicit CSDMs related to sexual initiation and refusal.

The paths from abuse experiences to cognitive mechanisms also need to be specified with greater precision. There are many dimensions to a trauma, not all of which would be expected to contribute equally to each type of cognitive adaptation. For example, our work to date suggests that a dissociative style may be especially adaptive when abuse is perpetrated by a caretaker. We believe that much more detailed and specific questions about all aspects of a traumatic experience must be asked, if we are to fully understand the resulting cognitive adaptations that can result in adult high-risk behavior.

Finally, we believe that it may be helpful to consider this mediational viewpoint when designing interventions. That is, if we can work directly on improving consensual sex decision making and decreasing dissociation about and during sex, we believe that a reduction in risky behaviors will result.

REFERENCES

Allers, C. T., Benjack, K. J., White, J., & Rousey, J. T. (1993). HIV vulnerability and the adult survivor of childhood sexual abuse. *Child Abuse and Neglect, 17,* 291–298.

American Academy of Pediatrics. (2000). Clinical practice guideline: Diagnosis and evaluation of the child with attention-deficit/hyperactivity disorder. *Pediatrics, 105,* 1158–1170.

American Psychiatric Association. (1994). *Diagnostic and statistical manual of mental disorders* (4th ed.). Washington, DC: Author.

Banyard, V. L. (1999). Childhood maltreatment and the mental health of low-income women. *American Journal of Orthopsychiatry, 69,* 161–171.

Becker, K. A. (2002). *Attention and traumatic stress in children.* Unpublished doctoral dissertation, University of Oregon, Eugene, OR.

Bernstein, E. M., & Putnam, F. W. (1986). Development, reliability, and validity of a dissociation scale. *Journal of Nervous and Mental Disease, 174,* 727–735.

Browne, A., & Finkelhor, D. (1986). Impact of child sexual abuse: A review of the research. *Psychological Bulletin, 99*, 66–77.

Cameron, C. (1993, April). *Recovering memories of childhood sexual abuse: A longitudinal report*. Paper presented at the meeting of the Western Psychological Association, Phoenix, AZ.

Chu, J., & Dill, D. (1990). Dissociative symptoms in relation to childhood physical and sexual abuse. *American Journal of Psychiatry, 147*, 887–892.

Cosmides, L., & Tooby, J. (1992). Cognitive adaptations for social exchange. In J. H. Barkow, L. Cosmides, & J. Tooby (Eds.), *The adapted mind: Evolutionary psychology and the generation of culture* (pp. 163–228). New York: Oxford University Press.

DePrince, A. P. (2001). *Trauma and posttraumatic symptoms: An examination of fear and betrayal*. Unpublished doctoral dissertation, University of Oregon, Eugene, OR.

DePrince, A. P., & Freyd, J. J. (1999). Dissociative tendencies, attention, and memory. *Psychological Science, 10*, 449–452.

DiTomasso, M. J., & Routh, D. K. (1993). Recall of abuse in childhood and three measures of dissociation. *Child Abuse and Neglect, 17*, 477–485.

Feldman-Summers, S., & Pope, K. S. (1994). The experience of "forgetting" childhood abuse: A national survey of psychologists. *Journal of Consulting and Clinical Psychology, 62*, 636–639.

Fergusson, D. M., Horwood, L. J., & Lynskey, M. T. (1997). Childhood sexual abuse, adolescent sexual behaviors and sexual revictimization. *Child Abuse and Neglect, 21*, 789–803.

Foa, E. B., Feske, U., Murdock, T. B., Kozak, M. J., & McCarthy, P. (1991). Processing of threat-related information in rape victims. *Journal of Abnormal Psychology, 100*, 156–162.

Freud, S. (1913). *The interpretation of dreams* (3rd ed.) (J. Riviera, Trans.). London: Allen & Unwin.

Freyd, J. J. (1994). Betrayal-trauma: Traumatic amnesia as an adaptive response to childhood abuse. *Ethics and Behaviour, 4*, 307–329.

Freyd, J. J. (1996). *Betrayal trauma: The logic of forgetting childhood abuse*. Cambridge, MA: Harvard University Press.

Freyd, J. J. (2002). Memory and dimensions of trauma: Terror may be "all-too-well remembered" and betrayal buried. In J. R. Conte (Ed.), *Critical issues in child sexual abuse: Historical, legal, and psychological perspectives* (pp. 139–173). Thousand Oaks, CA: Sage.

Freyd, J. J., DePrince, A. P., & Zurbriggen, E. L. (2001). Self-reported memory for abuse depends upon victim–perpetrator relationship. *Journal of Trauma and Dissociation, 2*(3), 5–17.

Freyd, J. J., Martorello, S. R., Alvarado, J. S., Hayes, A. E., & Christman, J. C. (1998). Cognitive environments and dissociative tendencies: Performance on the standard Stroop task for high versus low dissociators. *Applied Cognitive Psychology, 12*, S91–S103.

Fritz, R. B. (1998). AIDS knowledge, self-esteem, perceived AIDS risk, and condom use among female commercial sex workers. *Journal of Applied Social Psychology*, 28, 888–911.

Glass, J. M., Schumacher, E. H., Lauber, E. J., Zurbriggen, E. L., Gmeindl, L., Kieras, D. E., & Meyer, D. E. (2000). Aging and the psychological refractory period: Task-coordination strategies in young and old adults. *Psychology and Aging*, 15, 571–595.

Goleman, D. (1985). *Vital lies, simple truths: The psychology of self-deception*. New York: Simon & Schuster.

Green, L. (1992). *Ordinary wonders: Living recovery from sexual abuse*. Toronto, Ontario, Canada: Women's Press.

Greenson, R. R. (1967). *The technique and practice of psychoanalysis* (Vol. 1). New York: International Universities Press.

Hinshaw, S. P., March, J. S., Abikoff, H., Arnold, L. E., Cantwell, D. P., Conners, C. K., et al. (1997). Comprehensive assessment of childhood attention-deficit hyperactivity disorder in the context of a multisite, multimodal clinical trial. *Journal of Attention Disorders*, 1, 217–234.

Hollar, D. S., & Snizek, W. E. (1996). The influences of knowledge of HIV/AIDS and self-esteem on the sexual practices of college students. *Social Behavior and Personality*, 24, 75–86.

Janet, P. (1889). *L'Automatisme psychologique* [Psychological Automatism]. Paris: Felix Alcan.

Knutson, J. F. (1995). Psychological characteristics of maltreated children: Putative risk factors and consequences. *Annual Review of Psychology*, 46, 401–431.

Lisak, D., Hopper, J., & Song, P. (1996). Factors in the cycle of violence: Gender rigidity and emotional constriction. *Journal of Traumatic Stress*, 9, 721–743.

Low, G., Jones, D., MacLeod, A., Power, M., & Duggan, C. (2000). Childhood trauma, dissociation, and self-harming behaviour: A pilot study. *British Journal of Medical Psychology*, 73(Pt. 2), 269–278.

MacLeod, C. M. (1991). Half a century of research on the Stroop effect: An integrative review. *Psychological Bulletin*, 109, 163–203.

McKenna, F. P., & Sharma, D. (1995). Intrusive cognitions: An investigation of the emotional Stroop task. *Journal of Experimental Psychology: Learning, Memory, and Cognition*, 21, 1595–1607.

McNally, R. J., Kaspi, S. P., Riemann, B. C., & Zeitlin, S. B. (1990). Selective processing of threat cues in posttraumatic stress disorder. *Journal of Abnormal Psychology*, 99, 398–402.

Meyer, D. E., Kieras, D. E., Lauber, E., Schumacher, E. H., Glass, J., Zurbriggen, E., et al. (1995). Adaptive executive control: Flexible multiple-task performance without pervasive immutable response-selection bottlenecks. *Acta Psychologica*, 90, 163–190.

Miller, D. A. F., McCluskey-Fawcett, K., & Irving, L. M. (1993). The relationship between childhood sexual abuse and subsequent onset of bulimia nervosa. *Child Abuse and Neglect*, 17, 305–314.

Morokoff, P. J., Quina, K., Harlow, L. L., Whitmire, L., Grimley, D. M., Gibson, P. R., & Burkholder, G. J. (1997). Sexual Assertiveness Scale (SAS) for women: Development and validation. *Journal of Personality and Social Psychology, 73*, 790–804.

Putnam, F. W., & Trickett, P. K. (1997). Psychobiological effects of sexual abuse: A longitudinal study. In R. Yehuda (Ed.), *Psychobiology of posttraumatic stress disorder* (pp. 150–159). New York: New York Academy of Sciences.

Romans, S. E., Martin, J., & Mullen, P. (1996). Women's self-esteem: A community study of women who report and do not report childhood sexual abuse. *British Journal of Psychiatry, 169,* 696–704.

Sanders, B., & Giolas, M. H. (1991). Dissociation and childhood trauma in psychologically disturbed adolescents. *American Journal of Psychiatry, 148,* 50–54.

Schumacher, E. H., Lauber, E. J., Glass, J. M., Zurbriggen, E. L., Gmeindl, L., Kieras, D. E., & Meyer, D. E. (1999). Concurrent response-selection processes in dual-task performance: Evidence for adaptive executive control of task scheduling. *Journal of Experimental Psychology: Human Perception and Performance, 25,* 791–814.

Seal, A., Minichiello, V., & Omodei, M. (1997). Young women's sexual risk taking behaviour: Re-visiting the influences of sexual self-efficacy and sexual self-esteem. *International Journal of STD and AIDS, 8,* 159–165.

Stroop, J. R. (1935). Studies of interference in serial verbal reactions. *Journal of Experimental Psychology, 18,* 643–662.

Thompson, N. J., Potter, J. S., Sanderson, C. A., & Maibach, E. W. (1997). The relationship of sexual abuse and HIV risk behaviors among heterosexual adult female STD patients. *Child Abuse and Neglect, 21,* 149–156.

Urquiza, A. J., & Capra, M. (1990). The impact of sexual abuse: Initial and long-term effects. In M. Hunter (Ed.), *The sexually abused male: Vol. 1. Prevalence, impact, and treatment* (pp. 105–135). Lexington, MA: Lexington Books.

van der Kolk, B. A., Perry, J. C., & Herman, J. L. (1991). Childhood origins of self-destructive behavior. *American Journal of Psychiatry, 148,* 1665–1671.

Walser, R. D., & Kern, J. M. (1996). Relationships among childhood sexual abuse, sex guilt, and sexual behavior in adult clinical samples. *Journal of Sex Research, 33,* 321–326.

Williams, L. M. (1994). Recall of childhood trauma: A prospective study of women's memories of child sexual abuse. *Journal of Consulting and Clinical Psychology, 62,* 1167–1176.

Williams, L. M. (1995). Recovered memories of abuse in women with documented child sexual victimization histories. *Journal of Traumatic Stress, 8,* 649–674.

Zurbriggen, E. L. (2000). Social motives and cognitive power/sex associations: Predictors of aggressive sexual behavior. *Journal of Personality and Social Psychology, 78,* 559–581.

7

TOWARD A SOCIAL-NARRATIVE MODEL OF REVICTIMIZATION

STEVEN JAY LYNN, JUDITH PINTAR, RACHAEL FITE,
KAREN ECKLUND, AND JANE STAFFORD

Women who were sexually abused as children suffer an increased risk of being repeatedly victimized through their adult lives (e.g., see Chu, 1992; Kluft, 1990a, 1990b; van der Kolk, 1989). In the majority of studies investigating risk factors in adult sexual victimization, the most highly correlated variable is previous sexual victimization (Ellis, Atkeson, & Calhoun, 1982; Gidycz, Coble, Latham, & Layman, 1993; Hanson & Gidycz, 1993; Koss & Dinero, 1989; Wyatt, Guthrie, & Notgrass, 1992). Additionally, previous victimization figures prominently as a predictor of current and future likelihood of sexual assault (Koss & Dinero, 1989; Sandberg, Matorin, & Lynn, 1999).

Clearly, revictimization—that is, repeated sexual victimization—is a social problem that affects a particularly vulnerable group of women in society. To protect those at risk, it is necessary to understand the antecedents and mechanisms of revictimization. In this chapter we survey the most prominent theoretical approaches to this puzzling phenomenon, which we categorize into three major explanatory themes, following Sandberg, Lynn, and Green (1994): (a) the search for mastery and meaning, (b) dysfunctional

159

learning, and (c) cognitive defenses. Although each approach to understanding revictimization offers insight into the reasons why an abused woman might be at risk for future victimization, none has proven conclusive enough to be translated into widely accepted clinical techniques for intervention and prevention. We argue here that what is missing from all three approaches is a full acknowledgment of the intrinsically social nature of abuse, and we suggest that the key to revictimization may lie in the nature of the social contexts in which abuse survivors lived as children, and continue to live as adults. We take a first step toward articulating a social-narrative model of revictimization, suggest avenues for empirical verification, and conclude with a consideration of how such a social view might be integrated into clinical interventions.

REPETITION, COMPULSION, AND THE SEARCH FOR MASTERY AND MEANING

A prominent theory of revictimization (Chu, 1992; van der Kolk, 1989) is that an initial sexual assault constitutes a highly stressful circumstance that the individual is compelled to repeat, in whole or in part, to achieve a sense of mastery, reduce attendant anxiety, and find meaning related to the initial experience of victimization (Sandberg et al., 1994). Chu (1992) provided an apt example of a prostitute who was victimized as a child who stated: "When I do it, I'm in control. I can control them (men) through sex" (p. 261). As Sandberg et al. (1994) noted, Freud (1920/1954) coined the term *repetition compulsion* in "Beyond the Pleasure Principle" in his description of a case that was not specifically related to sexual victimization. Freud related his observations of his 18-month-old grandson, Ernst, who had experienced repeated separations from his (Ernst's) mother. The child had a wooden reel with a piece of string wound around it, which he would throw over the side of his cot time and again, making the reel disappear from view. Immediately after throwing the reel, Ernst would draw it back and cheerfully greet its reappearance. Freud linked the game to the child's recurrent separations from his mother. In essence, the child replicated the stressful loss experience, but in a manner that allowed him to master or control the outcome, thereby providing a satisfactory resolution to the experience of loss.

According to Freud, until the person is capable of "working through" the original trauma by remembering, reexperiencing, and mastering it, repressed elements will continue to compel the person to repeat the experience, despite the harm it may cause. If the tendency to repeat experiences to gain mastery over them—the repetition compulsion—could be demonstrated, it would provide an account for why some women are sexually revictimized at such astonishing rates (Sandberg et al., 1994).

Freud's description of the repetition compulsion perhaps implies a degree of "blaming the sexual assault victim" and leaves the relevance to the male perpetrator of sexual violence open to question. Clearly, there is no reason to believe that sexual abuse victims want to be victimized. Additionally, there is little in the way of convincing evidence to support Freud's contention that the repression of traumatic events is a robust phenomenon, and that repressed, as opposed to unexamined or incompletely processed, traumatic experiences account for a tendency to repeat or master traumatic experiences.

Horowitz (1975) restated Freud's ideas in terms of "cognitive operations" (p. 146) wherein repetition is conceptualized as a normal response to stress. Intrusive thoughts and memories—the repetitive element of this stress response—continue to be processed indefinitely until they are fully assimilated and accommodated into relevant cognitive schema and anxiety is reduced. Repetition can be conceptualized as a way of achieving extinction of anxiety-related responses related to the trauma, which can be expressed as behavioral reenactments of the event (Horowitz, 1975). Foa and her colleagues (Foa & Kozak, 1991) have argued that repeated reliving of traumatic memories is necessary for successful processing of traumatic events and recovery. Not surprisingly, a number of workers in the field (Chu, 1992; Gelinas, 1983; van der Kolk, 1989) have virtually equated sexual revictimization to behavioral reenactment.

Our discussion implies that activities that place a woman at risk for revictimization, and that have a repetitive and even compulsive quality, recur until effective extinction and mastery of trauma-related anxiety occurs. Romantic or sexual situations provide an important context for extinction and mastery. However, the rub is that the more sexual partners a woman has, the greater are her chances of encountering a perpetrator of sexual assault. Studies have shown that child sexual victimization is related to the number of reported consensual partners in adulthood (Maker, Kemmelmeier, & Peterson, 2001; Mandoki & Burkhart, 1989), which is a strong predictor of sexual victimization in adulthood (Koss & Dinero, 1989; Mandoki & Burkhart, 1989).

Another way that extinction can occur is by exposure to "risky" situations that were associated with the initial victimization (Sandberg et al., 1994). Unfortunately, women may be unaware of the fact that certain activities increase the risk of revictimization: alcohol consumption (Koss & Dinero, 1989; Miller & Marshall, 1987; Muehlenhard & Linton, 1987), the man's initiation of the date and paying of all expenses on a date (Muehlenhard & Linton, 1987), dating at a secluded location (Muehlenhard & Linton, 1987), and poor communication about sex (Byers, Giles, & Price, 1987; Muehlenhard & Linton, 1987).

The seemingly compulsive nature of behaviors associated with sexual revictimization has also been discussed by object-relations theorists who underline the importance of early interpersonal relationships and their impact on mental representations of the self and others (e.g., Fairbairn, 1954; Masterson & Klein, 1989). Alexander (1993) has argued that compulsive sexuality can arise in the context of certain personality disorders related to attachment styles that develop early in life. Sexual abuse can lead not only to a negative self-concept but also to unhealthy or insecure attachments in interpersonal relationships. These negative developmental influences set the stage for avoidant, dependent, self-defeating, and borderline personality disorders, which are thought to increase the risk of sexual assault and revictimization.

Alexander (1993) found that only 14% of female incest victims' self-descriptions reflected a secure attachment style (Alexander, 1993), in comparison with a rate of 55% based on reports of unselected college students (Bartholemew & Horowitz, 1991). However, 58% of the incest victims' self-descriptions were categorized as fearful, a style related to avoidant personality. According to Alexander, an avoidant personality style increases sexual assault risk insofar as women who are avoidant may compulsively engage in sexual relations with men on a short-term basis to avoid anxiety associated with long-term emotionally committed relationships. Compulsive sexual activity, in turn, increases the risk of encountering a man who will perpetrate sexual assault.

Object-relations theorists have linked compulsive sexuality and an increased risk of sexual abuse to *introjection*, whereby children come to view themselves in much the same way as they are treated by important people in their lives. Because of the threat to security associated with adopting a negative view of parents, whom children depend on for survival, children are prone to blame themselves for the maltreatment they experience, or they attempt to repress, suppress, or dissociate memories related to the maltreatment (see Freyd, 1996). To do otherwise, and fail to preserve the "all good" image of the needed objects (parents), would be tantamount to feeling unprotected in a threat-filled world (Sandberg et al., 1994). Because of their negative mental self-representations and the dependent or self-defeating personality style such children develop over time (Alexander, 1993), they are predisposed to tolerate, if not elicit, abusive interchanges with others (see Gelinas, 1983). In this way, they reenact the perpetrator–victim dynamic.

Psychodynamic theorists have also underscored the importance of guilt and unresolved conflicts as integral to revictimization. Sloane and Karpinski (1942) argued that unresolved conflict surrounding incestuous experiences elicits guilt feelings that lead abuse survivors to engage in compulsive sexual relations with men that serve to alleviate feelings of guilt. Passivity, fueled by conflicts regarding expressing hostile or angry feelings related to sexual abuse, may actually increase the likelihood the victim will become involved in abusive relationships in the future (Walker, 1981).

It is questionable whether mere repetition, or repeated occurrence, can be equated with truly compulsive activity associated with psychopathology such as obsessive–compulsive disorder. In the latter case, the tendency to repeat a given behavior is perpetuated by anxiety associated with the failure to perform the behavior. It is clear that research in this area suffers from a lack of operationalization of terms such as *compulsive, drive for mastery, introjection,* and *guilt,* as well as from a lack of understanding of the role of anxiety in seemingly repetitive behaviors (Sandberg et al., 1994). Additionally, little is known about (a) the extent to which hypothesized "drives for mastery," for example, are consciously articulated, and (b) the relationship among personality characteristics of at-risk women, their self-perceptions and relationship choices, and their participation in risky activities such as alcohol and drug consumption. In conclusion, much work needs to be done to fulfill the rich heuristic potential of theories related to the compulsive nature of revictimization.

DYSFUNCTIONAL LEARNING

Dysfunctional learning refers to maladaptive attitudes and beliefs about the self, others, and the world in general (Sandberg et al., 1994). Dysfunctional learning occurs in the context of intimate interpersonal relationships, so it is not surprising that problems in relational as well as cognitive domains of functioning are associated with revictimization (Briere, 1992; Chu, 1992; Gelinas, 1983; McCann, Sakheim, & Abrahamson, 1988; van der Kolk, 1989). Finkelhor and Browne (1985) identified four primary dynamics as relevant to dysfunctional learning and pertinent to psychological injury inflicted by abuse: traumatic sexualization, betrayal, powerlessness, and stigmatization.

Traumatic Sexualization

Traumatic sexualization refers to the way a child's cognitive and emotional development and sexuality are shaped in inappropriate and interpersonally dysfunctional ways by premature exposure to sexuality. Finkelhor and Browne (1985) proposed that this harmful exposure interferes with the normal development of sexuality and results in a variety of dysfunctional behaviors and cognitions. The child who is rewarded for sexual behavior learns that she can exchange sex for affection, attention, privileges, or love—"commodities" that are unconditionally provided in a healthy parent–child relationship. Such reinforcement socializes the child to use sex to manipulate others to ensure that important nonsexual needs are met. Clinical observations that child sexual abuse (CSA) victims frequently engage in precocious, inappropriate, repetitive, and compulsive sex play and masturbation with adults or peers (Finkelhor & Browne, 1985; Kendall-Tackett, Williams, & Finkelhor, 1993; Yates, 1983) are consistent with idea that the relationships of children who are subjected to inappropriate early sexual experiences are sexualized.

According to Finkelhor (1988), the repercussions of traumatic sexualization are legion and can include confusion regarding sexual morality and sexual identity, the association of frightening and unpleasant memories with sexuality, misunderstandings about the role of sex in interpersonal relationships, avoidance and fear of sexuality, and sexual dysfunctions. The use of force, enticing the child to participate in sexual activities, eliciting the child's sexual response, and the child's awareness of the inappropriateness of the situation are all hypothesized to increase the negative impact of traumatic sexualization.

Until recently, research on traumatic sexualization has been hampered by the lack of a measure of this construct. To respond to this need, Matorin and Lynn (1998) developed the Traumatic Sexualization Survey (TSS) based on Finkelhor and Browne's (1985) conceptualization of the effects of traumatic sexualization to assess cognitive and behavioral factors purportedly associated with CSA histories.

A factor analysis of the scale yielded four subscales: (a) Avoidance and Fear of Sexual and Physical Intimacy, (b) Thoughts About Sex, (c) Role of Sex in Relationships, and (d) Attraction/Interest in Sexuality. Among individuals with a history of CSA, all of the TSS factors were associated with sex guilt, dysfunctional sexual behavior (as defined by Briere & Runtz, 1988), sex drive, and attitudes regarding sexual behavior. Furthermore, sexually abused women scored higher than nonabused women on three TSS factors: Thoughts About Sex, Role of Sex in Relationships, and Attraction/Interest and Sexuality. Physically abused women differed from nonabused women on only one of the factors, Thoughts About Sex. It is interesting to note that sexually abused women did not score significantly higher than physically abused women on any of the TSS factors, indicating that what the TSS measures is not necessarily specific to sexual victimization.

In a prospective study of sexual assault (Fite & Lynn, 2001), the TSS was found to be more strongly predictive of future sexual assault than the variables of previous sexual victimization, drug and alcohol use, and psychological adjustment. Two of the TSS factors in particular played a dominant role in the prediction of subsequent sexual assault: Role of Sex in Relationships and Attraction/Interest in Sexuality. The first factor, Role of Sex in Relationships, reflects an attitude that sex is a means of attaining fulfillment of social and personal needs such as acceptance, self-confidence, and intimacy. The items that compose this factor are concerned with basing relationships on sex, using sex to avoid loneliness or rejection, and having sex to feel good about oneself. Examples include "My relationships with men are based on sex," "I use sex to avoid loneliness," "I avoid rejection by having sex," and "Men base their relationships with me on sex."

The second TSS factor, Attraction/Interest in Sexuality, reflects beliefs that the qualities of seductiveness and sexuality are the basis of personal attractiveness. Examples of items for this factor include "People are interested in me because I act seductively," "Men want to be with me because I am seductive," and "My sexuality is what attracts people to me." The female participants who scored high on these two TSS factors were at significantly greater risk for subsequent sexual assault. Even when previous sexual victimization was controlled for, the factors continued to be significant predictors of subsequent sexual assault. We believe that women who score high on the TSS may resemble so-called "hyperfeminine" women (Gold, Sinclair, & Balge, 1999; McKelvie & Gold, 1994; Murnen & Byrne, 1991) who (a) place a great deal of importance on relationships with men, (b) use sex to gain or maintain a romantic relationship, (c) make poor relationship choices, and (d) engage in brief sexual encounters to achieve intimacy and avoid feelings of loneliness.

Betrayal

Betrayal occurs when the CSA victim discovers that the person she depended on to protect and nurture her has caused her harm. This breach of trust engenders anger, sadness, and loss, along with feelings of disenchantment and depression (Finkelhor, 1988). Freyd (1996; see also chap. 6, this volume) has argued that profound amnesias for abuse and related events may occur when a betrayal of trust produces conflict between external reality and a necessary system of social dependence. Recent research with a newly developed instrument, the Betrayal Trauma Inventory, has shown that memory of sexual or physical abuse was related to caretaker status, with greater memory impairment related to abuse by a caretaker than a noncaretaker (Freyd, DePrince, & Zurbriggen, 2001). Freyd's (1996) reanalysis of a number of large data sets revealed that memories of incest were more likely to be forgotten and recovered than memories for non-incest-related abuse. Conceivably, the effects of betrayal can be expressed in terms of avoidance of intimate relationships, impaired judgment about the trustworthiness of others, and extreme dependency and clinging behaviors intended to achieve a sense of security (Finkelhor & Browne, 1985, p. 535; see also McCann et al., 1988). Accordingly, betrayal may motivate some women to initiate or continue relationships with unstable or abusive men.

Powerlessness

Powerlessness and attendant feelings of behavioral impotence, depression, and despair are common repercussions of feeling trapped in an abusive situation in which self-efficacy and coping skills are compromised (Finkelhor, 1988). Sinclair et al. (1999) noted that the negative sequelae of powerlessness include anxiety and tension (Briere & Runtz, 1988), sleep disturbances (Briere & Runtz, 1988), expectations of being victimized again (Russell, 1986), and dissociation. Finkelhor (1988) suggested that the passivity engendered by sexual abuse may result in women viewing themselves as incapable of protecting themselves and devoid of power to the point that they "give up" and do not consider escaping or extricating themselves from destructive relationships. In short, victims of sexual abuse are socialized to subordinate themselves to perpetrators of maltreatment.

A related possibility is that abusive early-life circumstances increase tolerance and acceptance of subsequent abuse, thereby engendering passivity in response to abusive treatment. A study in our laboratory (Kelder, McNamara, Carlson, & Lynn, 1991) indicated that individuals who reported being severely disciplined as children rated punishment in scenarios in which children were physically punished as more appropriate than individuals who reported being less severely disciplined. Further, participants who rated their own severe and abusive punishment in childhood as "deserved" rated physical punishment as more appropriate in general than those who perceived their experiences to be "less deserved." In all likelihood these findings apply to sexual abuse, although this has yet to be determined on an empirical basis.

Stigmatization

Stigmatization occurs when the victim of abuse perceives herself as "bad" as she gains awareness of the inappropriate treatment she has been subject to and her "differentness" from other children. Pressure for secrecy, knowledge of incest taboos, and demeaning comments made by the perpetrator can engender feelings of shame and guilt that persist into adulthood. Child victims may be further stigmatized by people who "blame the victim" or view them as "spoiled goods" (Finkelhor & Browne, 1985, p. 533). According to this line of thinking, victims internalize this negative view of the self, fail to recognize their own worth, and fail to protect themselves from abuse that is felt to be deserved.

Unfortunately, many of the hypotheses regarding traumatic sexualization, while reasonable and intuitively appealing, have garnered minimal or no empirical attention. The research in this area has been hampered by a lack of standardized measures for constructs such as betrayal and stigmatization. Recently, however, a number of retrospective and prospective studies, summarized below, which are potentially related to dysfunctional learning, have delineated antecedent conditions that moderate the occurrence of revictimization.

Maker et al. (2001) conducted a retrospective investigation of the predictors and consequences of sexual assault in a nonclinical sample of women. The authors studied the relationship among CSA, peer sexual abuse, and adult sexual assault after the age of 16 in an effort to develop a multirisk model of revictimization. Maker et al.'s model considered the possible impact of severity of sexual abuse, the victim–perpetrator age differential, physical abuse, parental substance abuse, and parental antisocial behaviors.

Maker et al.'s (2001) study indicated that CSA was the only predictor of adult sexual assault among the risk factors considered. Maker et al. contended that their findings were consistent with a specificity model of trauma such that CSA "places women on a unique developmental trajectory for sexual revictimization over time" (p. 366). To be more specific, the severity of CSA, the number of perpetrators, and the age at onset of CSA were not associated with an increase in sexual revictimization risk. Rather, less severe abuse by a single perpetrator appeared to be sufficient to increase the risk of sexual assault later in life.

Wind and Silvern (1992) conducted a retrospective study that examined the separate and combined effects of sexual and physical abuse on adult adjustment with a sample of 259 female staff members at a university. Measures used included assessments of child and adult sexual and physical abuse, posttrauma symptoms, depression, and self-esteem. Twenty-one percent of the sample reported a history of child sexual but not physical abuse, 19% reported a history of child physical but not sexual abuse, 8% reported a history of combined child sexual and physical abuse, and 53% reported no history of child abuse.

The combined abuse group reported more symptoms compared with nonabused participants as well as participants who experienced only one form of child abuse. Importantly, the combined abuse group reported a higher rate of both sexual and physical assault in adulthood as compared with the other groups. However, notable limitations of this study included the use of single questions to assess child and adult victimization, a lack of control for the effects of adult victimization on adjustment, and a failure to examine between-groups differences in the rates of posttraumatic stress disorder (PTSD).

In an effort to remedy these shortcomings, Schaaf and McCanne (1998) conducted a retrospective study in which they attempted to disentangle the separate and combined effects of child sexual and physical abuse on both sexual revictimization and PTSD symptoms in adulthood. The researchers studied 475 female college students who were categorized as having experienced (a) only child contact sexual abuse, (b) only child physical abuse, (c) combined child sexual and physical abuse, and (d) no child abuse. Participants with a history of combined sexual and physical abuse reported the highest rate of adult sexual victimization. Compared with participants with no abuse history, individuals who reported combined abuse reported higher rates of PTSD and trauma symptoms when adult victimization was statistically controlled. Schaaf and McCanne suggested that differences in the rates of adult victimization and PTSD found in many previous studies that were attributed to a history of sexual abuse might instead be attributable to the effects of combined physical and sexual abuse.

Prospective studies of revictimization are sorely needed to trace the developmental trajectory of dysfunctional learning and to tease apart the role of general dysfunctional family relational patterns from the specific posttraumatic effects of abuse and situational risk factors such as alcohol consumption. For example, Fergusson and his colleagues (Fergusson, Horwood, & Lynskey, 1997) reported that a history of CSA is associated with family characteristics such as social disadvantage, family instability, frequent or severe punishment, poor parental attachment, and parental substance abuse. The authors determined that each of these characteristics increased children's risk of sexual revictimization in later adolescence or adulthood. In the study of Navy recruits (Merrill, Newell, Gold, & Milner, 1999), both alcohol problems and number of sex partners predicted rape; however, the effects of these variables were independent of the effects of CSA, which increased the likelihood of rape nearly fivefold.

Alcohol and drug use figure prominently as risk factors in sexual assault and revictimization (see also chap. 8, this volume) and, not infrequently, occur in the context of involvement in delinquent activities. Social learning associated with a delinquent lifestyle that includes drug and alcohol use, and relatively early intercourse and initiating of sexual activity, can increase the risk of initial and subsequent sexual victimization (Mott & Haurin, 1988). Gold et al.'s (1999) multifactorial of revictimization includes delinquency and drug use as an important risk factor, in addition to the effects of traumatic sexualization, attachment styles, and hyperfemininity, which we have reviewed earlier, and coping styles, which we consider below under the rubric of dissociation as a cognitive defense.

Studies of vulnerability to revictimization are important insofar as only a minority of sexually abused children evidence apparent consequences of sexual abuse (e.g., sexualized behavior) that are hypothesized to increase revictimization risk (Rind, Tromovitch, & Bauserman, 1998). Additionally, some adults with no abuse history are at high risk for repeated sexual assault. Discriminating preexisting risk or vulnerability factors that are independent of child abuse from those that arise as a direct consequence of abuse is an important task for researchers, as is discriminating the effects of independent versus co-occurring physical, sexual, and emotional forms of abuse. Additionally, studies that pinpoint the role of social support in buffering the effects of abuse on the risk of revictimization would contribute to the literature.

DISSOCIATION AS A COGNITIVE DEFENSE

Numerous investigators have documented a link between dissociation and a variety of traumatic experiences (for reviews, see Lynn & Rhue, 1994; chap. 6, this volume). Dissociation is generally described as a normal psychological coping response that is used to reduce anxiety associated with overwhelming traumatic experiences by (a) disengaging from the traumatic event itself or events associatively linked to the event by way of fantasy, imagination, and other attention-regulating strategies (e.g., imagining floating above the body during abuse, being in another place, "spacing out"; Lynn, Neufeld, Green, Rhue, & Sandberg, 1996); (b) avoiding, disrupting, or compartmentalizing memories and affect related to traumatic events (see Eisen & Lynn, 2001); and (c) numbing in relation to events or memories associated with trauma (Beahrs, 1990; Putnam, 1989; Spiegel, 1986; Terr, 1991). Because these defensive operations are thought to operate on a largely unconscious basis, they preclude exposure to and extinction of anxiety and full resolution of the trauma-related emotions.

Dissociation is also believed to increase the risk of not recognizing or responding to "danger cues" that typically signal the need to escape or avoid a menacing situation (Chu, 1992; Gold et al., 1999; Kluft, 1990a, 1990b; Sandberg et al., 1994). Poor risk recognition is associated with revictimization (Meadows, Jaycox, Stafford, Hembree, & Foa, 1995), and numerous anecdotal reports link dissociation and subsequent revictimization (Chu, 1992; Kluft, 1990a, 1990b; van der Kolk, 1989). With the exception of Becker-Lausen, Sanders, and Chinsky's (1992) study, which found that dissociation but not depression mediated revictimization, very little empirical work has been devoted to examining the relation between dissociation and revictimization. Additionally, virtually no controlled research has investigated how dissociation affects information processing of stimuli preceding a sexual assault.

To better understand the link between dissociation and information processing, Sandberg, Lynn, and Matorin (2001) used an information-processing paradigm known as *unitization* (Newtson, 1973) in which participants who observe an interaction or a videotape press a button each time they perceive the occurrence of a significant or meaningful event. Unitization reflects the way an observer actively processes and regulates stimuli in the environment by dividing observed, ongoing behavior into greater or lesser meaningful units of action (Newtson, 1973).

Relatively high levels of arousal can lead to decreased memory for an event (Clifford & Scott, 1978) and lower rates of unitization (Newtson, Enquist, & Bois, 1977). Accordingly, poor memory or *dissociation* associated with an upsetting event may be mediated by an arousal-induced reduction in the perceiver's rate of unitization (Lassiter, Stone, & Rogers, 1988). Sandberg et al. (2001) compared the information-processing styles of three groups of undergraduate women: (a) 20 women who scored in the upper 10% on the Dissociative Experience Scale (DES; Bernstein & Putnam, 1986), a measure of trait dissociation; (b) 20 women with the same degree of general psychopathology as the high dissociating group but relatively few dissociative experiences; and (c) 27 women with relatively low levels of general psychopathology and relatively few dissociative experiences. Information-processing styles were examined in response to videotaped scenarios of the events leading up to an acquaintance rape and a nonthreatening control situation. To assess unitization, participants pressed a button every time they perceived a significant or meaningful event.

The results indicated that trait dissociation was negatively correlated with unitization of the acquaintance rape videotape, unitization was positively correlated with the ability to identify danger cues associated with possible rape in the tape, and a measure of state dissociation was negatively correlated with perceptions of how dangerous the male was rated in the tape. Combined, these findings bolster the hypothesis that dissociation is related to the way information relevant to a sexual assault is processed. Further research is needed to examine how dissociation influences various aspects of information processing, including attention, arousal, encoding, storage, activation, and retrieval, and whether specific information-processing deficits place a woman at risk for sexual victimization.

A SOCIAL-NARRATIVE MODEL

We (Lynn & Pintar, 1997a, 1997b; Lynn, Pintar, & Rhue, 1997) have begun to sketch a social-narrative model of dissociation that has some bearing on understanding revictimization. Traditional conceptualizations of dissociation conceive of it as an intrapsychic phenomenon, a disturbance of feeling, cognition, and memory. Dissociation is theorized to occur and to persist as a dysfunctional symptom of abuse or as a functional defense mechanism that outlives its usefulness (see Lynn & Rhue, 1994). In either case, the dissociation is understood to originate in response to traumatic events. While not disputing the phenomenon of dissociation as subjectively experienced by certain victims of abuse or its function as a defense mechanism, we suggest that the phenomenon does not result from traumatic violence the way a bump follows a hit on the head, but that it arises as a result of the social conditions in which victims live and are abused, and as a reflection of intolerably conflicted social relations.

Unlike betrayal trauma theory (Freyd, 1996), which fixes its attention on one particular emotional dynamic of the disjunctive relationship between victims and perpetrators, our model is more general in scope. Unlike prevailing theories of dissociation (see Lilienfeld et al., 1999; Spanos, 1994, for exceptions), which are not particularly social in focus and locate dysfunctional dissociation in the individual, the social-narrative model's focus is on contradictory or dissociative social relations.

What do we mean when we say that social conditions and relations generate dissociation? We begin with the assertion that traumatic interpersonal violence is a jarring contradiction of cultural norms as expressed in shared social narratives. In most cases, CSA is a socially anomalous, secretive event, one that is not mirrored in children's books or cartoons or the experience of other children in the neighborhood. Victims cannot rely on traditional cultural stories to explain what is happening to them. A child who is raped by her father, for example, has little help from the social world in understanding what has happened to her. The rape may contradict her prior experience of who her father is, but more significantly, it also bears no resemblance to what the dominant social narratives have taught her about what fathers are supposed to do and to be. There are no fathers like hers portrayed on Saturday morning television.

The narrative explanation of the abuse offered by the perpetrator is also likely to contradict the child's experience sharply. He may tell her she liked it, or wanted it, or deserved it, or imagined it, or even that it did not happen at all. The child may try to hold out against the powerful meaning-making force of her father's version of the events and to create a narrative that more accurately describes what she has experienced. Storytelling, however, is a social event by definition. Children who are threatened into silence, or are socialized in such a way as to suppress angry feelings and enact the role of the stereotypic, passive "good girl" who does not make trouble (Walker, 1981), rarely have anyone to whom they can freely share their stories.

The dreadful aloneness experienced by some sexually abused children also causes painful contradictions in other important social relations. Our culture suggests to children that they can tell their mothers and their best friends "anything," because these are the people who will do anything to protect and defend them. At the crucial moment in their lives when abused children really need that protection, they frequently find themselves protecting these others with their silence instead, and protecting for them the shared social assumption that all is normal and well. When the victim's narrative of abuse is wholly private and individual, it is necessarily distorted, because it develops independent of shared social reflection.

It should not be surprising that even the memories of a child who has been assaulted are confused and lack narrative coherence, or that her sense of self and her place in the world are equally chaotic. Indeed, it may be her inability or unwillingness to disclose her experience to anyone that ensures that the unrehearsed traumatic events will be relegated to the background of experience or manifest as intrusive and recurrent memories with no coherent narrative thread. The idea that traumatic events can compromise the coherence of memory and narrative production is consistent with the following findings: (a) Rape narratives are more ambiguous than narratives related to nonrape events (Tromp, Koss, Figueredo, & Tharan, 1995), (b) the level of articulation of trauma narratives is inversely related to chronic PTSD (Amir, Stafford, Freshman, & Foa, 1998), and (c) reductions in trauma-related anxiety during therapy for PTSD are associated with a decrease in the fragmentation of rape narratives (Foa, Monlar, & Cashman, 1995). These findings are consonant with the hypothesis that emotional processing involves the creation of an organized, unfragmented, and more articulated narrative related to the traumatic event (Amir et al., 1998; Foa & Riggs, 1994).

We may describe the tenuous relationship of an abuse victim to her past as dissociative, but what must be noted is that her mental state directly reflects the social reality that faces her: There is an irreconcilable opposition between life as she experienced it and the life that the social world and everyone in it told her that she should be experiencing. She is trapped between her experience of being assaulted by her own father and a broad social narrative that says, "Fathers care for their daughters and don't hurt them." It is the social world of an abused child that is incoherent and dissociated, and she must learn to dissociate in turn, if she is to survive the violence of its contradictions.

We refer to the extreme discrepancy between personal narrative and shared social narratives as *social incoherence*, a concept that recalls some features of Festinger's (1957) cognitive dissonance and Bateson's (Bateson, Jackson, Haley, & Weakland, 1956) double-bind theory. Dissociation functions as a defense mechanism, but what it is defending against is more than abuse or even the fear of future abuse: It is also an adaptation to continuing social incoherence. The social-narrative model converges with a more purely cognitive model in the sense that abuse is posited to affect beliefs, expectations, and cognitive schemas for relationships. However, in the social-narrative model, the problem is not so much that the individual's cognitive expectations do not match the social world but the opposite—that the world's expectations (generally expressed as shared cultural and social narratives) do not match the individual's experience of what the world was and is. It is perhaps a subtle point, but a purely cognitive model locates the dysfunction more in the victim, whereas the social-narrative view locates the dysfunction in the social world.

The social world remains dissociated for an abused child long after the abuse has ended, if the shared social narrative and the private internal narrative are never reconciled—if, for example, the child never tells anyone what happened to her; if she tells her family but they refuse to believe her; if they take the side of the perpetrator or force her to interact with him in ways that make her uncomfortable; and if her experience is minimized or trivialized by those she finally chooses to tell. In other words, an abuse survivor is limited in her ability to recover from the abuse if the dissociated social conditions remain in place. By distinguishing the social conditions from any particular act of traumatizing abuse, the chronic and long-term effects of trauma are seen to be located in the social world, not merely as persistent or posttraumatic symptoms within a victim.

This shift of focus from event to context is important to the analysis of revictimization. It is the time in between a child and an adult assault that begs explanation. Because the dissociated social conditions and relations that give rise to violence and abuse may precede and will certainly outlast any particular abusive event, it follows that personal dissociation can occur both when a woman is being abused and also when she is only in danger of being abused. The evidence clearly demonstrates that women abused in childhood are at risk of being assaulted again; they are never, in a manner of speaking, "out of danger." Instead of locating that danger solely in the victims—in their self-destructiveness, compulsiveness, or poor judgments, and in their socializations, adaptations, or defense mechanisms—we look for it in their relationship to the social worlds that they inhabit and, most importantly, to the perpetrators who live there too.

Ironically, being revictimized may have the effect, for some women, of bringing shared social narratives in line with their private knowledge of the "true" nature of the world. Messman and Long (1996) contended that repeated victimization is not unusual for some women who, abused as children, associate sexuality with pain, punishment, and other negative consequences to the point that they create the impression of having a "masochistic tendency" (Herman & Hirschman, 1971; van der Kolk, 1989). When a woman who was victimized as a child marries a man who abuses her, her commitment to him will seem incomprehensible to those who grew up in nondissociated social worlds. For her, the marriage may be oddly comfortable, or at least familiar, verifying for her what she learned as a child to be true: "Men who are supposed to love me will hurt me." By this reckoning, it does not seem so strange that women not infrequently have relationships with men who resemble their molesters (Tsai & Wagner, 1978).

Relationships with nonabusive men may be uncomfortable for the same reason: Their love may seem untrustworthy, their kindness illusory, a reminder of those childhood friends and family members who failed to recognize the abuse. It is familiar enough to be a cultural cliché, that women may love a good man "like a friend" but only fall in love with the bad ones, but this trend seems to be exacerbated in survivors of child abuse, who may find potential abusers subjectively "more real" than nonabusers who do not and cannot inhabit the dissociated social world shared so intimately by perpetrators and their victims.

These women may also be hoping that they can achieve social coherence in the opposite direction: If a dangerous man turns out not to be a perpetrator, if an abuser chooses not to abuse, it seems as though, by some sort of sympathetic magic, this can erase the abuse experienced in the past. It sometimes looks to observers as if these women actively put themselves in the path of danger, as if they are waiting to see what will happen to them. It is not so inexplicable when we realize that either outcome, positive or negative, provides a sort of temporary relief to the chronic discomfort of social incoherence. Ironically, the repeated victimization is dysfunctionally functional, lessening the contradiction between private experience and social expectation. It is more difficult (though not impossible) for a woman who is assaulted as an adult to keep that experience completely to herself. If others find about what has happened to her, the inner and outer worlds may actually, for once, cohere because publicly recurring violence validates the private experience of childhood trauma. Now there is not one abuser, but three or seven, and with each new violation, more people can see what is happening; with each revictimization the violence becomes more socially real. It is this communicative component that may be the key: Revictimization can sometimes operate as a kind of performance, a way of narrating past abuse for others to see, not by telling the story in words but by enacting it, again and again, until somebody sees, somebody understands, somebody finally steps in and helps the victim to experience a different ending this time.

These repetitions are not compulsive so much as they may be increasingly desperate, the way our voices will get louder each time we call for help if no one answers the first time. In this view, the victim is not recreating the past trauma to gain a sense of mastery over those old experiences and the pain and anxiety that they cause, but rather to alter the social relations of the present and the pain and anxiety that come from knowing she is still in danger. The statistics tell us that this is so: Past victims of abuse are more likely to be abused again for a variety of complicated reasons that this chapter has detailed. What we want to underscore is that only some of these are under women's direct control. The fear is not imaginary, and it is not irrational. The world is a dangerous place, and there are perpetrators enough to go around opportunistically revictimizing; they are compulsively replaying socially incoherent dramas of their own.

The challenge that faces us now is to operationalize and evaluate some of the theory's loosely defined central constructs. We might hypothesize that a sexually abused child who shared her story to a sympathetic listener in childhood may be less likely to "dissociate" and less likely to be revictimized as an adult, because her private suffering had been reflected and acknowledged in the external world. Sinclair and Gold (1997) have found that trauma symptoms were increased when women with a history of child abuse "held back" from disclosing the abuse when they would have liked to disclose it to others.

Hypothesizing a correlation between revictimization and social coherency, we would predict that revictimization events would occur more frequently to women whose personal and social worlds remain most dissociated from one another. An instrument to assess the presence and degree of social coherency would need to include questions about both the past, including whether a woman abused in childhood received any social support in the form of adult intervention, an unusually well-informed child friend, or media sources communicating the idea that child abuse is wrong, and the present, including how many family members know about the abuse now, what their reactions were when they found out, the level and quality of adult contact with the perpetrator, the necessity of still maintaining silence about the abuse and protecting family members, the quality and intimacy of an individual's current relationships, and the extent to which these people know of the individual's abuse history and are able to offer active support.

The literature we have reviewed implies that important steps can be taken to reduce the risk of revictimization: (a) sensitize women to situational risk factors (e.g., excessive alcohol consumption) and danger cues that have been empirically demonstrated to be associated with sexual assault risk; (b) educate women about the connection between previous abuse and revictimization; (c) increase women's self-esteem, self-respect, and repertoire of assertive, social, communication, and limit-setting skills in sexual and nonsexual situations; (d) encourage the examination of relationship choices and the use of sex to fulfill nonsexual needs (e.g., avoid loneliness, rejection, achieve intimacy) and mitigate excessive impulsivity; and (e) facilitate the emotional processing of past traumatic events and the creation of a coherent narrative in the context of a supportive relationship in which disclosure is valued and rewarded.

We hasten to add that, of course, it is not enough to narrate events differently solely as a cognitive task. Social incoherence is not a posttraumatic symptom that lives within a person; rather, the concept reflects a particular social condition that continues to traumatize the victim long after the initial traumatic episodes have passed. Therapists who embrace a traditional cognitive view might see the primary therapeutic task as changing the victim's false beliefs and dysfunctional expectations. Of course, it would be good for the victim to live in a world in which the men who love her do not hurt her. However, according to the social-narrative model, she is only going to believe that after the men in her life stop hurting her. It makes little sense, in our view, to try to have the victim make the change internally as a cognitive task in therapy, so that she now believes that "men who love me don't hurt me," unless that is actually true in the world. If it is not true, then the victim might actually be "set up" to experience continued social incoherence, and she may instinctively "know better." In an odd and ironic way, being revictimized might be safer, or at least more in line with her perceptions of "the way the world is." At any rate, achieving social coherence is decidedly not a cognitive task but a social one, because it is the world that needs to achieve consistency, not the victim.

From the social-narrative perspective, the goal of intervention is to help abuse survivors achieve social coherence before they find themselves victimized once again. They accomplish this not by attempting to gain mastery over historic events but by recognizing the persistent traumas of the present. Those at risk of revictimization will have to find active ways to protect themselves from current and future threats, not by narrating the danger away but by acknowledging and responding to it in concrete ways.

These women must also see the social world around themselves changing: If a victim changes but the world does not, her "new self" may well be just another dissociation in a continuingly incoherent world. What it means to "change the social world" will be different in every circumstance. It will be appropriate to alter or sever dangerous relationships with potential perpetrators and others as well, most notably those who contribute to the incoherence by rationalizing or denying past violence, minimizing current threats, or encouraging high-risk behavior such as excessive alcohol consumption. For others, these personal solutions may not be enough. Some women will only find therapeutic relief in reaching out to other victims or those at risk, by sharing their own experiences through publishing their writing or speaking publicly about what they have experienced, or in a more informal way through peer counseling or participation in support group-type activities. Others will be moved to go further still. When those who experience a loss or are the victims of a terrible crime testify about the event to change legislation or to raise money for preventative efforts, they are also effectively and dramatically reducing social incoherence, because they ensure that their private and social worlds overlap completely with one another. There is no need to recreate the original trauma, if the world witnesses and acknowledges that such things have occurred and may happen again. The recognition that personal tragedy reflects larger social issues is a key insight for survivors of abuse. It means they no longer have to inhabit their traumatic world alone.

REFERENCES

Alexander, P. C. (1993). The differential effects of abuse characteristics and attachment in the prediction of long-term effects of sexual abuse. *Journal of Interpersonal Violence, 8*, 346–362.

Amir, N., Stafford, J., Freshman, M. S., & Foa, E. B. (1998). Relationship between trauma narratives and trauma pathology. *Journal of Traumatic Stress, 11*, 385–393.

Bartholomew, K., & Horowitz, L. M. (1991). Attachment styles among young adults: A test of a four-category model. *Journal of Personality and Social Psychology, 51*, 226–244.

Bateson, G., Jackson, D. D., Haley, J., & Weakland, J. (1956). Towards a theory of schizophrenia. *Behavioural Science, 1*, 251–264.

Beahrs, J. O. (1990). The evolution of post-traumatic behavior: Three hypotheses. *Dissociation, 3*, 15–21.

Becker-Lausen, E., Sanders, B., & Chinsky, J. M. (1992, August). *A structural analysis of child abuse and negative life experiences.* Paper presented at the 100th Annual Convention of the American Psychological Association, Washington, DC.

Bernstein, E. M., & Putnam, F. W. (1986). Development, reliability, and validity of a dissociation scale. *Journal of Nervous and Mental Disease, 174*, 727–735.

Briere, J. N. (1992). *Child abuse trauma: Theory and treatment of the lasting effects.* Newbury Park, CA: Sage.

Briere, J., & Runtz, M. (1988). Symptomatology associated with childhood sexual victimization in a nonclinical adult sample. *Child Abuse and Neglect, 12*, 51–59.

Byers, E. S., Giles, B. L., & Price, D. L. (1987). Definiteness and effectiveness of women's responses to unwanted sexual advances: A laboratory investigation. *Basic and Applied Social Psychology, 8*, 321–338.

Chu, J. A. (1992). The revictimization of adult women with histories of childhood abuse. *Journal of Psychotherapy Practice and Research, 1, 259–269.*

Clifford, B. R., & Scott, J. (1978). Individual and situational factors in eyewitness testimony. *Journal of Applied Psychology, 63, 352–359.*

Eisen, M., & Lynn, S. J. (2001). Memory, suggestibility, and dissociation in children and adults. *Applied Cognitive Psychology, 15, 49–73.*

Ellis, E. M., Atkeson, B. M., & Calhoun, K. S. (1982). An examination of differences between multiple- and single-incident victims of sexual assault. *Journal of Abnormal Psychology, 91, 221–224.*

Fairbairn, W. R. D. (1954). Observations on the nature of hysterical states. *British Journal of Medical Psychology, 27, 105–125.*

Fergusson, D. M., Horwood, L. J., & Lynskey, M. T. (1997). Childhood sexual abuse, adolescent sexual behaviors and sexual revictimization. *Child Abuse and Neglect, 21, 789–803.*

Festinger, L. A. (1957). *A theory of cognitive dissonance.* Stanford, CA: Stanford University Press.

Finkelhor, D. (1988). The trauma of child sexual abuse: Two models. *Journal of Interpersonal Violence, 2, 348–366.*

Finkelhor, D., & Browne, A. (1985). The traumatic impact of child sexual abuse: A conceptualization. *American Journal of Orthopsychiatry, 55, 530–541.*

Fite, R., & Lynn, S. J. (2001). *Sexual assault in college women: A prospective, cognitive-behavioral model.* Unpublished manuscript, Binghamton University.

Foa, E. B., & Kozak, M. J. (1991). Emotional processing: Theory, research and clinical implications for anxiety disorders. In J. Safran & L. S. Greenberg (Eds.), *Emotion, psychotherapy and change* (pp. 21–49). New York: Guilford Press.

Foa, E. B., Molnar, C., & Cashman, L. (1995). Changes in rape narratives during exposure therapy for posttraumatic stress disorder. *Journal of Traumatic Stress, 8, 675–690.*

Foa, E.B., & Riggs, D. S. (1994). Post-traumatic stress disorder and rape. In R. S. Pynoos (Ed.) *Post-traumatic stress disorder: A clinical review* (pp. 133–163). Lutherville, MD: Sidran Press.

Freud, S. (1954). Beyond the pleasure principle. In J. Strachey (Trans. and Ed.), *Complete psychological works* (Standard ed., Vol. 18). London: Hogarth Press. (Original work published 1920)

Freyd, J. J. (1996). *Betrayal trauma: The logic of forgetting childhood abuse.* Cambridge, MA: Harvard University Press.

Freyd, J. J., DePrince, A. P., & Zurbriggen, E. L. (2001). Self-reported memory for abuse depends upon victim–perpetrator relationship. *Journal of Trauma and Dissociation, 2, 5–17.*

Gelinas, D. J. (1983). The persistent negative effects of incest. *Psychiatry, 46, 312–332.*

Gidycz, C. A., Coble, C. N., Latham, L., & Layman, M. J. (1993). Sexual assault experience in adulthood and prior victimization experiences: A prospective analysis. *Psychology of Women Quarterly, 17, 151–168.*

Gold, S. R., Sinclair, B. B., & Balge, K. A. (1999). Risk of sexual revictimization: A theoretical model. *Aggression and Violent Behavior, 4*, 457–470.

Hanson, K. A., & Gidycz, C. A. (1993). An evaluation of a sexual assault prevention program. *Journal of Consulting and Clinical Psychology, 61*, 1046–1052.

Herman, J., & Hirschman, L. (1971). Father–daughter incest. *Signs: Journal of Women in Culture and Society, 2*, 735–756.

Horowitz, M. J. (1975). Intrusive and repetitive thoughts after experimental stress. *Archives of General Psychiatry, 32*, 1457–1463.

Kelder, L. R., McNamara, J., Carlson, B., & Lynn, S. J. (1991). Perceptions of physical punishment. *Journal of Interpersonal Violence, 6*, 432–445.

Kendall-Tackett, K. A., Williams, L. M., & Finkelhor, D. (1993). Impact of sexual abuse on children: A review and synthesis of recent empirical studies. *Psychological Bulletin, 113*, 164–180.

Kluft, R. P. (1990a). Dissociation and subsequent vulnerability: A preliminary study. *Dissociation, 3*, 167–173.

Kluft, R. P. (1990b). Incest and subsequent revictimization: The case of therapist–patient sexual exploitation, with a description of the sitting duck syndrome. In R. P. Kluft (Ed.), *Incest-related syndromes of adult psychopathology* (pp. 263–287). Washington, DC: American Psychiatric Press.

Koss, M. P., & Dinero, T. E. (1989). Discriminant analysis of risk factors for sexual victimization among a national sample of college women. *Journal of Consulting and Clinical Psychology, 57*, 242–250.

Lassiter, D. G., Stone, J. I., & Rogers, S. L. (1988). Memorial consequences of variation in behavior perception. *Journal of Experimental Social Psychology, 24*, 229–239.

Lilienfeld, S., Lynn, S. J., Kirsch, I., Chaves, J., Sarbin, T., Ganaway, G., & Powell, R. (1999). Dissociative identity disorder and the sociocognitive model: Recalling the lessons of the past. *Psychological Bulletin, 125*, 507–523.

Lynn, S. J., Neufeld, V., Green, J., Rhue, J., & Sandberg, D. (1996). Daydreaming, fantasy, and psychopathology. In R. Kunzendorf, N. Spanos, & B. Wallace (Eds.), *Hypnosis and imagination* (pp. 67–98). Amityville, NY: Baywood Press.

Lynn, S. J., & Pintar, J. (1997a). The social construction of multiple personality disorder. In D. Read & S. Lindsay (Eds.), *Recollections of trauma: Scientific studies and clinical practice* (pp. 483–492). New York: Plenum Press.

Lynn, S. J., & Pintar, J. (1997b). A social narrative model of dissociative identity disorder. *Australian Journal of Clinical and Experimental Hypnosis, 25*, 1–7.

Lynn, S. J., Pintar, J., & Rhue, J. W. (1997). Fantasy proneness, dissociation, and narrative construction. In S. Powers & S. Krippner (Eds.), *Broken selves: Dissociative narratives and phenomena* (pp. 274–304). New York: Bruner/Mazel.

Lynn, S. J., & Rhue, J. (Eds.). (1994). *Dissociation: Clinical and theoretical perspectives*. New York: Guilford Press.

Maker, A. H., Kemmelmeier, M., & Peterson, C. (2001). Child abuse, peers sexual abuse, and sexual assault in adulthood: A multi-risk model of revictimization. *Journal of Traumatic Stress, 14*, 351–368.

Mandoki, C. A., & Burkhart, B. R. (1989). Sexual victimization: Is there a vicious cycle? *Violence and Victims, 4,* 179–190.

Masterson, J. F., & Klein, R. (1989). *Psychotherapy of the disorders of the self: The Masterson approach.* New York: Brunner/Mazel.

Matorin, A. I., & Lynn, S. J. (1998). The development of a measure of correlates of child sexual abuse: The Traumatic Sexualization Survey. *Journal of Traumatic Stress, 11,* 261–280.

McCann, I. L., Sakheim, D. K., & Abrahamson, D. J. (1988). Trauma and victimization: A model of psychological adaptation. *The Counseling Psychologist, 16,* 531–549.

McKelvie, M., & Gold, S. R. (1994). Hyperfemininity: Further definition of the construct. *Journal of Sex Research, 31,* 91–98.

Meadows, E. A., Jaycox, L. H., Stafford, J., Hembree, E. A., & Foa, E. B. (1995, November). *Recognition of risk of assault in revictimized women.* Poster presented at the annual meeting of the Association for Advancement of Behavior Therapy, Washington, DC.

Merrill, L. L., Newell, C. E., Gold, S. R., & Milner, J. S. (April, 1999). Childhood abuse and sexual revictimization in a female Navy recruit sample. *Journal of Traumatic Stress, 12,* 211–225.

Messman, T. L., & Long, P. J. (1996). Child abuse and its relationship to revictimization in adult women: A review. *Clinical Psychology Review, 16,* 397–420.

Miller, B., & Marshall, J. C. (1987). Coercive sex on the university campus. *Journal of College Student Personnel, 28,* 38–47.

Mott, F. L., & Haurin, R. J. (1988). Linkages between sexual activity and alcohol and drug use among American adolescents. *Family Planning Perspectives, 20,* 128–136.

Muehlenhard, C. L., & Linton, M. A. (1987). Date rape and sexual aggression in the dating situation: Incidence and risk factors. *Journal of Counseling Psychology, 34,* 186–196.

Murnen, S. K., & Byrne, D. (1991). Hyperfemininity: Measurement and initial validation of the construct. *Journal of Sex Research, 28,* 479–489.

Newtson, D. (1973). Attribution and the unit of perception of ongoing behavior. *Journal of Personality and Social Psychology, 28,* 28–38.

Newtson, D., Enquist, G., & Bois, J. (1977). The objective basis of behavior units. *Journal of Personality and Social Psychology, 35,* 847–862.

Putnam, F. W. (1989). *Diagnosis and treatment of multiple personality disorder.* New York: Guilford Press.

Rind, B., Tromovitch, P., & Bauserman, R. (1998). A meta-analytic examination of assumed properties of child sexual abuse using college samples. *Psychological Bulletin, 124,* 22–53.

Russell, D. (1986). *The secret trauma: Incest in the lives of girls and women.* New York: Basic Books.

Sandberg, D., Lynn, S. J., & Green, J. (1994). Sexual abuse and revictimization: Mastery, dysfunctional learning, and dissociation. In S. J. Lynn & J. Rhue (Eds.), *Dissociation: Clinical and theoretical perspectives* (pp. 242–267). New York: Guilford Press.

Sandberg, D., Lynn, S. J., & Matorin, A. I. (2001). Information processing of an acquaintance rape scenario among high and low dissociating college women. *Journal of Traumatic Stress, 14*, 585–603.

Sandberg, D., Matorin, A., & Lynn, S. J. (1999). Dissociation, posttraumatic symptomatology, and sexual revictimization: A prospective examination of mediator and moderator effects. *Journal of Traumatic Stress, 12*, 127–138.

Schaaf, K. K., & McCanne, T. R. (1998). Relationship of childhood sexual, physical, and combined sexual and physical abuse to adult victimization and posttraumatic stress disorder. *Child Abuse and Neglect, 22*, 1119–1133.

Sinclair, B. B., & Gold, S. R. (1997). The psychological impact of withholding disclosure of child sexual abuse. *Violence and Victims, 12*, 125–133.

Sinclair, B. B., Merrill, L. L., Thomsen, C. J., & Gold, S. R. (1999). *Predicting the impact of child sexual abuse in women: A model of severity, support, attachment, and coping.* NHRC Report No. 99-25. San Diego, CA: Naval Health Research Center.

Sloane, P., & Karpinski, E. (1942). Effects of incest on the participants. *American Journal of Orthopsychiatry, 12*, 666–673.

Spanos, N. P. (1994). Multiple identity enactments and multiple personality disorder: A sociocognitive perspective. *Psychological Bulletin, 116*, 143–165.

Spiegel, D. (1986). Dissociating damage. *American Journal of Clinical Hypnosis, 29*, 123–131.

Terr, L. C. (1991). Childhood traumas: An outline and overview. *American Journal of Psychiatry, 148*, 10–20.

Tromp, S., Koss, M., Figueredo, A. J., & Tharan, M. (1995). Are rape memories different? A comparison of rape, other unpleasant, and pleasant memories among employed women. *Journal of Traumatic Stress, 4*, 607–627.

Tsai, M., & Wagner, N. (1978). Therapy groups for women sexually molested as children. *Archives of Sexual Behavior, 7*, 417–427.

van der Kolk, B. A. (1989). The compulsion to repeat the trauma: Re-enactment, revictimization, and masochism. *Psychiatric Clinics of North America, 12*, 389–411.

Walker, L. E. (1981). Battered women: Sex roles and clinical issues. *Professional Psychology, 12*, 81–91.

Wind, T. W., & Silvern, L. E. (1992). Type and extent of child abuse as predictors of adult functioning. *Journal of Family Violence, 7*, 261–281.

Wyatt, G. E., Guthrie, D., & Notgrass, C. M. (1992). Differential effects of women's child sexual abuse and subsequent sexual revictimization. *Journal of Consulting and Clinical Psychology, 60*, 167–173.

Yates, A. (1983). Children eroticized by incest. *American Journal of Psychiatry, 139*, 482–485.

8

CHILD SEXUAL ABUSE AND ALCOHOL USE AMONG WOMEN: SETTING THE STAGE FOR RISKY SEXUAL BEHAVIOR

SHARON C. WILSNACK, RICHARD W. WILSNACK,
ARLINDA F. KRISTJANSON, NANCY D. VOGELTANZ-HOLM,
AND T. ROBERT HARRIS

Child sexual abuse (CSA) has been associated with increased risk for a variety of negative sexual and reproductive health outcomes, among them high-risk sexual behavior and its sequelae, including unintended pregnancy and sexually transmitted diseases such as HIV infection (Bensley, Van Eenwyk, & Simmons, 2000; M. Cohen et al., 2000; Thompson, Potter, Sanderson, & Maibach, 1997; Zierler et al., 1991). Although many studies show that CSA is associated with risky sexual behavior in adulthood, it is still unclear *how* CSA is connected with risky sex.

The national longitudinal survey reported in this chapter was supported by Research Grant R37 AA04610 from the National Institute on Alcohol Abuse and Alcoholism, National Institutes of Health. We are grateful to the late Albert D. Klassen and to Sara R. Murphy and Woody Carter of the National Opinion Research Center (NORC), University of Chicago, for their collaboration in developing the child sexual abuse measure used in this study; to NORC field staff and interviewers for their sensitivity and expertise in conducting the personal interviews; to Perry Benson for assistance with computer data analysis; and to Louise Diers and Loraine Olson for administrative support and editorial assistance. An earlier version of this chapter was presented at the Conference on Childhood Sexual Abuse and HIV Risk: Breaking the Link, sponsored by the Centers for Disease Control and Prevention and the National Institute of Mental Health, Decatur, Georgia, November 1998.

Various biological, psychological, and social processes have been identified that may lead from CSA to unsafe sexual behavior, including developing attitudes about sex that encourage early onset of voluntary sexual activity (Browning & Laumann, 1997), learning to trade sex for rewards (leading to prostitution; Widom & Kuhns, 1996; Zierler et al., 1991), and developing unstable and multiple sexual relationships because CSA has reduced the ability to trust a sexual partner or to be psychologically intimate (Kirkham & Lobb, 1998; Mullen, Martin, Anderson, Romans, & Herbison, 1994). The hypothetical process discussed in this chapter is that the experience of CSA may lead women to use alcohol (and other psychoactive substances) in ways that make them more likely to engage in risky sexual behavior or that make them more vulnerable to the imposition of risky sex. This chapter focuses on women because (a) the large majority of research on CSA has included only female participants, and (b) the national survey whose data are used to evaluate connections among CSA, alcohol use, and sex later in this chapter sampled only women. Analyses focus on women's alcohol use rather than on substance abuse more broadly, because the data set analyzed contains much more detailed and extensive measures of alcohol use than of other drug use and abuse.

CHILD SEXUAL ABUSE AND SUBSTANCE USE

What is the evidence to support a hypothesis that CSA leads to substance use/abuse that then leads to risky sexual behavior, at least among women? Numerous studies of adolescents and adults have found that a history of CSA is associated with the use of alcohol and illicit substances (Harrison, Fulkerson, & Beebe, 1997; Jantzen, Ball, Leventhal, & Schottenfeld, 1998; Johnsen & Harlow, 1996; S. C. Wilsnack, Vogeltanz, Klassen, & Harris, 1997; Wingood & DiClemente, 1997) and is also associated with the development of substance abuse or dependence (Clark, Lesnick, & Hegedus, 1997; Fergusson, Horwood, & Lynskey, 1996; Galaif, Stein, Newcomb, & Bernstein, 2001; Goodman & Fallot, 1998; McCauley et al., 1997; Miller, Downs, & Testa, 1993; Spak, Spak, & Allebeck, 1998). The link between CSA and substance abuse appears to be stronger for more severe forms of CSA (Fergusson et al., 1996; Kendler et al., 2000; Mullen, Martin, Anderson, Romans, & Herbison, 1993) and may be mediated by psychological distress related to CSA, such as depression, anxiety, and post-traumatic stress disorder (Downs & Harrison, 1998; Epstein, Saunders, Kilpatrick, & Resnick, 1998; Schuck & Widom, 2001).

The consistent association of CSA with later substance use is remarkable because of the diversity of the groups studied and the diversity of ways that substance use and CSA have been measured. Furthermore, in several large studies the relationships between CSA and subsequent alcohol/

substance abuse have remained statistically significant after controlling for a variety of childhood and family background variables, such as parental substance abuse, physical and emotional abuse, and parental divorce or separation (see Kendler et al., 2000; Vogeltanz-Holm, 2002).

SUBSTANCE USE AND HIGH-RISK SEXUAL BEHAVIOR

Research on relationships between substance use and unsafe sex has found less consistent patterns, perhaps because of the several different ways that substance use and sexual activity may be connected. Most studies of alcohol use during specific sexual events find no connection between drinking and unprotected sexual intercourse (Harvey & Beckman, 1986; Lauchli et al., 1996; Perry et al., 1994; Temple, Leigh, & Schafer, 1993; Testa & Collins, 1997). When studies have found risky sex to be associated with drinking at the time, these have generally been studies of adolescents (Cooper, Peirce, & Huselid, 1994; Robertson & Plant, 1988) or of first-time sexual encounters with a new sexual partner (Graves & Hines, 1997; Halpern-Felsher, Millstein, & Ellen, 1996).

Research has more consistently found that people who use alcohol and other substances, and in particular people who use alcohol or other substances frequently or in large quantities, are more likely to engage in risky sexual activities, such as not using condoms and having multiple sexual partners (Anderson & Dahlberg, 1992; Hingson, Strunin, Berlin, & Heeren, 1990; Lauchli et al., 1996; Leigh, Temple, & Trocki, 1994; McEwan, McCallum, Bhopal, & Madhok, 1992; Molitor, Truax, Ruiz, & Sun, 1998; Parker, Harford, & Rosenstock, 1994; Potthoff et al., 1998; Sly, Quadagno, Harrison, Eberstein, & Riehman, 1997; Wingood & DiClemente, 1998). The idea that this association may result from a general personality pattern of risk taking or sensation seeking is not consistently supported (Fenaughty & Fisher, 1998; Sly et al., 1997), but no alternative general explanation has yet emerged.

It is also possible that alcohol consumption by couples may serve as a signal (at least to men) that sexual overtures are acceptable. Drinking on dates may lead to risky sexual imposition for reasons other than intoxication. Evidence suggesting this effect includes (a) associations of date rape with drinking by dating partners beforehand (Abbey, McAuslan, & Ross, 1998) and (b) laboratory research on hypothetical dating situations, in which a woman's drinking was perceived to indicate her sexual interest or availability (Garcia & Kushnier, 1987; George, Cue, Lopez, Crowe, & Norris, 1995; George et al., 1997) and observers interpreted drinking by either partner as indicating a greater likelihood of subsequent sexual intercourse (Corcoran & Bell, 1990; Corcoran & Thomas, 1991).

Finally, both CSA and heavy use of alcohol or other drugs may increase women's risks of having sex with a high-risk partner, for example, one who refuses to use a condom (Johnsen & Harlow, 1996; Kalichman, Williams, Cherry, Belcher, & Nachimson, 1998; Wingood & DiClemente, 1997) or who is physically or sexually abusive (M. Cohen et al., 2000). Hypothetically, effects of CSA may predispose women to develop sexual relationships with men over whom they have little control, and effects of drinking or drug use may reduce women's ability to resist sexual imposition or to insist on condom use.

LIMITATIONS OF EXISTING RESEARCH

The available research evidence for the connections from CSA to substance use to risky sex has several major limitations. First, most of the research is cross-sectional rather than longitudinal, making it difficult to determine whether alcohol use is an antecedent of risky sex rather than an accompaniment or consequence. Second, most studies do not include analyses in which use of alcohol or other drugs is examined as an intervening variable, mediating or modifying the effects of CSA on later risky sexual activity. And, finally, most studies have been based on clinical, institutional, or convenience samples. As a consequence, it is unclear to what extent observed effects of CSA on substance use, and observed effects of substance use on risky sex, are contingent on special characteristics of these samples.

TESTING THE CONNECTIONS: CHILD SEXUAL ABUSE, ALCOHOL USE, AND RISKY SEX

Some evidence that partially overcomes the three limitations above is available from the National Study of Health and Life Experiences of Women, a continuing longitudinal study of antecedents and consequences of women's drinking behavior in the general U.S. population. The first wave of survey data was collected in 1981; the fifth 5-year wave of data was collected in 2001. Details of the sample design and survey methodology can be found in S. C. Wilsnack, Klassen, Schur, and Wilsnack (1991) and R. W. Wilsnack, Wilsnack, Kristjanson, and Harris (1998).

Sample

The findings presented here are based on a nationally representative sample of 709 women age 21 to 49 in 1991, who were interviewed in 1991 and again in 1996. The total 1991 sample (N = 1,099) included both women initially interviewed in 1981 (now age 31–96) and women age 21 to 30 added to the sample in 1991. The 1996 sample was age restricted, both for economic reasons (husbands or cohabiting partners were also interviewed, substantially increasing survey costs) and for epidemiological-based reasons (younger women were more likely both to be heavier drinkers and to have marital or cohabiting partners). Ninety percent of eligible women completed interviews in 1996. For data analysis, respondents were weighted to adjust for stratified sampling and subgroup variation in response rates. The upper age limit of 54 years in 1996 should not exclude many women who would be at risk for HIV infection. A limitation of the sample is that it does not include adolescents or women under age 26 in 1996.

Measures

Child Sexual Abuse

A detailed series of questions asked about experiences before age 18 of eight specific sexual activities (exposure of respondent's or other person's genitals, touching/fondling, sexual kissing, oral-genital activity [as initiator and recipient], anal intercourse, and vaginal intercourse) with follow-up questions about ages of onset, participants, and the respondent's feelings about each experience at the time it first occurred. These questions enabled us to determine whether a respondent had experienced CSA according to criteria developed in previous research (Wyatt, 1985). Safeguards against bias included asking only whether certain described events occurred and in what circumstances, without asking respondents to judge whether these events were abusive. The questions were asked late in the interviews (conducted by female interviewers), after rapport and trust had been established between interviewers and respondents; this may have contributed to a high completion rate (99%) of the CSA questions.

For the analyses reported here, CSA was defined (after Wyatt, 1985) as (a) any intrafamilial sexual activity before age 18 that was unwanted by the respondent or involved a family member 5 or more years older than the respondent and (b) any extrafamilial activity that occurred before age 18 and was unwanted or that occurred before age 13 and involved another person 5 or more years older than the respondent. In the total 1991 sample of 1,099 women, 21.4% of women reported CSA, 67.9% reported no CSA, 9.6% provided insufficient information to determine CSA, and 1.1% provided no information on childhood sexual experiences. (For additional details about CSA measures, see S. C. Wilsnack et al., 1997; for information about CSA prevalence and correlates, see Vogeltanz et al., 1999.)

Drinking Behavior

In both the 1991 and 1996 surveys, respondents who had consumed any alcohol in the preceding 12 months answered questions about their typical drinking patterns (frequencies and quantities per drinking day), their frequencies of intoxication and of having six or more drinks in a day, and their recent and lifetime experiences with a set of adverse behavioral outcomes of drinking and a set of drinking patterns potentially symptomatic of alcohol dependence. Each respondent also reported the age at which she began drinking, as part of a lifetime drinking history. The analyses here used the measures of drinking versus abstaining, typical quantity of alcohol consumed per drinking day, frequency of days of having six or more drinks (heavy episodic drinking), and symptoms of potential alcohol dependence (e.g., memory lapses while drinking, morning drinking, loss of control over drinking). The measures of typical quantity, heavy episodic drinking, and symptoms of potential alcohol dependence were all log-transformed to reduce effects of skewness. Detailed descriptions of all drinking measures are provided in R. W. Wilsnack et al. (1998).

Alcohol-Related Risky Sexual Behavior

On the basis of factor analysis, a four-item index of alcohol-related risky sexual behavior included (a) frequency of drinking just before or during sexual activity with the respondent's current or most recent partner (*never, rarely, sometimes, usually*) and any experience in the past 12 months of (b) becoming sexually forward when drinking, (c) becoming less particular about sexual partners when drinking, and (d) experiencing sexually aggressive behavior from someone who had been drinking (Cronbach's α for 1991 index = .57, for 1996 index = .49). Respondents also reported the number of partners with whom they had sexual activity in the past 12 months. In addition, respondents reported their age of first sexual intercourse after puberty, as an experience separate from questions about CSA.

Background and Early Onset Variables

Background variables included the respondent's age and several characteristics of family life during the respondent's childhood: father's drinking (abstainer vs. drinker), mother's drinking (abstainer vs. light drinker vs. moderate-to-heavy drinker), rules against drinking (yes/no) in the religion in which the respondent was raised, the respondent's perception of her father and of her mother as loving or rejecting (on 5-point scales, with higher scores indicating rejection), and stability/disruption of the biological family (indicated by whether the respondent was or was not living with both biological parents at age 16). The respondent's reported age when she first began to drink and when she first had sexual intercourse were subtracted from age 18, so that higher scores indicate earlier onset.

Data Analysis

Imputation of Missing Values

The first step of data analysis was to impute missing values for several key variables. Missing values were imputed using multiple imputation (MI)

methods and software developed by Schafer (1997a, 1997b). Multiple imputations are several sets of imputed values that are deliberately caused to vary
so as to reflect the amount of uncertainty that exists about the true values of
the missing data. The MI software was designed to be used with panel data
and with cluster samples. To reflect the multistage sampling design, the imputation method used a multivariate mixed effects linear model. In this model,
the dependent variables were those with missing data, the fixed effects were
a set of variables with no missing values used to predict the dependent variables, and the random effect was based on sampling clusters. Multiple imputation creates wider confidence intervals for estimated values and lower risks
of Type I errors than other imputational methods based more simply on variable means or on single regression equations.

For the analyses presented here, values were imputed for those variables missing more than 20 data points. Mother's drinking pattern, age of
onset of drinking, and age of first intercourse were imputed simultaneously in
one MI procedure, and the eight components used to determine a history of
CSA were imputed in another procedure. Each procedure created 10 imputed data sets by iterations (10,000 iterations for the first data set, and an
additional 1,000 iterations for each successive data set). The imputed values
(and variation thereof) were derived from these data sets. In diagnostic tests
for possible biases across the iterations, time series plots for each parameter
showed no trend, and autocorrelation plots showed autocorrelations decreasing to zero at sufficiently large lags. (Further details of the imputation procedures are available from the authors on request.)

Path Analysis

After examining bivariate relationships, we analyzed multivariate relationships using path analysis. Path analysis is the simplest procedure for analyzing and describing time-ordered relationships among multiple variables in
a single causal model. It builds on multiple regression analysis and has been
widely used for many years in social research with large samples (J. Cohen &
Cohen, 1983; Pedhazur, 1997), including research on women's alcohol use/
abuse (R. W. Wilsnack, Wilsnack, & Klassen, 1987; Woldt & Bradley, 1996)
and on links between CSA and adult alcohol use/abuse (Epstein et al., 1998).
A major advantage of path analysis is that it can estimate both direct and
indirect effects of independent variables.

To carry out a path analysis, one must arrange all the variables to be
analyzed in a time sequence (a path model), with each independent variable assumed to have its effects before, after, or at the same time as specific
other variables. Path analysis also assumes that relationships between time-
ordered variables are one-directional and that all relationships between
variables are linear. With these assumptions, a hierarchical series of multiple regression equations can be used to construct a path diagram, with

arrows showing how each variable is connected to the other variables, and with the standardized regression coefficients (path coefficients) showing how strong the connection is from one variable to a later one, controlling for the effects of all other antecedent and simultaneous independent variables.

The path model for our analyses (see Figure 8.1) had four time-ordered stages: (a) background characteristics, including reported characteristics of the respondent's parents and upbringing; (b) CSA history (present or absent), age of onset of drinking, and age of first sexual intercourse; (c) 1991 drinking and risky sexual behavior; and (d) 1996 drinking and risky sexual behavior. The equation predicting each variable in a subsequent stage was derived by stepwise backward elimination from the set of all antecedent variables, until removal of another variable would significantly reduce ($p < .05$) the explanatory power of the equation. From each derived equation the model retained only the paths with statistically significant coefficients ($p < .05$, two-tailed). We had no theoretical basis for constructing a model with non-linear relationships and no theoretical basis for creating latent variables (i.e., combining variables used in the model in Figure 8.1). However, we did modify conventional path analysis by using logistic regression rather than ordinary least squares regression to predict CSA experience (as a dichotomous variable) from background variables; because of this modification, the resulting path diagram indicates the direction of statistically significant paths (with inverse relationships indicated by a negative sign) but does not provide estimates of numerical path coefficients.

In the model presented here, CSA experience, age of onset of drinking, and age of first sexual intercourse are entered in the same stage, without assumptions about time ordering among these variables. The time orders of these variables varied among respondents. For example, onset of CSA did not always precede the onset of drinking or first non-CSA intercourse, although this was the pattern among 85% of the respondents who reported CSA. The model used here allowed us to make maximum use of information about early experiences from the maximum number of respondents. However, we also compared patterns in this model with patterns in five other variations of the model: (a) eliminating imputations, with listwise exclusion of respondents with missing data; (b) requiring that CSA precede onset of drinking and voluntary sexual intercourse, that is, excluding those women who first experienced CSA after the onset of drinking or sexual intercourse; (c) limiting analyses to those women who were drinkers in 1991 or 1996, and including 1991 and 1996 measures of heavy episodic drinking and symptoms of potential alcohol dependence; (d) treating CSA, early drinking, and early sexual intercourse as a syndrome, using a single measure of the number of these three experiences that the respondent reported; and (e) introducing possible interaction effects of CSA with early onsets of drinking and sexual intercourse.

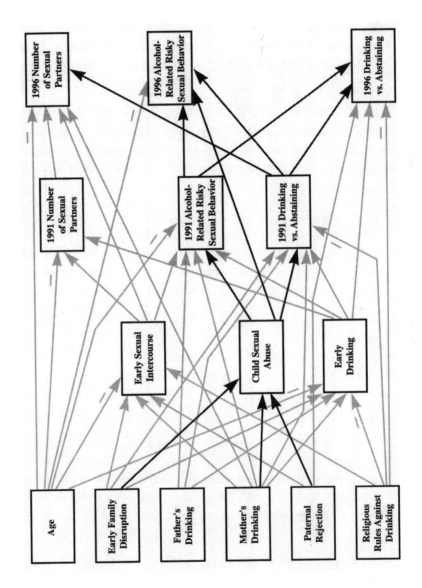

Figure 8.1. A model of child sexual abuse (CSA) and adult drinking and risky sexual behavior. Negative signs indicate inverse relationship. Predictors and effects of CSA are shown in darker-line paths to highlight the relationships that are the most important given the CSA focus of this chapter.

Bivariate Relationships

For the total sample, CSA was associated with an earlier age of first sexual intercourse and with alcohol-related risky sexual behavior in 1991 and 1996 ($rs = .15$, $ps < .001$) but was more weakly associated with the number of sexual partners ($rs = .11$, $p < .05$ only in 1996). Family background characteristics associated with CSA included mother's drinking, father's rejection, and separation from one or both biological parents by age 16 ($rs = .15$, $ps < .001$); CSA was also weakly associated with father's drinking versus abstaining ($r = .08$, $p < .05$).

Child sexual abuse was weakly associated with earlier onset of drinking and with alcohol use in 1991 and 1996 ($rs = .11$, $ps < .05$), but among women drinkers CSA generally was not associated with frequency of heavy episodic drinking (six or more drinks in a day) or with symptoms of potential alcohol dependence. The one significant association was with dependence symptoms in 1991 ($r = .15$, $p < .01$).

Among women drinkers, heavy episodic drinking and alcohol dependence symptoms were both strongly associated (cross-sectionally) with alcohol-related risky sexual behavior in 1991 and in 1996 (rs ranging from .30 to .51, $ps < .001$). Heavy episodic drinking and dependence symptoms were also moderately associated with the number of sexual partners in 1991 ($rs = .33$ and .29, respectively) and to a lesser extent in 1996 ($rs = .16$ and .17, respectively, all $ps < .001$).

Path Analyses

Predictors of Child Sexual Abuse and Early Onsets of Drinking and Sexual Intercourse

Figure 8.1 shows the statistically significant results of multivariate analyses using our main four-stage path model, with CSA and ages of onset of drinking and sexual intercourse entered simultaneously in the second stage. Predictors of CSA, and both direct and indirect effects of CSA, are shown as darker-line paths to highlight the relationships that are the most important given the CSA focus of this chapter. Women reporting histories of CSA and early intercourse were more likely to report having rejecting fathers, drinking mothers, and childhood separation from their biological parents. Having drinking mothers or drinking fathers, and being separated from biological parents, were associated with early drinking. Earlier onset of drinking and of sexual intercourse were more likely to be reported by younger women. If women had been taught religious rules against drinking, onset of drinking was delayed but first sexual intercourse occurred at a younger age. After age and family background variables were controlled for, early sexual intercourse was weakly associated with CSA and early onset of drinking (partial correlations of .09 and .11, respectively; $ps < .05$), but there was no association between CSA and early onset of drinking.

Predictors of Drinking, Risky Sex, and Number of Sexual Partners, in 1991

In 1991, women reported more sexual partners, and were more likely to have engaged in alcohol-related risky sexual activity, if they were young and if they had begun to drink and to have sexual intercourse at early ages. A history of CSA also increased the likelihood of alcohol-related risky sexual activity, as did a background of drinking by mother or by father. Women were more likely to be drinkers in 1991 (rather than abstainers) not only if their fathers or their mothers were drinkers and if they had begun drinking at an early age, but also if they had experienced CSA and early separation from one or both biological parents.

Predictors of Drinking, Risky Sex, and Number of Sexual Partners, in 1996

Alcohol-related risky sexual behavior in 1991 predicted such behavior in 1996, and the number of sexual partners in 1991 predicted the number of sexual partners in 1996. After controlling for 1991 drinking and sexual behavior, and all earlier experiences, CSA experience still directly increased the risks of women's alcohol-related risky sexual behavior in 1996. Being younger and being a drinker in 1991 were associated with both alcohol-related risky sex and number of sexual partners in 1996. Early onset of sexual activity and having a drinking mother predicted having a greater number of sexual partners in 1996. Women were more likely to be drinkers in 1996 if they had experienced rejection by their fathers and early onset of drinking, and if in 1991 they had been drinkers and had engaged in alcohol-related risky sexual activity. Religious rules against drinking learned in childhood made it less likely that women would drink in 1991 or in 1996.

Alternative Models

To analyze the path model presented in Figure 8.1, we made several assumptions about missing data, linear relationships, the time ordering of variables, and the appropriate group of women to be included. To evaluate the consequences and justification for making those assumptions, we also analyzed and evaluated five possible modifications of the main path model. These are discussed below.

Listwise Deletion

Instead of using multiple imputation to estimate missing values of key variables, we constructed a model based on listwise deletion of respondents with missing data on any variables in the model. The model produced by this procedure lost nine paths from the main model and gained only two (associating younger age with a history of CSA and associating early sexual intercourse directly with alcohol-related risky sex in 1996). There were no changes in directions of other paths. In general, this procedure weakened the analyses in a potentially biasing way (because the respondents eliminated by listwise deletion were not a random subset of the total sample).

Requiring Child Sexual Abuse Before Onset of Drinking or Sexual Intercourse

Using the imputed data, we required the onset of CSA to precede the onset of drinking and first sexual intercourse, excluding respondents who did not meet this stipulation. The aim was to reveal any direct influences of CSA on early drinking and early intercourse that might indirectly affect adult drinking and sexual behavior. No such influences of CSA were discovered, nor were any other new paths revealed. Instead, six paths in the main model disappeared, including paths connecting father's drinking and childhood separation from biological parents to early drinking, and connecting CSA to alcohol-related risky sex in 1991. The procedure weakened analyses in a potentially biasing way (by excluding 63 respondents who experienced CSA that did not clearly precede the onset of drinking and sexual intercourse) without uncovering any new influences of CSA.

Analyses of Drinkers Only

We reanalyzed the model with imputed data but using responses only from women who were drinkers rather than abstainers in 1991 or in 1996. We also introduced 1991 and 1996 measures of heavy episodic drinking and symptoms of potential alcohol dependence into these analyses. It was possible that this procedure might reveal links between sexual and drinking experience that were obscured by including abstainers in the analyses. However, among women drinkers, early onset of drinking no longer had any connection with alcohol-related risky sex. CSA experience no longer had any connection with 1991 sexual or drinking behavior, but early intercourse predicted higher rates of heavy episodic drinking in 1991 and 1996. Neither heavy episodic drinking nor dependence symptoms in 1991 had any connection with alcohol-related risky sex or the number of sexual partners reported in 1996, indicating that effects of 1991 drinking in the original model are not dependent on exceptionally heavy or hazardous drinking patterns. The lack of evidence for any enhanced effects of drinking experience on risky sexual activity, coupled with the biasing effect of systematically excluding nondrinking women, limits the utility of analyzing data only from women who drink.

Child Sexual Abuse/Early Intercourse/Early Drinking "Syndrome"

It is possible that experiences of CSA, early intercourse, and early drinking are signs of some underlying syndrome of childhood vulnerability or dysfunctional family environment. In that case, the number and diversity of such early experiences might affect adult behavior more than which specific experiences a woman had had. We reanalyzed the model with imputed data but using a single variable for the sum of three childhood experiences (CSA, early intercourse, and early drinking) instead of treating these experiences as separate variables. This simplified model did not improve the prediction of sexual and drinking behavior in 1991 or 1996. It did produce three new significant paths: direct influences of early family disruption and father's drinking on the number of sexual partners in 1991, as well as direct effects of father's drinking on 1996 drinking, separate from any effects of the "syndrome" of childhood experiences. However, the simplified model also eliminated early effects of religious rules against drinking (negative for early drinking, positive for early intercourse in the original model) and effects of father's drinking on early drinking; it eliminated effects of early drinking on 1996 drinking and effects of early intercourse on the number of sexual partners in 1996; and it eliminated the association of young age with alcohol-related risky sexual activity in 1996. In short, reducing the measures of early experiences to an additive measure of a "syndrome" did not improve the explanatory power of the model, added few new paths (none to or from the syndrome) while removing more paths (some from syndrome experiences), and generally reduced the amount of information provided by the model.

Interactions Among Child Sexual Abuse, Early Drinking, and Early Intercourse

Finally, we evaluated how the model would be modified by including interaction effects from experiencing combinations of CSA with early drinking or with early intercourse. (This version of the model did not use backward elimination because of the need to retain both direct and interaction effects of variables in the model.) Combinations of CSA with early drinking or early intercourse had no significant interaction effects on 1991 variables. For 1996 variables, the interaction of CSA and early intercourse experience increased the likelihood of drinking rather than abstaining and increased the number of sexual partners, whereas the interaction of CSA and early drinking experience increased the likelihood of alcohol-related risky sexual activity. Inclusion of interaction effects eliminated any direct effects of CSA (perhaps because of multicollinearity), but in 1991 early drinking still increased the likelihood of drinking, and early intercourse was still associated with more sexual partners and more risky sexual activity. Including the interaction effects neither added nor eliminated significant paths from other variables in the model.

CONCLUSION

Summary of Findings

The path analyses reported here indicate that in the general population, women who have experienced CSA report greater involvement in alcohol-related risky sexual behavior as adults. Women who have experienced CSA are also more likely to be drinkers rather than abstainers, which in turn increases their likelihood of engaging in alcohol-related risky sexual behavior and having larger numbers of sexual partners. However, such effects of CSA are not mediated by how heavily women drink. The data do not suggest that CSA leads women in general to consume so much alcohol that they become more reckless in their sexual activities or more unable to resist sexual imposition.

Sexual intercourse at an early age also predicts that a woman in adulthood will engage in more alcohol-related risky sexual activity and will have more sexual partners. Drinking at an early age predicts that women will continue to drink in adulthood (and will have more sexual partners and engage in more alcohol-related sexual activity). If CSA leads to early sexual intercourse and early drinking, it could thus indirectly lead to sexual behavior with higher risks of HIV infection. However, among women who experienced CSA prior to any drinking or sexual intercourse, we found no evidence that CSA accelerated the onsets of drinking and sexual intercourse, and no evidence that CSA mediated family influences on these early experiences. Furthermore, in all the models we tested, family characteristics not only influenced multiple childhood experiences (including CSA) but also continued to influence women's adult sexual and drinking behavior, separate from effects of CSA and early drinking and intercourse. These findings suggest that CSA is only one of several important childhood influences on adult risks of HIV infection.

It is possible that CSA may more strongly affect women's adult sexual risks when it occurs together with early drinking or early sexual intercourse. Simply summing how many of these experiences had occurred did not improve the predictions of adult drinking and sexual behavior. However, CSA in combination with early drinking was associated with more risky sexual behavior, and CSA in combination with early sexual intercourse was associated with drinking and a larger number of sexual partners, to a greater extent than could be accounted for by just adding together the separate effects of the two experiences.

Implications for Future Research and Intervention

Research Needs

Contrary to expectations based on clinical experience and opinion, CSA in this study was only one of several early experiences that predicted increased likelihood of high-risk sexual behavior. CSA was neither a mediator of earlier family experiences on later drinking or sexual behavior nor a major predictor of early onset of drinking and sexual intercourse. Future research should attempt to replicate these findings using other samples of women (e.g., including women younger than 26 and older than 54 and larger subsamples of women of color), additional measures of CSA characteristics including severity, and measures specifically developed to assess various patterns of high-risk sexual behavior.

It is possible that effects of CSA are contingent on childhood conditions and subsequent adult experiences not included in the present analyses, for example, women's experience with marriage or other intimate relationships (see, e.g., Jennison & Johnson, 2001) and women's use of substances other than alcohol. Future research designed to analyze such complex interactions of CSA with other childhood and adult experiences may help to explicate how CSA may lead some women to engage in high-risk sexual activity, whereas other women may be more immune or resilient to such effects of CSA.

Possible Implications for Prevention and Treatment

If future research supports the findings here that CSA combines with other early experiences (e.g., early alcohol use and sexual intercourse) to predict subsequent patterns of sexual risk-taking, these findings may suggest approaches to prevention of high-risk sexual behavior. Identification of target groups and prevention messages may be more effective if they address young women who have had any of a number of related experiences, including histories of CSA, early drinking, and early sexual activity. This "clustered" rather than behavior-specific prevention approach might include an abuse awareness and support component for young women with CSA histories, together with individual- and peer-oriented strategies to delay the onset of alcohol use and sexual intercourse. Secondary prevention or treatment of women already exhibiting high-risk sexual behavior might benefit from efforts to increase women's awareness of a variety of possible contributing factors (including family characteristics such as early family disruption, parental drinking, and parental rejection; CSA history; and experiences of early alcohol use or sexual intercourse) and how these experiences may be affecting a woman's current choices about her sexual behavior.

Finally, the finding that family background characteristics such as parental drinking, family disruption, and parental rejection not only predict the likelihood of CSA but also continue to influence women's drinking behavior and sexual risk-taking in adulthood, independent of other early experiences, has several potential implications. First, an increased understanding of family background characteristics associated with increased likelihood of CSA may offer clues for eventual efforts to reduce the societal prevalence of CSA. Second, as noted earlier, interventions with women already engaging in high-risk sexual behavior should include attention to early family experiences as possible sources of social learning or psychological distress that may contribute to a woman's current choices about her sexual partners and sexual behavior. Third, education and training designed to improve women's (and men's) parenting skills, in addition to their potential value in many other areas, may also have a positive intergenerational effect of reducing daughters' risks of experiencing CSA, early alcohol use and sexual behavior, and subsequent high-risk sexual behavior. Taken as a whole, greater understanding of the complex interactions of variables—family background characteristics, CSA and other early experiences, and substance use and other adult experiences—that increase high-risk sexual behavior can inform the design of better-focused interventions to increase resilience and reduce the damaging effects of CSA for women who experience early sexual victimization.

REFERENCES

Abbey, A., McAuslan, P., & Ross, L. T. (1998). Sexual assault perpetration by college men: The role of alcohol, misperception of sexual intent, and sexual beliefs and experiences. *Journal of Social and Clinical Psychology, 17*, 167–195.

Anderson, J. E., & Dahlberg, L. L. (1992). High-risk sexual behavior in the general population: Results from a national survey, 1988–1990. *Sexually Transmitted Diseases, 19*, 320–325.

Bensley, L. S., Van Eenwyk, J., & Simmons, K. W. (2000). Self-reported childhood sexual and physical abuse and adult HIV-risk behaviors and heavy drinking. *American Journal of Preventive Medicine, 18*, 151–158.

Browning, C. R., & Laumann, E. O. (1997). Sexual contact between children and adults: A life course perspective. *American Sociological Review, 62*, 540–560.

Clark, D. B., Lesnick, L., & Hegedus, A. M. (1997). Traumas and other adverse life events in adolescents with alcohol abuse and dependence. *Journal of the American Academy of Child and Adolescent Psychiatry, 36*, 1744–1751.

Cohen, J., & Cohen, P. (1983). *Applied multiple regression/correlation analysis for the behavioral sciences* (2nd ed.). Hillsdale, NJ: Erlbaum.

Cohen, M., Deamant, C., Barkan, S., Richardson, J., Young, M., Holman, S., et al. (2000). Domestic violence and childhood sexual abuse in HIV-infected women and women at risk for HIV. *American Journal of Public Health, 90*, 560–565.

Cooper, M. L., Peirce, B. S., & Huselid, R. F. (1994). Substance use and sexual risk-taking among Black adolescents and White adolescents. *Health Psychology, 13*, 251–262.

Corcoran, K. J., & Bell, B. G. (1990). Opposite sex perceptions of the effects of alcohol consumption on subsequent sexual activity in a college dating situation. *Psychology: A Journal of Human Behavior, 27*(2), 7–11.

Corcoran, K. J., & Thomas, L. R. (1991). The influence of observed alcohol consumption on perceptions of initiation of sexual activity in a college dating situation. *Journal of Applied Social Psychology, 21*, 500–507.

Downs, W. R., & Harrison, L. (1998). Childhood maltreatment and the risk of substance problems in later life. *Health and Social Care in the Community, 6*, 35–46.

Epstein, J. N., Saunders, B. E., Kilpatrick, D. G., & Resnick, H. S. (1998). PTSD as a mediator between childhood rape and alcohol use in adult women. *Child Abuse and Neglect, 22*, 223–234.

Fenaughty, A. M., & Fisher, D. G. (1998). High-risk sexual behavior among drug users: The utility of a typology of alcohol variables. *Sexually Transmitted Diseases, 25*, 38–43.

Fergusson, D. M., Horwood, L. J., & Lynskey, M. T. (1996). Childhood sexual abuse and psychiatric disorder in young adulthood: II. Psychiatric outcomes of childhood sexual abuse. *Journal of the American Academy of Child and Adolescent Psychiatry, 35*, 1365–1374.

Galaif, E. R., Stein, J. A., Newcomb, M. D., & Bernstein, D. P. (2001). Gender differences in the prediction of problem alcohol use in adulthood: Exploring the influence of family factors and childhood maltreatment. *Journal of Studies on Alcohol, 62*, 486–493.

Garcia, L. T., & Kushnier, K. (1987). Sexual inferences about female targets: The use of sexual experience correlates. *Journal of Sex Research, 23*, 252–256.

George, W. H., Cue, K. L., Lopez, P. A., Crowe, L. C., & Norris, J. (1995). Self-reported alcohol expectancies and postdrinking sexual inferences about women. *Journal of Applied Social Psychology, 25*, 164–186.

George, W. H., Lehman, G. L., Cue, K. L., Martinez, L. J., Lopez, P. A., & Norris, J. (1997). Postdrinking sexual inferences: Evidence for linear rather than curvilinear dosage effects. *Journal of Applied Social Psychology, 27*, 629–648.

Goodman, L. A., & Fallot, R. D. (1998). HIV risk-behavior in poor urban women with serious mental disorders: Association with childhood physical and sexual abuse. *American Journal of Orthopsychiatry, 68*, 73–83.

Graves, K. L., & Hines, A. M. (1997). Ethnic differences in the association between alcohol and risky sexual behavior with a new partner: An event-based analysis. *AIDS Education and Prevention, 9*, 219–237.

Halpern-Felsher, B. L., Millstein, S. G., & Ellen, J. M. (1996). Relationship of alcohol use and risky sexual behavior: A review and analysis of findings. *Journal of Adolescent Health, 19*, 331–336.

Harrison, P. A., Fulkerson, J. A., & Beebe, T. J. (1997). Multiple substance use among adolescent physical and sexual abuse victims. *Child Abuse and Neglect, 21*, 529–539.

Harvey, S. M., & Beckman, L. J. (1986). Alcohol consumption, female sexual behavior and contraceptive use. *Journal of Studies on Alcohol, 47*, 327–332.

Hingson, R. W., Strunin, L., Berlin, B. M., & Heeren, T. (1990). Beliefs about AIDS, use of alcohol and drugs, and unprotected sex among Massachusetts adolescents. *American Journal of Public Health, 80*, 295–299.

Jantzen, K., Ball, S. A., Leventhal, J. M., & Schottenfeld, R. S. (1998). Types of abuse and cocaine use in pregnant women. *Journal of Substance Abuse Treatment, 15*, 319–323.

Jennison, K. M., & Johnson, K. A. (2001). Parental alcoholism as a risk factor for DSM–IV-defined alcohol abuse and dependence in American women: The protective benefits of dyadic cohesion in marital communication. *American Journal of Drug and Alcohol Abuse, 27,* 349–374.

Johnsen, L. W., & Harlow, L. L. (1996). Childhood sexual abuse linked with adult substance use, victimization, and AIDS-risk. *AIDS Education and Prevention, 8,* 44–57.

Kalichman, S. C., Williams, E. A., Cherry, C., Belcher, L., & Nachimson, D. (1998). Sexual coercion, domestic violence, and negotiating condom use among low-income African American women. *Journal of Women's Health, 7,* 371–378.

Kendler K. S., Bulik, C. M., Silberg, J., Hettema, J. M., Myers, J., & Prescott, C. A. (2000). Childhood sexual abuse and adult psychiatric and substance use disorders in women: An epidemiological and cotwin control analysis. *Archives of General Psychiatry, 57,* 953–959.

Kirkham, C. M., & Lobb, D. J. (1998). The British Columbia Positive Women's Survey: A detailed profile of 110 HIV-infected women. *Canadian Medical Association Journal, 158,* 317–323.

Lauchli, S., Heusser, R., Tschopp, A., Gutzwiller, F., Hornung, R., Twisselmann, W., et al. (1996). Safer sex behavior and alcohol consumption. *Annals of Epidemiology, 6,* 357–364.

Leigh, B. C., Temple, M. T., & Trocki, K. F. (1994). The relationship of alcohol use to sexual activity in a U.S. national sample. *Social Science and Medicine, 39,* 1527–1535.

McCauley, J., Kern, D. E., Kolodner, K., Dill, L., Schroeder, A. F., DeChant, H. K., et al. (1997). Clinical characteristics of women with a history of childhood abuse: Unhealed wounds. *Journal of the American Medical Association, 277,* 1362–1368.

McEwan, R. T., McCallum, A., Bhopal, R. S., & Madhok, R. (1992). Sex and the risk of HIV infection: The role of alcohol. *British Journal of Addiction, 87,* 577–584.

Miller, B. A., Downs, W. R., & Testa, M. (1993). Interrelationships between victimization experiences and women's alcohol use. *Journal of Studies on Alcohol, Supplement 11,* 109–117.

Molitor, F., Truax, S. R., Ruiz, J. D., & Sun, R. K. (1998). Association of methamphetamine use during sex with risky sexual behaviors and HIV infection among non-injection drug users. *Western Journal of Medicine, 168,* 93–97.

Mullen, P. E., Martin, J. L., Anderson, J. C., Romans, S. E., & Herbison, G. P. (1993). Childhood sexual abuse and mental health in adult life. *British Journal of Psychiatry, 163,* 721–732.

Mullen, P. E., Martin, J. L., Anderson, J. C., Romans, S. E., & Herbison, G. P. (1994). The effect of child sexual abuse on social, interpersonal and sexual function in adult life. *British Journal of Psychiatry, 165,* 35–47.

Parker, D. A., Harford, T. C., & Rosenstock, I. M. (1994). Alcohol, other drugs, and sexual risk-taking among young adults. *Journal of Substance Abuse, 6,* 87–93.

Pedhazur, E. J. (1997). *Multiple regression in behavioral research* (3rd ed.). New York: Harcourt Brace.

Perry, M. J., Solomon, I. J., Winett, R. A., Kelly, J. A., Roffman, R. A., Desiderato, L. L., et al. (1994). High risk sexual behavior and alcohol consumption among bar-going gay men. *AIDS, 8,* 1321–1324.

Potthoff, S. J., Bearinger, L. H., Skay, C. L., Cassuto, N., Blum, R. W., & Resnick, M. D. (1998). Dimensions of risk behaviors among American Indian youth. *Archives of Pediatrics and Adolescent Medicine, 152,* 157–163.

Robertson, J. A., & Plant, M. A. (1988). Alcohol, sex, and risks of HIV infection. *Drug and Alcohol Dependence, 22,* 75–78.

Schafer, J. L. (1997a). *Analysis of incomplete multivariate data.* London: Chapman & Hall.

Schafer, J. L. (1997b). *Imputation of missing covariates under a multivariate linear mixed model.* University Park: Pennsylvania State University, Department of Statistics. Retrieved February 13, 1997, from http://www.stat.psu.edu/~jls

Schuck, A. M., & Widom, C. S. (2001). Childhood victimization and alcohol symptoms in females: Causal inferences and hypothesized mediators. *Child Abuse and Neglect, 25,* 1069–1092.

Sly, F., Quadagno, D., Harrison, D. F., Eberstein, I., & Riehman, K. (1997). The association between substance use, condom use and sexual risk among low-income women. *Family Planning Perspectives, 29,* 132–136.

Spak, L., Spak, F., & Allebeck, P. (1998). Sexual abuse and alcoholism in a female population. *Addiction, 93,* 1365–1373.

Temple, M. T., Leigh, B. C., & Schafer, J. (1993). Unsafe sexual behavior and alcohol use at the event level: Results of a national survey. *Journal of Acquired Immune Deficiency Syndromes, 6,* 393–401.

Testa, M., & Collins, R. L. (1997). Alcohol and risky sexual behavior: Event-based analyses among a sample of high-risk women. *Psychology of Addictive Behaviors, 11,* 190–201.

Thompson, N. J., Potter, J. S., Sanderson, C. A., & Maibach, E. W. (1997). The relationship of sexual abuse and HIV risk behaviors among heterosexual adult female STD patients. *Child Abuse and Neglect, 21,* 149–156.

Vogeltanz, N. D., Wilsnack, S. C., Harris, T. R., Wilsnack, R. W., Wonderlich, S. A., & Kristjanson, A. F. (1999). Prevalence and risk factors for childhood sexual abuse in women: National survey findings. *Child Abuse and Neglect, 23,* 579–592.

Vogeltanz-Holm, N. D. (2002). Childhood sexual abuse and risk for psychopathology. In N. J. Smelser & P. B. Baltes (Eds.), *International encyclopedia of the social and behavioral sciences, Vol. 3* (pp. 1712–1716). London: Elsevier Science.

Widom, C. S., & Kuhns, J. B. (1996). Childhood victimization and subsequent risk for promiscuity, prostitution, and teenage pregnancy: A prospective study. *American Journal of Public Health, 86,* 1607–1612.

Wilsnack, R. W., Wilsnack, S. C., & Klassen, A. D. (1987). Antecedents and consequences of drinking and drinking problems in women: Patterns from a U.S. national survey. In P. C. Rivers (Ed.), *Nebraska Symposium on Motivation: Vol.*

34. Alcohol and addictive behavior (pp. 85–158). Lincoln: University of Nebraska Press.

Wilsnack, R. W., Wilsnack, S. C., Kristjanson, A. F., & Harris, T. R. (1998). Ten-year prediction of women's drinking behavior in a nationally representative sample. *Women's Health: Research on Gender, Behavior, and Policy, 4*, 199–230.

Wilsnack, S. C., Klassen, A. D., Schur, B. E., & Wilsnack, R. W. (1991). Predicting onset and chronicity of women's problem drinking: A five-year longitudinal analysis. *American Journal of Public Health, 81*, 305–318.

Wilsnack, S. C., Vogeltanz, N. D., Klassen, A. D., & Harris, T. R. (1997). Childhood sexual abuse and women's substance abuse: National survey findings. *Journal of Studies on Alcohol, 58*, 264–271.

Wingood, G. M., & DiClemente, R. J. (1997). Child sexual abuse, HIV sexual risk, and gender relations of African-American women. *American Journal of Preventive Medicine, 13*, 380–384.

Wingood, G. M., & DiClemente, R. J. (1998). The influence of psychosocial factors, alcohol, drug use on African-American women's high-risk sexual behavior. *American Journal of Preventive Medicine, 15(1)*, 54–59.

Woldt, B. D., & Bradley, J. R. (1996). Precursors, mediators and problem drinking: Path analytic models for men and women. *Journal of Drug Education, 26*, 1–12.

Wyatt, G. E. (1985). The sexual abuse of Afro-American and white-American women in childhood. *Child Abuse and Neglect, 9*, 507–519.

Zierler, S., Feingold, L., Laufer, D., Velentgas, P., Kantrowitz-Gordon, I., & Mayer, K. (1991). Adult survivors of childhood sexual abuse and subsequent risk of HIV infection. *American Journal of Public Health, 81*, 572–575.

9

TRANSLATING TRAUMATIC EXPERIENCES INTO LANGUAGE: IMPLICATIONS FOR CHILD ABUSE AND LONG-TERM HEALTH

JAMES W. PENNEBAKER AND LORI D. STONE

Traumatic experiences in childhood, especially those that cannot openly be discussed with others, place individuals at higher risk for illness. In the last several years, multiple laboratories have provided compelling evidence that traumatic childhood traumas, especially sexual traumas, are associated with much higher rates of a variety of major and minor illnesses (Pennebaker & Susman, 1988), higher usage of medical facilities in general, and diagnoses of various problems such as irritable bowel syndrome (Drossman, 1997; Pennebaker & Susman, 1988). In exploring some of the links between traumatic sexual experiences and health, we proposed that actively not talking about major life upheavals constituted a form of behavioral inhibition. The work of inhibition, we reasoned, was stressful and resulted in a number of measurable autonomic, hormonal, and immune changes linked to greater incidence of illness (e.g., Pennebaker, 1989, 1997).

Preparation of this chapter was aided by Grant No. MH52391 from the National Institutes of Health.

The evidence for the increased health risk of long-term inhibition is now solidly established. Various researchers have contributed converging evidence to suggest that keeping long-term secrets is unhealthy. Results from projects with inhibited children (e.g., Kagan et al., 1994), students induced to inhibit emotions (e.g., Gross & Levenson, 1997), and even individuals who are chronically inhibited (e.g., Jamner, Schwartz, & Leigh, 1988) have shown that inhibited individuals are more likely to exhibit elevated autonomic levels, higher resting cortisol, and suppressed immune function. In addition, gay men who keep their sexual orientation secret have higher rates of cancer and, if they are HIV-positive, are more prone to early death. Indeed, the link between concealing gay status is related to health problems in a dose–response relationship (Cole, Kemeny, Taylor, & Visscher, 1996; Cole, Kemeny, Taylor, Visscher, & Fahey, 1996).

In recent years, we have begun examining ways by which to improve the health and functioning of individuals who have experienced traumatic events in their lives. We have been most interested in those who have had traumas about which they have not spoken to others. As discussed below, an increasing body of work indicates that translating upsetting experiences into words has a significant health impact. A guiding assumption of the present work is that the act of constructing stories is a natural human process that helps individuals to understand their experiences and themselves. This process allows one to organize and remember events in a coherent fashion while integrating thoughts and feelings. In essence, this gives individuals a sense of predictability and control over their lives. Once an experience has structure and meaning, it would follow that the emotional effects of that experience would be more manageable. Constructing stories facilitates a sense of resolution, which results in less rumination and eventually allows disturbing experiences gradually to subside from conscious thought. Painful events that are not structured into a narrative format may contribute to the continued experience of negative thoughts and feelings. Indeed, one of the most prevalent reasons why people begin therapy is because they report suffering from emotional distress (Mahoney, 1995). Disclosure is unequivocally at the core of therapy. Psychotherapy usually involves putting together a story that will explain and organize major life events that cause distress.

Extensive research has revealed that when people put their emotional upheavals into words, their physical and mental health improve markedly. The first author (Pennebaker) began work in this area over a decade ago. In the initial studies, students were asked to write about their deepest thoughts and feelings about traumatic experiences as part of a laboratory experiment. The mere act of writing about traumatic experiences had surprising and striking results. The writing exercise improved the students' physical health, resulted in better grades, and often changed their lives.

The basic technique was straightforward (Pennebaker, 1997). Students were brought into the laboratory and were told that they would be participating in a study wherein they would write about an assigned topic for 4 consecutive days, for 15 minutes each day. They were assured that their writing would be anonymous and that they would not receive any feedback on it. As far as they knew, the purpose of the project was to learn more about writing and psychology. The only rule about the writing assignment was that once they began writing, they were to continue to do so without stopping and without regard to spelling, grammar, or sentence structure. Participants were then randomly assigned to either an experimental group or a control group.

Those randomly assigned to the experimental group were asked to spend each session writing about one or more traumatic experiences in their lives. *Trauma* was not further defined but rather was left to the subjective judgment of participants. Following are instructions and guidance from the experimenter:

> For the next 4 days, I would like you to write about your very deepest thoughts and feelings about the most traumatic experience of your entire life. In your writing, I would like you to really let go and explore your very deepest emotions and thoughts. You might tie your topic to your relationships with others, including parents, lovers, friends, or relatives, to your past, your present, or your future, or to who you have been, who you would like to be, or who you are now. You may write about the same general issues or experiences on all days of writing or on different traumas each day. All of your writing will be completely confidential.

Those who were assigned to the control condition were asked to write about nonemotional topics for 15 minutes on all 4 days of the study. Examples of their assigned writing topics included describing the laboratory room in which they were seated or their own living room. One group, then, was encouraged to delve into their emotions whereas the other was to describe objects and events dispassionately.

The first writing study yielded astounding results (Pennebaker & Beall, 1986). Most striking was that beginning college students immediately took to the task of writing. Those in the experimental condition averaged writing 340 words during each 15-minute session. Although many cried, the vast majority reported that they found the writing to be extremely valuable and meaningful. Indeed, 98% of the experimental participants said that, if given the choice, they would participate in the study again (Pennebaker, 1989, 1993). Most surprising was the nature of the writing itself. The students, who tended to come from upper-middle-class backgrounds, described a painful array of tragic and depressing stories. Rape, family violence, suicide attempts, drug problems, and other horrors were common topics. Indeed, approximately half of the students wrote about experiences that any clinician would agree were truly traumatic.

What made this first experiment so compelling, however, was not just the narratives themselves. Rather, we were primarily interested in how the writing exercise influenced physical health. During the school year, we followed the students' illness visits to the university health center in the months before and after the experiment. We discovered that those who had written about their thoughts and feelings drastically reduced their doctor visit rates after the study compared with our control participants who had written about trivial topics. Confronting traumatic experiences had a salutary effect on physical health.

Over the last decade, more than two dozen studies from multiple laboratories around the world have confirmed and extended the basic findings. Some of the general results include the following.

1. *Benefits are found across different populations.* Writing benefits a variety of groups of individuals beyond undergraduate college students. Positive health and behavioral effects have been found with maximum-security prisoners, medical students, community-based samples of distressed crime victims, arthritis and chronic pain sufferers, men laid off from their jobs, and women who have recently given birth to their first child. These effects have been found in all social classes and major racial/ethnic groups in the United States as well as in samples in Mexico City, New Zealand, French-speaking Belgium, and the Netherlands (Dominguez et al., 1995; Petrie, Booth, Pennebaker, Davison, & Thomas, 1995; Richards, Pennebaker, & Beal, 1995; Rimé, 1995; Schoutrop, Lange, Brosschot, & Everaerd, 1997; Spera, Buhrfeind, & Pennebaker, 1994).

2. *Short- versus long-term mood effects of writing.* Despite the clear health and behavioral effects, writing about traumatic experiences tends to make people feel more unhappy and distressed in the hours after writing. These emotions, in many ways, can be viewed as appropriate to the topics the individuals are confronting. When questionnaires are administered to participants at least 2 weeks after the studies, however, experimental volunteers report being as happy as or happier than control participants. It is interesting that among highly distressed samples, such as the unemployed male engineers, writing about losing their jobs produced immediate improvements in moods compared with controls. Emotional state after writing depends on how participants are feeling prior to writing: The better they feel before writing, the worse they feel afterward and vice versa (Pennebaker, 1997; Pennebaker, Colder, & Sharp, 1990).

3. *Talking versus writing.* Although most experiments have focused primarily on writing, a few studies have compared writ-

ing with talking into a tape recorder. Overall, writing and talking have produced comparable effects. Additional experiments by Murray and his colleagues (Donnelly & Murray, 1991; Murray, Lamnin, & Carver, 1989) at the University of Miami suggest that writing about traumatic experiences brings about comparable changes to talking to a psychotherapist, at least among a psychologically healthy sample. Additional research should be conducted to examine the efficacy of doing the emotional writing task verbally—perhaps privately into a tape recorder, to most closely match our current paradigm—in a wide variety of samples.

4. *Differences as a function of personality*. There are no strong indications that some personality types benefit more from writing than others do. An analysis of several writing studies by Smyth (1998) suggests that men may benefit somewhat more than women may. This effect, however, still must be tested in future studies. Although traditional measures of neuroticism, depression-proneness, and extraversion are unrelated to the benefits of writing, an experiment by Christensen and Smith (1993) indicates that individuals who are particularly hostile and suspicious benefited more from writing than people who were low in these traits.

5. *The audience*. The effects of writing are not related to the presumed audience. In most studies, participants turn in their writing samples with the understanding that only the experimenters will examine what they have written. Other experiments, however, have allowed participants to keep their writing samples, or in one master's thesis by Czajka (1987), students wrote on a child's magic pad where their writing was erased as soon as they lifted the plastic sheet on the writing tablet.

6. *Time parameters*. Although the original studies required participants to write on 4 consecutive days for 15 minutes each day, later studies have varied the number of sessions from 1 to 5 days from 15 minutes to 30 minutes each session. The summary project by Smyth (1998) hints that the longer time the study lasts, the better. Again, this effect needs to be examined experimentally.

7. *The writing topic*. A variety of writing topics produce comparable health benefits. Although the earlier studies asked volunteers to write about traumas, more recent experiments have had new students write about their thoughts and feelings about coming to college or, in the case of the unemployed male engineers, about the experience of being laid off (Spera et al.,

1994). Most impressive is a study by Greenberg, Stone, and Wortman (1997) wherein previously traumatized students were asked to write about an imaginary trauma rather than something that they had experienced directly. Their results indicated that writing about someone else's trauma as though they had lived through it produced health benefits comparable with a separate group who wrote about their own traumas. What is critical in all of these studies, however, is that people are encouraged to explore their emotions and thoughts no matter what the content might be.

WHAT ARE THE UNDERLYING MECHANISMS RESPONSIBLE FOR THESE BENEFITS?

Why does writing or talking about emotional experiences influence health? More recent efforts have been aimed at understanding the precise mechanisms underlying these changes. This has been the central question that has guided our research over the last several years. Three general research directions have provided a number of answers.

One possibility is that by writing about emotional experiences, people simply become more health conscious and change their behaviors accordingly. Very little evidence supports this. As indicated by Smyth's (1998) meta-analysis, most experiments find that after writing about emotional topics, participants continue to smoke, exercise, diet, and socialize in ways similar to those in the control conditions. The one exception may be alcohol intake. In two studies with adults, people who wrote about emotional topics later reported a drop in the amount of alcohol they were drinking each day. This pattern has not held up for college students or prisoners.

A second possible explanation for the value of writing is that it allows people to express themselves. If the driving process is self-expression, one could argue that both verbal and nonverbal forms of expression would provide comparable benefits. Dance, music, and art therapists, for example, assume that the expression of emotion through nonverbal means is therapeutic. It should be noted, however, that traditional research on catharsis or the venting of emotions has failed to support the clinical value of emotional expression in the absence of cognitive processing (Lewis & Bucher, 1992).

In our own lab, we have attempted to determine the degree to which language is necessary for physical and mental health improvement. In an experiment, Krantz and Pennebaker (1995) sought to learn if the disclosure of a trauma through dance or bodily movement would bring about health improvements in ways comparable with writing. In the study, students were asked to express a traumatic experience using bodily movement, to express an experience using movement and then to write about it, or to exercise in a

prescribed manner for 3 days, 10 minutes per day. Whereas the two movement expression groups reported that they felt happier and mentally healthier
in the months after the study, only the movement-plus-writing group evidenced significant improvements in physical health and grade point average.
The mere expression of a trauma is not sufficient to bring about long-term
physiological changes. Health gains appear to require translating experiences
into language.

A third broad explanation for the effects of writing is that the act of
converting emotions and images into words changes the way the person or-
ganizes and thinks about the trauma. Further, part of the distress caused by
the trauma lies not just in the events but also in the person's emotional reactions to them. By integrating thoughts and feelings, then, the person can
more easily construct a coherent narrative of the experience. Once formed,
the event can now be summarized, stored, and forgotten more efficiently.
Tests of this general idea are still in progress. However, preliminary findings
are encouraging.

One of our first systematic approaches to understanding the potential
cognitive benefits of writing was to examine the essays themselves. Independent raters initially compared the writing samples of people whose health subsequently improved after the experiment with those whose health remained
unchanged. Essays from those who improved were judged more self-reflective,
emotionally open, and thoughtful. Not being content with clinical evaluations, we decided to subject the essays to computer text analyses to learn if
language use could predict improvements in health among people who had
written about emotional topics.

No standard computer programs existed that specifically measured emotional and cognitive categories of word usage. We spent 3 years developing a
computer program called LIWC (Linguistic Inquiry and Word Count) that
analyzed essays in text format. LIWC was developed by having groups of
judges evaluate the degree to which over 2,000 words or word stems were
related to each of several dozen categories (Pennebaker & Francis, 1996).
Although there are now over 70 word categories in the most recent version
of the LIWC program (LIWC2001, from Pennebaker, Francis, & Booth,
2001), only 4 categories were of primary interest to us. Two of the categories
were emotion dimensions and the other 2 were cognitive. The emotion categories included negative emotion words (e.g., *sad, angry*) and positive emotion words (e.g., *happy, laugh*). The two cognitive categories, causal and insight words, were intended to capture the degree to which participants were
actively thinking in their writing. The causal words (e.g., *because, reason*)
were included because they implied people were attempting to put together
causes and reasons for the events and emotions that they were describing.
The insight words (e.g., *understand, realize*) reflected the degree to which
individuals were specifically referring to cognitive processes associated with
thinking. For each essay that a person wrote, we were able to quickly com-

pute the percentage of total words that these and other linguistic categories represented.

The LIWC program allowed us to go back to previous writing studies and link word usage among individuals in the experimental conditions with various health and behavioral outcomes. To date, the most extensive re-analysis of data concerns six writing studies: two studies involving college students writing about traumas in which blood immune measures were collected, two studies in which first-year college students wrote about their deepest thoughts and feelings about coming to college, one study by maximum-security prisoners in a state penitentiary, and one study using professionals who had unexpectedly been laid off from their jobs after over 20 years of employment.

In an analysis of the use of negative and positive emotion words, two important findings were revealed (Pennebaker, Mayne, & Francis, 1997). First, the more that people used positive emotion words, the more their health improved. Second, negative emotion word use also predicted health changes but in an unexpected way. Individuals who used a moderate number of negative emotions in their writing about upsetting topics evidenced the greatest drops in physician visits in the months after writing. That is, those people who used a very high rate of negative emotion words and those who used very few were the most likely to have continuing health problems after participating in the study. In many ways, these findings are consistent with other literatures. Individuals who tend to use very few negative emotion words are undoubtedly most likely to be characterized as repressive copers—people who Weinberger, Schwartz, and Davidson (1979) have defined as poor at being able to identify and label their emotional states. Those who overuse negative emotion words may well be the classic high neurotic or high negative affect (Watson & Clark, 1984) individuals. These individuals are people who ponder their negative emotions in exhaustive detail and who may simply be in a recursive loop of complaining without attaining closure. Indeed, this may be exacerbated by the inability of these individuals to develop a story or narrative.

Although the findings concerning emotion words use were intriguing, the results surrounding the cognitive word categories were even more robust. Recall that in our studies, people wrote for 3 to 5 days, 15 to 30 minutes per day. As they wrote, they gradually changed what they said and how they said it. The LIWC analyses showed strong and consistent effects for changes in insight and causal words over the course of writing. Specifically, people whose health improved, who got higher grades, and who found jobs after writing went from using relatively few causal and insight words to using a high rate of them by the last day of writing. In reading the essays of people who showed this pattern of language use, it became apparent that they were constructing a story over time. Building a narrative, then, seemed to be critical in reaching understanding. It is interesting to note that those people who started the study with a coherent story that explained some past experience did not benefit from writing (see Gergen & Gergen, 1988; Mahoney, 1995; Meichenbaum & Fong, 1993).

These findings are consistent with current views on narrative and psychotherapy in suggesting that it is critical for clients to confront their anxieties and problems by creating a story to explain and understand past and current life concerns. The story can be in the form of an autobiography or even a third-person narrative. It is interesting that our data indicate that merely having a story may not be sufficient to assure good health. A story that may have been constructed when the person was young or in the midst of a trauma may be insufficient later in life when new information is discovered or broader perspectives are adopted. In our studies, as in narrative therapies, the act of constructing the stories is associated with mental and physical health improvement. A constructed story, then, is a type of knowledge that helps to organize the emotional effects of an experience as well as the experience itself.

WHY DO PEOPLE FORM STORIES ABOUT THEIR EXPERIENCES?

One basic question in our research concerns why people tell stories. Where does this motivation to write come from? Part of it may arise from conflicted childhoods, adolescent tragedies, or other unexpected turns in life.

Within the psychological literature, there is a broadly accepted belief that humans—and perhaps most organisms with at least a moderately complex nervous system—seek to understand the world around them. If one feels pain or hears a strange noise, one tries to learn the cause of it. Once an individual understands how and why an event has occurred, he or she is more prepared to deal with it should it happen again. By definition, then, people will be far more motivated to learn about events that have unwanted or, on the contrary, very desired consequences than about common or predictable events that do not affect them. Similarly, events with large and significant personal consequences will be examined to a greater degree than relatively superficial events (see Kelley, 1967; Kohler, 1947).

Over the course of a normal day, people are constantly surveying and analyzing their worlds. The person in the car behind honks the horn while another sits at a red light. Automatically, the latter asks questions such as, "Is the person honking at me?" "Is the light green?" "Do I know this person?" As soon as the individual comes to some understanding as to the meaning of the horn honk, he or she adjusts his or her behavior (one goes if the light is green, waves if it is a friend) or returns to his or her private world if the honk was not relevant. As soon as this brief episode is over, the individual will probably put it out of his or her mind forever.

Whereas the search for the meaning of a honking horn is a brief, relatively automatic process, major life events are far more difficult to comprehend. If one's lover leaves, a close friend dies, or one faces a significant career setback, one generally mulls the event over in one's mind trying to understand the causes and consequences of it. To complicate matters, a major life event usually consists of many interrelated events and experiences. If one's lover has gone, it will affect one's relationships with others, finances, self-image, and even daily eating, sleeping, talking, and sexual habits. In trying to understand this experience, individuals will naturally attempt to ask themselves why this happened and how they can cope with it. To the degree that the event is unresolved, they will think, dream, obsess, and talk about it for days, weeks, or years.

Exactly what constitutes meaning or understanding is far less clear. Philosophers, psychologists, poets, and novelists have noted that a single event can have completely different meaning for different individuals. Following the death of a very close friend, some may find meaning in religion ("God has a plan"), others in understanding the cause of the death ("he smoked, what can you expect?"), and others in exploring the implications for their own lives ("he would have wanted me to change my life"). Simple analyses relying on a single causal explanation may be useful in explaining some aspects of the death but probably will not be helpful in all aspects. We may have a straightforward explanation on why the friend died, but we still must deal with a change in our friendship network, our daily routine of talking with our friend, and so on. The beauty of a narrative is that it allows us to tie all of the changes in our life into a broad comprehensive story. That is, in the same story we can talk both about the cause of the event and its many implications. Much as in any story, there can be overarching themes, plots, and subplots—many of them arranged logically or hierarchically. Through this process, then, the many facets of the presumed single event are organized into a more coherent whole.

Drawing on research on conversation and language, Clark (1993) pointed out that conveying a story to another person requires that the speech act be coherent. Linguistic coherence subsumes several characteristics, including structure, use of causal explanation, repetition of themes, and an appreciation of the listener's perspective. Referring to the work of Labov and Fanshel (1977), Clark emphasized that conversations virtually demand the conveying of stories or narratives that require an ordered sequence of events.

Once a complex event is put into a story format, it is simplified. The mind does not need to work as hard to bring structure and meaning to it. As the story is told over and over again, it becomes shorter with some of the finer detail gradually leveled. The information that is recalled in the story is that which is congruent with the story. Whereas the data (or raw experiences) were initially used to create the story, once the story is fixed in the person's mind only story-relevant data are conjured up. Further, as time passes, people have the tendency to fill in gaps in their story to make the story more cohesive and complete. The net effect of constructing a good narrative is that our recollection of emotional events is efficient—in that we have a relatively short, compact story—and undoubtedly biased (Novales, 1997; Pennebaker, Paez, & Rimé, 1997).

IMPLICATIONS OF WRITING FOR COMMUNITIES AT RISK

Despite the fact that writing studies are conducted predominantly with college students, the findings have been replicated on a variety of populations, as previously discussed. While the extension of this work to clinical populations and at-risk groups such as child sexual abuse (CSA) survivors or HIV-infected individuals is in the early stages, recent findings are certainly relevant. We discuss some of them below.

Impact on the Immune System

Writing influences more than just physician visits. Several studies have found that writing or talking about emotional topics influences immune function in beneficial ways, including T-helper cell growth (Pennebaker, Kiecolt-Glaser, & Glaser, 1988), antibody response to the Epstein-Barr virus (Esterling, Antoni, Fletcher, Margulies, & Schneiderman, 1994), and antibody response to hepatitis B vaccinations (Petrie et al., 1995). A recent study examining HIV viral load and CD4$^+$ lymphocyte counts in HIV-infected individuals found that emotional writing contributed to increases in CD4$^+$ lymphocyte counts and lower HIV viral loads, compared with those HIV-infected individuals who wrote about a nonemotional topic (Fontanilla, Thomas, Booth, Pennebaker, & Petrie, 2003). These immunological benefits were most dramatic in the assessments immediately following the writing intervention. It remains unknown whether the beneficial effects of the writing task are long-lasting or whether occasional "boosters" would be necessary to maintain the improved immunological functioning associated with emotional writing.

Writing and Social Stigma

Being a member of a stigmatized group can play a profound role in a person's life. How might writing about group membership affect attitudes and behavior? A recent study found that among members of stigmatized groups, writing about being a group member changes one's level of collective self-esteem (the sense of self-worth one derives from a group membership). People who had a visible stigmatized identity (e.g., Latino, being overweight) benefited more from writing about being a member of the general community (as opposed to writing about being a member of their in-group of others who share that identity). In contrast to this, those with a nonvisible identity (e.g., gay, lesbian, Jewish) benefited more when writing about being a member of the stigmatized group. These groups stated that it was harder for them to write over the 3 days, but they reported that writing had more long-lasting benefits, and they felt less sad and depressed a month later than people who were in the other writing conditions (those with a visible identity who wrote about being a member of a stigmatized group and those with a nonvisible identity who wrote about being a member of the general community) and relative to the control group (Pennebaker & Seagal, 1999). The implications for these findings are numerous. One could tentatively argue that therapists working with clients who are members of stigmatized groups may decide to focus on a person's commonalities versus differences with the larger community, depending on the type of stigma. Writing may also affect prejudicial attitudes and behaviors, although this notion has not been tested empirically to our knowledge.

These issues of stigmatized identity are relevant for CSA survivors and HIV-infected individuals. Because many stigmatized groups (gay men, intravenous drug users, and CSA survivors) are also among those at greatest risk for HIV infection, a writing intervention designed to focus the individual's experience and story in a positive direction may be an important element to consider in efforts to reduce risky sexual behavior. In other words, because sexual orientation and history of CSA are nonvisible stigmas, helping these individuals to develop a story that connects them to the stigmatized community may be a useful approach to consider.

Writing and Severe Trauma

There is some evidence that writing may not always work by itself in samples that may have disordered cognitive processing or relatively severe depression. For instance, a recent large-scale study in the Netherlands on recently bereaved older adults failed to find benefits of writing (Stroebe & Stroebe, 1996). Similarly, in a study conducted in Israel among a group of 14 posttraumatic stress disorder (PTSD) patients, the half assigned to write and orally expand about their traumas slightly worsened compared with controls. The authors suggested that writing may not benefit PTSD patients in the absence of cognitive or coping skills training (Gidron, Peri, Connolly, & Shalev, 1996). Further, severe cases of PTSD may be associated with the inability to cognitively organize traumatic experiences despite the continuous ruminating and emotional responses to thoughts of the precipitating traumas.

In another application of the writing paradigm to adults with serious traumatic backgrounds, Batten and colleagues (Batten, Follette, Rasmussen Hall, & Palm, 2002) recruited adult women who reported a CSA history. In that study, women in the experimental condition received instructions directing them to focus on sensory details of their CSA on the 2nd day of writing, and the consequences of the CSA on the 3rd day. This represents an important variation on the standard writing instructions, which emphasize focusing on deepest thoughts, feelings, and emotions. The results of this study diverged from the standard findings; women in the experimental condition did not exhibit the psychological or physical health benefits that are typically found in a writing study. Batten et al. proposed that survivors of truly traumatic experiences such as CSA may need more than three or four times writing to achieve the benefits of this type of intervention.

DISCUSSION

Where does writing fit within the context of therapy? Can writing change behavior? Do people begin to interact differently with others or perhaps see themselves in a new light after writing about an emotional topic? Although little research has thus far looked at whether a clinical population benefits from writing, it appears to be the case that writing would be a useful accompaniment. Having clients keep a journal may facilitate the process of forming a narrative about their experiences, as well as reinforce progress and support the change of maladaptive behaviors.

Forming a story about one's experiences in life is associated with improved physical and mental health across a variety of populations. Current evidence points to the value of having a coherent, organized format as a way to give meaning to an event and manage the emotions associated with it. In this way, having a narrative is similar to completing a job, allowing one essentially to forget the event.

Whether in written or spoken form, putting personal experiences into a story is associated with both physical and mental benefits across diverse samples. The topic may be general emotional concerns or may be domain specific. Research has further found that neither personality variables of the author nor qualities of the audience to whom the writing is directed matter in predicting benefits. An analysis of the writings that people produce has revealed that copious use of positive emotion words, a moderate use of negative emotion words, and an increase in the use of insight and causal words are associated with a variety of physical and emotional benefits. This is perhaps the most promising and direct evidence that benefiting from writing is linked to forming a story about one's experiences.

People have a tendency to seek out meaning in their environment, although sometimes this is more difficult in some situations, and for some people. Psychotherapy is a more formal venue that often involves putting a story together. Regardless of how narratives are formed, they serve a critical function in people's lives that has important implications for health and general well-being.

REFERENCES

Batten, S. V., Follette, V. M., Rasmussen Hall, M., & Palm, K. M. (2002). Physical and psychological effects of written disclosure among sexual abuse survivors. *Behavior Therapy, 33,* 107–122.

Christensen, A. J., & Smith, T. W. (1993). Cynical hostility and cardiovascular reactivity during self-disclosure. *Psychosomatic Medicine, 55,* 193–202.

Clark, L. F. (1993). Stress and the cognitive–conversational benefits of social interaction. *Journal of Social and Clinical Psychology, 12,* 25–55.

Cole, S. W., Kemeny, M. E., Taylor, S. E., & Visscher, B. R. (1996). Elevated physical health risk among gay men who conceal their homosexual identity. *Health Psychology, 15,* 243–251.

Cole, S. W., Kemeny, M. E., Taylor, S. E., Visscher, B. R., & Fahey, J. L. (1996). Accelerated course of human immunodeficiency virus infection in gay men who conceal their homosexual identity. *Psychosomatic Medicine, 58,* 219–231.

Czajka, J. A. (1987). *Behavioral inhibition and short term physiological responses.* Unpublished master's thesis, Southern Methodist University, Dallas.

Dominguez, B., Valderrama, P., Meza, M., Perez, S. L., Silva, A., Martinez, G., et al. (1995). The roles of disclosure and emotional reversal in clinical practice. In J. W. Pennebaker (Ed.), *Emotion, disclosure, and health* (pp. 255–270). Washington, DC: American Psychological Association.

Donnelly, D. A., & Murray, E. J. (1991). Cognitive and emotional changes in written essays and therapy interviews. *Journal of Social and Clinical Psychology, 10,* 334–350.

Drossman, D. (1997). Irritable bowel syndrome and sexual/physical abuse history. *European Journal of Gastroenterology and Hepatology, 9,* 327–330.

Esterling, B. A., Antoni, M. H., Fletcher, M. A., Margulies, S., & Schneiderman, N. (1994). Emotional disclosure through writing or speaking modulates latent Epstein-Barr virus reactivation. *Journal of Consulting and Clinical Psychology, 62,* 130–140.

Fontanilla, I., Thomas, M., Booth, R. J., Pennebaker, J. W., & Petrie, K. J. (2003). *Effect of written emotional expression on CD4 and viral load in HIV positive individuals.* Manuscript submitted for publication.

Gergen, K. J., & Gergen, M. M. (1988). Narrative and the self as relationship. In L. Berkowitz (Ed.), *Advances in experimental social psychology* (Vol. 21, pp. 17–56). New York: Academic Press.

Gidron, Y., Peri, T., Connolly, J. F., & Shalev, A. Y. (1996). Written disclosure in posttraumatic stress disorder: Is it beneficial for the patient? *Journal of Nervous and Mental Disease, 184,* 505–507.

Greenberg, M. A., Stone, A. A., & Wortman, C. B. (1997). Health and psychological effects of emotional disclosure: A test of the inhibition-confrontation approach. *Journal of Personality and Social Psychology, 71,* 588–602.

Gross, J. J., & Levenson, R. W. (1997). Hiding feelings: The acute effects of inhibiting negative and positive emotion. *Journal of Abnormal Psychology, 106,* 95–103.

Jamner, L. D., Schwartz, G. E., & Leigh, H. (1988). The relationship between repressive and defensive coping styles and monocyte, eosinophile, and serum glucose levels: Support for the opioid peptide hypothesis of repression. *Psychosomatic Medicine, 50,* 567–575.

Kagan, J., Arcus, D., Snidmna, N., Feng, W. Y., Hendler, J., & Greene, S. (1994). Reactivity in infants: A cross-national comparison. *Developmental Psychology, 30,* 342–345.

Kelley, H. H. (1967). Attribution theory in social psychology. In D. Levine (Ed.), *Nebraska Symposium on Motivation: Vol. 15* (pp. 192–238). Lincoln: University of Nebraska Press.

Kohler, W. (1947). *Gestalt psychology.* New York: Liveright.

Krantz, A., & Pennebaker, J. W. (1995). *Bodily versus written expression of traumatic experience.* Unpublished manuscript.

Labov, W., & Fanshel, D. (1977). *Therapeutic discourse.* New York: Academic Press.

Lewis, W. A., & Bucher, A. M. (1992). Anger, catharsis, the reformulated frustration-aggression hypothesis, and health consequences. *Psychotherapy, 29,* 385–392.

Mahoney, M. J. (Ed.). (1995). *Cognitive and constructive psychotherapies: Theory, research, and practice.* New York: Springer.

Meichenbaum, D., & Fong, G. T. (1993). How individuals control their own minds: A constructive narrative perspective. In D. M. Wegner & J. W. Pennebaker (Eds.), *Handbook of mental control* (pp. 473–490). Englewood Cliffs, NJ: Prentice Hall.

Murray, E. J., Lamnin, A. D., & Carver, C. S. (1989). Emotional expression in written essays and psychotherapy. *Journal of Social and Clinical Psychology, 8,* 414–429.

Novales, B. (1997). *Elements of successful fiction: The linguistic and psychological factors of a good story.* Unpublished master's thesis, Southern Methodist University, Dallas.

Pennebaker, J. W. (1989). Confession, inhibition, and disease. In L. Berkowitz (Ed.), *Advances in experimental social psychology* (Vol. 22, pp. 211–244). New York: Academic Press.

Pennebaker, J. W. (1993). Putting stress into words: Health, linguistic, and therapeutic implications. *Behaviour Research and Therapy, 31,* 539–548.

Pennebaker, J. W. (1997). *Opening up: The healing power of emotional expression.* New York: Guilford Press.

Pennebaker, J. W., & Beall, S. K. (1986). Confronting a traumatic event: Toward an understanding of inhibition and disease. *Journal of Abnormal Psychology, 95,* 274–281.

Pennebaker, J. W., Colder, M., & Sharp, L. K. (1990). Accelerating the coping process. *Journal of Personality and Social Psychology, 58,* 528–537.

Pennebaker, J. W., & Francis, M. (1996). Cognitive, emotional, and language processes in disclosure. *Cognition and Emotion,10,* 601–626.

Pennebaker, J. W., Francis, M. E., & Booth, R. J. (2001). *Linguistic Inquiry and Word Count, LIWC2001: A computerized text analysis program*. Mahwah, NJ: Erlbaum.

Pennebaker, J. W., Kiecolt-Glaser, J. K., & Glaser, R. (1988). Disclosure of traumas and immune function: Health implications for psychotherapy. *Journal of Consulting and Clinical Psychology, 56*, 239–245.

Pennebaker, J. W., Mayne, T. J., & Francis, M. E. (1997). Linguistic predictors of adaptive bereavement. *Journal of Personality and Social Psychology, 72*, 863–871.

Pennebaker, J. W., Paez, D., & Rimé, B. (Eds.). (1997). *Collective memories of political events: Social psychological perspectives*. Mahwah, NJ: Erlbaum.

Pennebaker, J. W., & Seagal, J. (1999). Forming a story: The health benefits of narrative. *Journal of Clinical Psychology, 55*, 1243–1254.

Pennebaker, J. W., & Susman, J. R. (1988). Disclosure of traumas and psychosomatic processes. *Social Science and Medicine, 26*, 327–332.

Petrie, K. J., Booth, R. J., Pennebaker, J. W., Davison, K. P., & Thomas, M. (1995). Disclosure of trauma and immune response to Hepatitis B vaccination program. *Journal of Consulting and Clinical Psychology, 63*, 787–792.

Richards, J. M., Pennebaker, J. W., & Beal, W. E. (1995, May). *The effects of criminal offense and disclosure of trauma on anxiety and illness in prison inmates*. Paper presented at the annual meeting of the Midwest Psychological Association, Chicago.

Rimé, B. (1995). Mental rumination, social sharing, and the recovery from emotional exposure. In J. W. Pennebaker (Ed.), *Emotion, disclosure, and health* (pp. 271–291). Washington, DC: American Psychological Association.

Schoutrop, M. J. A., Lange, A., Brosschot, J., & Everaerd, W. (1997). Overcoming traumatic events by means of writing assignments. In A. Vingerhoets, F. van Bussel, & J. Boelhouwer (Eds.), *The (non)expression of emotions in health and disease* (pp. 279–289). Tilburg, the Netherlands: Tilburg University Press.

Smyth, J. M. (1998). Written emotional expression: Effect sizes, outcome types, and moderating variables. *Journal of Consulting and Clinical Psychology, 66*, 174–184.

Spera, S. P., Buhrfeind, E. D., & Pennebaker, J. W. (1994). Expressive writing and coping with job loss. *Academy of Management Journal, 37*, 722–733.

Stroebe, M., & Stroebe, W. (1996, June). *Writing assignments and grief*. Paper presented at The (Non)Expression of Emotions and Health and Disease Conference, Tilburg, the Netherlands.

Watson, D., & Clark, L. A. (1984). Negative affectivity: The disposition to experience aversive emotional states. *Psychological Bulletin, 96*, 465–490.

Weinberger, D., Schwartz, G. E., & Davidson, R. J. (1979). Low-anxious, high-anxious, and repressive coping styles: Psychometric patterns and behavioral and physiological responses to stress. *Journal of Abnormal Psychology, 88*, 369–380.

IV

INTERVENTIONS TO PROMOTE HEALTHIER SEXUAL OUTCOMES AMONG CHILD SEXUAL ABUSE SURVIVORS

10

INTEGRATING HIV/AIDS PREVENTION ACTIVITIES INTO PSYCHOTHERAPY FOR CHILD SEXUAL ABUSE SURVIVORS

JOHN BRIERE

Child sexual abuse (CSA) is both common in U.S. culture and potentially associated with a wide variety of psychological symptoms and difficulties. Approximately 30% of women and 15% of men report sexual victimization experiences in childhood or adolescence (Briere & Elliott, in press; Finkelhor, Hotaling, Lewis, & Smith, 1990). These experiences, in turn, have been linked to later posttraumatic stress, anxiety, depression, cognitive distortions, sexual disturbance, relationship problems, substance abuse, dissociative symptoms, inadequate emotional regulation capacities, and dysfunctional personality traits (see reviews by Berliner & Elliott, 2001; Neumann, Houskamp, Pollock, & Briere, 1996). Although not all of those who are sexually abused as children appear to experience significant effects later in life (Finkelhor, 1990), CSA appears to be a major risk factor for subsequent psychological distress and disorder in society.

Especially relevant to the ongoing epidemic of HIV/AIDS in North America is the frequently reported association between CSA and a variety of factors known to increase HIV risk. These include more numerous sex part-ners (Rotheram-Borus, Mahler, Koopman, & Langabeer, 1996; Thompson, Potter, Sanderson, & Maibach, 1997; Wyatt, 1988); low self-esteem, hope-lessness, and associated self-destructiveness (Bowser, Fullilove, & Fullilove, 1990; Rotheram-Borus et al., 1996); unsafe sexual practices, including un-protected sex (Carballo-Diéguez & Dolezal, 1995; Rotheram-Borus et al., 1996; Wingood & DiClemente, 1997); use of recreational substances (in-cluding alcohol) that decrease vigilance to HIV prevention and, in the case of some drugs, may involve injection administration (Kalichman, Adair, Somlai, & Weir, 1995; Longshore & Anglin, 1995; chap. 8, this volume); dissociation, denial, or other avoidance symptoms that can impair danger awareness (Becker, Rankin, & Rickel, 1998); prostitution and other sex work (Bartholow et al., 1994; Zierler et al., 1991); and increased likelihood of being sexually coerced or assaulted by others (Briere, Woo, McRae, Foltz, & Sitzman, 1997; Russell, 1986) that, in turn, is associated with a concomitant decreased likelihood of condom use (Biglan, Noell, Ochs, Smolkowski, & Metzler, 1995). The presence of these abuse-related risk factors for HIV prob-ably explains the finding of significantly greater HIV infection rates among sexual abuse survivors than those without abuse histories (Bartholow et al., 1994; Zierler et al., 1991). Although some might argue that the reported relationship between male-to-male sexual contact and a history of CSA (e.g., Keane, Young, Boyle, & Curry, 1995) also is an important factor, it is not sexual orientation, per se, that determines risk of HIV infection but rather specific factors (e.g., unsafe sexual practices) that increase the likelihood of HIV/AIDS.

The fact that sexual abuse is associated with a variety of risk factors for HIV, however, does not necessarily mean that treatment for abuse-related distress is an effective way to reduce HIV risk in the general population. Such an intensive, case-by-case approach is highly inefficient from a public health standpoint, given the millions of individuals with sexual abuse histo-ries. In addition, not all cultures, subcultures, or socioeconomic groups may find psychotherapy a useful or valid endeavor, nor is such intensive treat-ment typically available to those in poverty or with limited economic re-sources. This later fact is especially unfortunate because conditions of pov-erty and social oppression seem integrally associated with HIV risk.

Despite these concerns, there are many sexual abuse survivors who are currently in treatment or who would be, given the opportunity. And, prob-ably by virtue of their symptomatology, some abuse survivors are relatively nonresponsive to more broad-based public health messages regarding safer sex (Belcher et al., 1998; Kalichman, Carey, & Johnson, 1996). Thus, al-though abuse-focused treatment should not be considered a primary approach to HIV risk in the general population, specific attention to risk variables during abuse-focused psychotherapy is a worthwhile endeavor.

Given the above, in what areas might one expect abuse-focused therapy to reduce HIV risk? Some of these areas are addressed in this chapter; a nonexhaustive list is presented below.

ALTERING COGNITIVE DISTORTIONS AND IMPROVING SELF-ESTEEM

The relationship between child maltreatment (including CSA) and enduring helplessness, self-blame, and low self-esteem has been demonstrated in various studies (e.g., Briere, 2000a; Jehu, Gazan, & Klassen, 1984/1985). Because these cognitive distortions are likely to increase HIV risk by reducing the survivor's interest in self-preservation or by supporting his or her assumption that HIV prevention activities will not work, or even that negative outcomes like AIDS are deserved (Becker et al., 1998: Bowser et al., 1990), successful treatment of negative cognitions is likely to affect the risk of contracting HIV among symptomatic abuse survivors. Most modern survivor treatment models include a strong cognitive component, with foci on self-esteem, self-blame, and helplessness. Such approaches have been shown to be effective in reducing survivors' cognitive distortion in several studies (e.g., Chard, Weaver, & Resick, 1997; Jehu, 1989).

Many survivors of severe sexual abuse see themselves as abnormal, both because they believe themselves to have been selected for abuse—usually by virtue of their alleged "seductiveness" or other negative characteristics—and because their current responses to the world sometimes are seen as deviant or pathological by others (Courtois, 1988). In response, many therapeutic approaches to abuse trauma focus on *normalization* as a primary technique. Normalization refers to therapist interventions that help the CSA survivor to understand that his or her current behavior is not irrational or abnormal but rather an understandable reaction to his or her childhood experiences.

One of the most direct forms of normalization occurs when the therapist shares information with the client regarding (a) the relative commonness of abuse in our society, and thus the fact that he or she is not alone or particularly "selected out" for abuse; (b) the abuser's and society's (not the victim's) general culpability regarding the molestation and its impact; and (c) the common psychological effects of sexual abuse, as opposed to the survivor's assumed intrinsic pathology. This information can reduce some of the shame and guilt the CSA survivor feels regarding his or her victimization, thereby potentially reducing his or her tendency to engage in self-punitive or self-destructive activities (Briere, 1996; Courtois, 1988). Such interventions also serve to increase the client's awareness of the relationship between self-hatred or shame and activities associated with increased HIV risk, so that he or she may be more able to identify and break the chain of catastrophizing and self-stigmatizing cognitions that lead to dangerous activities.

In addition to providing normalizing information, the clinician may choose to engage in more formal cognitive therapy regarding the client's feelings of abnormality, shame, and isolation. Among other things, this involves asking the client to concretely describe those thoughts or interpretations of memories that cause him or her to feel intrinsically bad or different from others. When these cognitions are disclosed, the therapist gently works with the survivor to disentangle the connection between bad things happening to him or her and being "bad" as a person. This process does not, however, involve the therapist lecturing the client on his or her "illogical thinking" as much as it reflects (a) exploration of ways in which the survivor came to understand himself or herself in the context of being treated badly and (b) the inaccuracy of this understanding as it relates to the survivor's current life, capacities, and entitlements. The intent of such clarification is the client's growing awareness of the negative assumptions he or she has made regarding the meaning of the abuse—both in terms of his or her self-perceptions and how he or she construes his or her value to others. In this process, the therapist respectfully and gently challenges the client's abuse-related assumptions and provides the necessary questions and feedback to permit the CSA survivor to reexamine these beliefs.

In a similar vein, the perceived helplessness of some CSA survivors can be addressed in cognitive therapy. This may be accomplished through discussions of the client's underlying, often childhood-based, assumptions that, for example, bad things just happen and one is powerless to stop them, and that one has only marginal control over one's own behavior. Among the targets of such interventions may be the beliefs that the client is helpless to change HIV-risky behaviors, that he or she is unworthy of a less chaotic life, and that his or her sexual behavior is uncontrollable or under the control of others.

Finally, cognitive interventions may occur implicitly during the process of relationship-based psychotherapy. In the context of sustained therapist nonjudgment and positive regard, the survivor may slowly come to view himself or herself more positively and as more entitled to respect and positive treatment from others. In combination with normalization and formal cognitive restructuring, such interventions may increase the survivor's willingness to engage in self-care and self-protection, and consequently to decrease contact with those who might maltreat (sexually or otherwise) him or her.

REDUCING THE NEED FOR EXTERNAL TENSION REDUCTION AND SUBSTANCE ABUSE

A central concept in some modern analyses of abuse-related disturbance is that of *tension reduction behavior* (Briere, 1992, 2001). It is suggested that the emotional ("affect") regulation problems reported in several studies of abuse survivors (Briere, 2000b; Elliott, 1994; Herman, Perry, & van der Kolk, 1989) preclude sufficient internal reduction of painful abuse-related emotional states, thereby motivating the use of external behaviors that soothe, distract, or otherwise reduce overwhelming dysphoria. Tension reduction behaviors that have been linked to inadequate affect regulation include intentional self-injury (Briere & Gil, 1998), binge–purge activities (Stice, Nemeroff, & Shaw, 1996), and, especially relevant to this chapter, repetitive or indiscriminant sexual behavior (e.g., Becker et al., 1998; Brennan & Shaver, 1995). Similarly, substance abuse has been shown to correlate with inadequate affect regulation skills (Grilo et al., 1997; Verheul, van den Brink, & Geerlings, 1999), suggesting that those with diminished capacity to soothe internal distress may turn to anesthetizing or distracting substances as a way of reducing abuse-related dysphoria.

To the extent that the tension reduction and substance abuse model is accurate, two aspects of abuse-focused therapy may be especially helpful in decreasing the likelihood of indiscriminate sexual behavior and chemical dependency in sexual abuse survivors: reducing abuse-related posttraumatic stress and increasing affect regulation skills. Each approach is presented below.

Reducing Posttraumatic Stress

Resick and Schnicke's (1993) and Foa and Rothbaum's (1998) cognitive–behavioral approaches to rape victims—found in outcome studies to effectively reduce victimization-related posttraumatic stress—also are helpful in treating the posttraumatic symptoms of some sexual abuse survivors (see, e.g., adaptations by Chard et al., 1997; Smucker, Dancu, Foa, & Niederee, 1995). These (and related) approaches generally involve (a) repetitive exposure to trauma-related memories through verbal discussions, (b) activation of associated negative emotions and cognitions, (c) habituation and extinction of activated distress, and (d) cognitive processing of beliefs and assumptions associated with the victimization experience.

Such interventions typically result in less powerful negative affective responses to triggers in the interpersonal environment, thereby requiring less use of risky tension reduction behaviors or substance abuse to down-regulate distress. For individuals who are especially likely to respond to certain triggered memories with HIV risk behaviors, it may be helpful to "work backward"—first identifying risky behaviors that appear to arise from activated traumatic stress, then providing cognitive–behavioral approaches that address those trauma-related memories and emotions that motivate such behaviors.

In the specific case of the abuse survivor, such exposure and activation should be carefully titrated to match existing levels of his or her (often diminished) affect regulation capacity (Briere, 2001). For example, especially prolonged or intensive exposure to abuse memories in an individual with diminished abilities to self-soothe, modulate, or tolerate emotional pain might prove overwhelming (Chemtob, Novaco, Hamada, Gross, & Smith, 1997; Cloitre, Koenan, Cohen, & Han, 2002). Instead, it is suggested that therapeutic exposure to abuse-related psychological material be neither so minimal that there is inadequate emotional activation and processing nor so powerful that the client's affect regulation capacity is exceeded and further distress ensues (Briere, 2001).

Increasing Affect Regulation

If the imbalance between posttraumatic dysphoria and affect regulation capacity motivates some proportion of CSA survivors' involvement in indiscriminant sexual contacts or substance abuse, interventions that increase the survivor's emotional regulation repertoire and capacity to tolerate negative affects also might be helpful in reducing such HIV risk factors. In this regard, Linehan (1993) noted that distress tolerance and emotional regulation are both internal behaviors that can be learned during therapy. Among the specific skills taught by Linehan's empirically validated dialectical behavior therapy, many of which may also be considered a form of stress inoculation, are strategic distraction, self-soothing procedures, and activities that "improve the moment" (e.g., relaxation activities during stress). The survivor also learns to, for example, identify and label feelings, avoid catastrophizing cognitions, reduce vulnerability to hyper-emotionality (i.e., through self-care activities that decrease stress), and develop the ability to experience emotions without judging or rejecting them.

Affect tolerance and modulation also may be learned implicitly during effective abuse-focused therapy (Briere, 2001). Because, as outlined in the last section, trauma-focused interventions involve the repeated evocation and processing of distressing but nonoverwhelming emotions, such treatment slowly teaches the survivor to become more "at home" with some level of distress and to develop whatever skills are necessary to deescalate moderate levels of emotional arousal. This growing ability to move in and out of strong emotional states, in turn, fosters a reduced need for risky tension reduction behaviors or psychoactive substances in the service of affect regulation.

ADDRESSING RELATIONSHIP-LEVEL ISSUES

It is likely that abuse survivors who engage in dysfunctional sexual behavior are responding to, in part, activated negative relational schema involving expectations and beliefs about self as bad or unworthy and others as inevitably hurtful, abandoning, or dangerous (Baldwin, Fehr, Keedian, Seidel, & Thompson, 1993). Usually associated with negative early parent–child attachment experiences, these schema may, in turn, foster feelings of unwanted isolation and desperate needs for love and, yet, fear of intimacy and expectations of abandonment (Briere, 2001). In this regard, many survivors describe repetitive, short-term, but intense sexual relationships that, for one reason or another, do not endure. In such relationships sex may be a primary vehicle through which the survivor strives to feel close (attached) to, nurtured, or loved by another person. At the same time, however, many survivors describe feelings of anxiety or distress in the context of emotional proximity, because they may associate intimacy with danger (Courtois, 1988). Unfortunately, some survivors are essentially correct to fear such connection, given that their choice of exploitive or aggressive sexual partners may in some way replicate or "reenact" their child abuse experiences. This complex, pull–push process may lead to repetitive interpersonal conflict and, as a result, chaotic, rapidly terminated, or superficial relationships.

Abuse-focused therapy addresses this problem in a somewhat indirect manner. In treatment, aspects of the client–therapist relationship often become triggers for reexperiencing unprocessed childhood trauma at the relationship level. Such "transference" reactions are thought to be a reliving experience, in the same way that intrusive sensory images (flashbacks) or nightmares may be, albeit experienced as a gestalt of cognitive and emotional responses to a relational interaction (Briere, 2001). From this perspective, the process of "working through" the transference described by analysts is approximated in abuse-focused psychotherapy through cognitive–behavioral processing of relational schema involving isolation, abandonment, unlovability, and so on. As the distress associated with these relational schema is activated in the context of a safe, nonexploitive therapeutic relationship, such fears are no longer reinforced by actual rejection, devaluation, or exploitation and often are replaced by more positive feeling states.

As a result of this desensitization and counterconditioning process, the survivor client may have fewer triggered negative responses to interpersonal stimuli and, as a result, may be able to tolerate intimacy long enough to sustain longer term sexual and romantic relationships. Further, as his or her emotional needs are met via more appropriate relationships, and his or her cognitions are updated via positive adult interactions, the survivor may have less need to seek out love and connection through multiple short-term sexual relationships or, for example, the chaotic, dissociative attachments often fostered among chronic drug abusers.

TARGETED INTERVENTIONS FOR HIV RISK THAT COULD BE ADDED TO ABUSE-FOCUSED TREATMENT

In addition to the treatment components outlined above, there are several existing intervention approaches for HIV risk factors that can be adapted to an abuse treatment model. In fact, some of these have been informally included by clinicians working with abuse survivors who are especially at risk for sexually transmitted diseases, substance abuse, and sexual victimization. As noted earlier, for some abuse survivors, these HIV risk interventions are likely to be most successful to the extent that they are embedded in the context of ongoing psychotherapy.

Intervention in Substance Abuse

As described at the outset of this chapter, as well as in chapter 8 (this volume), the link between substance abuse and child sexual victimization is significant. For example, Briere and Runtz (1987) found that sexually abused female crisis center clients had 10 times the likelihood of a drug addiction history and over 2 times the likelihood of alcoholism as compared with a group of nonabused female clients from the same center. At least one research group has found an even more unfortunate relationship—that of sexual abuse history with injection drug abuse (Bartholow et al., 1994), a major risk factor for HIV. Although substance abuse issues are often included in abuse-focused psychotherapy, it is not clear that such unstructured approaches have much efficacy in reducing drug dependence or use. In contrast, 12-step programs (e.g., Alcoholics Anonymous) have been shown to be helpful for some patient populations (Emerick, Tonigan, Montgomery, & Little, 1993), as have focused cognitive–behavioral interventions (Carroll et al., 1994; Maude-Griffin et al., 1998). For this reason, some clinicians recommend that chemically dependent CSA survivors attend 12-step programs concomitantly with abuse-focused treatment. Although this approach has merit, not all abuse survivors appreciate a 12-step focus, some 12-step groups advocate perspectives incongruent with abuse-focused treatment, and the nonclinical approach of such programs may not allow much integration with the goals and methods of abuse-focused therapy.

On the other hand, cognitive–behavioral substance abuse modules are relatively congruent with modern abuse treatment approaches, especially to the extent that the abuse-focused treatment already includes cognitive interventions. Maude-Griffin et al. (1998), for example, outlined a cognitive–behavioral intervention that reduces crack cocaine usage (and associated depression) beyond that of a comparison 12-step approach. According to the authors, this treatment involves "strengthening commitment to abstinence, dealing effectively with urges and high risk situations, identifying and modifying irrational thoughts, managing negative moods, intervening after a relapse to prevent a full-blown relapse, and increasing positive mood and social support" (Maude-Griffin et al., 1998, p. 833)—many of the same goals of some abuse-focused treatment approaches.

Increasing Assertiveness and Sexual Boundaries

A frequent finding in the child sexual victimization literature is the relationship between CSA and subsequent revictimization, typically via coerced sexual contact or sexual assault, as an adult (e.g., Briere et al., 1997; Russell, 1986). In fact, a meta-analysis revealed that later rape experiences had the largest association (average effect size) to sexual abuse of all examined psychosocial outcomes (Neumann et al., 1996). As reported by Biglan et al. (1995), forced sexual contact is associated with an increased risk of HIV infection, probably because such contacts are more likely to produce tissue injury, less frequently involve condoms, and may involve repeated nonmonogamous contacts for women who are less able to resist sexual aggression or coercion.

Because, as noted by Becker et al. (1998), "intimidation, coercion, and violence by partners often make it problematic for women to engage in protective behavior around sexual activity" (p. 118), HIV prevention approaches for frequently victimized individuals may be unsuccessful to the extent that they rely solely on the assumptions of voluntary behavior implicit in "safe sex" education. Further, the dissociation and other avoidance strategies used by many survivors to cope with threatening material may preclude their full attention to didactic information, perhaps especially when the information intrinsically contradicts their cognitive schema that sex rarely is, in fact, safe.

Instead, potentially more effective approaches stress direct (e.g., via role-playing and coaching) training in assertiveness, sexual limit-setting, and sexual boundary issues. Although even strong limit-setting is unlikely to protect most women from a truly predatory male, it is more helpful in other situations (e.g., dating and ongoing relationships) in which an active position against being coerced or manipulated typically has more impact. Apropos of this notion, one successful HIV risk-reduction program includes role-playing and interactive didactic information on interpersonal assertiveness and limit-setting in sexual situations (Belcher et al., 1998). Such skill-development activities are a valuable addition to abuse-focused treatment, especially for clients who are repeatedly coerced or otherwise revictimized sexually. In fact, for those who have a long or severe victimization history, such learning may best occur in the context of a therapeutic relationship in which exposure to painful material that arises from role-playing activities can be titrated and in which avoidance can be more closely monitored and addressed.

Individualized Counseling on HIV Issues

Although information on HIV transmission and the relative risk of various sexual behaviors is an important component of almost all HIV prevention programs, merely presenting such information in a didactic form is not especially useful in work with some traumatized individuals. Instead, research suggests that HIV information is best retained by CSA survivors when it is (a) delivered in a small-group format or on a one-to-one basis; (b) tailored for the specific needs, culture, and clinical functioning (e.g., level of dissociative avoidance or denial) of the individuals receiving it; (c) delivered in such a way that it motivates the individual by providing feedback on the actual, real-world risks associated with his or her behavior; and (d) focused on the development of specific skills and behavior change as opposed to mere attitude change (Becker et al., 1998; Belcher et al., 1998; Kalichman et al., 1996). To the extent that these guidelines hold true, it is likely that one-to-one, abuse-focused therapy that includes tailored AIDS information, real-world pragmatic feedback, and skills training will more directly impact potentially high-risk behavior.

SUMMARY

The treatment of sexual abuse-related distress and disorder is often a complex and time-consuming process. Unlike some successful treatment approaches to less complicated acute traumas, intervention in severe sexual abuse sequelae often requires a diverse set of intervention strategies and must take into account the unique vulnerabilities of this client population. Within this complicated context, unfortunately, is the additional reality that severe abuse trauma places the survivor at risk for a variety of negative outcomes, many of which are chronic, painful, and sometimes dangerous. Tragically, in the era of the HIV virus, the abuse victim's "survival" strategies even may result in infection and death. As a result, the clinician is compelled to intervene.

For this reason, responsible clinicians have become more attuned to HIV/AIDS issues and increasingly seek to include HIV prevention components in their treatment of sexual abuse trauma. At the anecdotal level, this approach can be helpful: Clinical experience suggests that sexual abuse survivors who have completed a successful regimen of risk-relevant, abuse-focused therapy often have reduced reliance on substance abuse or externalizing behaviors and are less chaotic and impulsive in their choice of partners. Empirical support for this impression, however, has yet to be determined.

Unfortunately, despite the potentially critical importance of integrating HIV prevention into therapy for abuse survivors, most clinicians (abuse-specialized or otherwise) have received no specific training in this area. Although a few states now require psychologists to attend a continuing education course on HIV/AIDS, most others have no such requirements. Even when continuing education is available, often it is limited to generic "consciousness-raising" workshops on HIV transmission and risk factors, as opposed to information on how to integrate prevention activities into the actual context of psychotherapy. Given studies showing that some abuse survivors need special, customized prevention education and that some abuse-related responses increase HIV risk, training clinicians to provide safer-sex public health information is rarely enough. Instead, such training should be clinically relevant and focused on actual clinical practice, and undertaken as a licensure prerequisite for mental health professionals rather than as an optional learning experience.

Although the broadening of treatment goals to include HIV prevention is important, perhaps even critical, at the same time it is clear that the primary approach to HIV prevention will have to be focused on groups rather than individuals. Ultimately, one of the most basic and powerful HIV intervention strategies may extend beyond changing the CSA survivor's behavior. In the final analysis, the most effective interventions for HIV, substance abuse, self-destructiveness, and a number of other major problems in our culture will be to change the way we, as a society, treat those with lesser social power, including our children.

REFERENCES

Baldwin, M. W., Fehr, B., Keedian, E., Seidel, M., & Thompson, D. W. (1993). An exploration of the relational schemata underlying attachment styles: Self-report and lexical decision approaches. *Personality and Social Psychology Bulletin, 19,* 746–754.

Bartholow, B. N., Joy, D., Douglas, J. M., Bolan, G., Harrison, J. S., Moss, P. M., & McKirnan, D. (1994). Emotional, behavioral, and HIV risks associated with sexual abuse among adult homosexual and bisexual men. *Child Abuse and Neglect, 9,* 747–761.

Becker, E., Rankin, E., & Rickel, A. U. (1998). *High risk sexual behavior: Interventions with vulnerable populations.* New York: Plenum.

Belcher, L., Kalichman, S., Topping, M., Smith, S., Emshoff, J., Norris, F., & Nurs, J. (1998). A randomized trial of a brief HIV risk reduction counseling intervention for women. *Journal of Consulting and Clinical Psychology, 66,* 856–861.

Berliner, L., & Elliott, D. M. (2001). Sexual abuse of children. In J. E. B. Myers, L. Berliner, J. Briere, C. T. Hendrix, T. Reid, & C. Jenny (Eds.), *The APSAC handbook on child maltreatment* (2nd ed., pp. 55–78). Newbury Park, CA: Sage.

Biglan, A., Noell, J., Ochs, L., Smolkowski, K., & Metzler, C. (1995). Does sexual coercion play a role in the high-risk sexual behavior of adolescent and young adult women? *Journal of Behavioral Medicine, 18,* 549–568.

Bowser, B. P., Fullilove, M. T., & Fullilove, R. E. (1990). African-American youth and high risk AIDS behavior: The social context and barriers to prevention. *Youth and Society, 22,* 54–66.

Brennan, K. A., & Shaver, P. R. (1995). Dimensions of adult attachment, affect regulation, and romantic relationship functioning. *Personality and Social Psychology Bulletin, 21,* 267–283.

Briere, J. (1992). *Child abuse trauma: Theory and treatment of the lasting effects.* Newbury Park, CA: Sage.

Briere, J. (1996). *Therapy for adults molested as children* (2nd ed.). New York: Springer.

Briere, J. (2000a). *Cognitive Distortions Scale (CDS) professional manual*. Odessa, FL: Psychological Assessment Resources.

Briere, J. (2000b). *Inventory of Altered Self-Capacities (IASC) professional manual*. Odessa, FL: Psychological Assessment Resources.

Briere, J. (2001). Treating adult survivors of severe childhood abuse and neglect: Further development of an integrative model. In J. E. B. Myers, L. Berliner, J. Briere, C. T. Hendrix, T. Reid, & C. Jenny (Eds.). *The APSAC handbook on child maltreatment* (2nd ed., pp. 175–203). Newbury Park, CA: Sage.

Briere, J., & Elliott, D. M. (in press). Prevalence and symptomatic sequels of self-reported childhood physical and sexual abuse in a general population sample of men and women. *Child Abuse and Neglect*.

Briere, J., & Gil, E. (1998). Self-mutilation in clinical and general population samples: Prevalence, correlates, and functions. *American Journal of Orthopsychiatry, 68*, 609–620.

Briere, J., & Runtz, M. R. (1987). Post-sexual abuse trauma: Data and implications for clinical practice. *Journal of Interpersonal Violence, 2*, 367–379.

Briere, J., Woo, R., McRae, B., Foltz, J., & Sitzman, R. (1997). Lifetime victimization history, demographics, and clinical status in female psychiatric emergency room patients. *Journal of Nervous and Mental Disease, 185*, 95–101.

Carballo-Diéguez, A., & Dolezal, C. (1995). Association between history of childhood sexual abuse and adult HIV-risk sexual behavior in Puerto Rican men who have sex with men. *Child Abuse and Neglect, 19*, 595–605.

Carroll, K. M., Rounsaville, B. J., Niche, C., Gordon, L. T., Wirtz, P. W., & Gawin, F. H. (1994). One-year follow-up of psychotherapy and pharmacotherapy for cocaine dependence: Delayed emergence of psychotherapy effects. *Archives of General Psychiatry, 51*, 989–997.

Chard, K. M., Weaver, T. L., & Resick, P. A. (1997). Adapting cognitive processing therapy for child sexual abuse survivors. *Cognitive and Behavioral Practice, 4*, 31–52.

Chemtob, C. M., Novaco, R. W., Hamada, R. S., Gross, D. M., & Smith, G. (1997). Anger regulation deficits in combat-related posttraumatic stress disorder. *Journal of Traumatic Stress, 10*, 17–35.

Cloitre, M., Koenan, K. C., Cohen, C. R., & Han, H. (2002). Skills training in affective and interpersonal regulation followed by exposure: A phase-based treatment for PTSD related to childhood abuse. *Journal of Consulting and Clinical Psychology, 70*, 1067–1074.

Courtois, C. A. (1988). *Healing the incest wound: Adult survivors in therapy*. New York: Norton.

Elliott, D. M. (1994). Impaired object relationships in professional women molested as children. *Psychotherapy, 31*, 79–86.

Emerick, C. D., Tonigan, J. S., Montgomery, H., & Little, L. (1993). Alcoholics Anonymous: What is really known? In B. S. McCrady & W. R. Miller (Eds.), *Research on Alcoholics Anonymous: Opportunities and alternatives* (pp. 41–76).

New Brunswick, NJ: Rutgers—The State University of New York, Center of Alcoholic Studies.

Finkelhor, D. (1990). Early and long-term effects of child sexual abuse: An update. *Professional Psychology: Research and Practice, 21*, 325–330.

Finkelhor, D., Hotaling, G., Lewis, I. A., & Smith, C. (1990). Sexual abuse in a national survey of adult men and women: Prevalence, characteristics, and risk factors. *Child Abuse and Neglect, 14*, 19–28.

Foa, E. B., & Rothbaum, B. O. (1998). *Treating the trauma of rape: Cognitive–behavioral therapy for PTSD.* New York: Guilford Press.

Grilo, C. M., Martino, S., Walker, M. L., Becker, D. F., Edell, W. S., & McGlashan, T. H. (1997). Controlled study of psychiatric comorbidity in psychiatrically hospitalized young adults with substance use disorders. *American Journal of Psychiatry, 154*, 1305–1307.

Herman, J. L., Perry, C., & van der Kolk, B. A. (1989). Childhood trauma in borderline personality disorder. *Amercian Journal of Psychiatry, 146*, 490–494.

Jehu, D. (1989). *Beyond sexual abuse: Therapy with women who were childhood victims.* Chichester, UK: Wiley.

Jehu, D., Gazan, M., & Klassen, C. (1984/1985). Common therapeutic targets among women who were sexually abused in childhood. *Journal of Social Work and Human Sexuality, 3*, 25–45.

Kalichman, S. C., Adair, V., Somlai, A. M., & Weir, S. S. (1995). The perceived social context of AIDS: Study of inner-city sexually transmitted disease clinic patients. *AIDS Education and Prevention, 7*, 298–307.

Kalichman, S. C., Carey, M. P., & Johnson, B. T. (1996). Prevention of sexually transmitted HIV infection: A meta-analytic review and critique of the theory-based intervention outcome literature. *Annals of Behavioral Medicine, 18*, 6–15.

Keane, F. E. A., Young, S. M., Boyle, H. M., & Curry, K. M. (1995). Prior sexual assault reported by male attenders at a department of genitourinary medicine. *International Journal of STD and AIDS, 6*, 95–100.

Linehan, M. M. (1993). *Cognitive–behavioral treatment of borderline personality disorder.* New York: Guilford Press.

Longshore, D., & Anglin, M. D. (1995). Number of sex partners and crack cocaine use: Is crack an independent marker for HIV risk behavior? *Journal of Drug Issues, 25*, 1–10.

Maude-Griffin, P. M., Hohenstein, J. M., Humfleet, G. L., Reilly, P. M., Tusel, D. J., & Hall, S. M. (1998). Superior efficacy of cognitive behavioral therapy for urban crack cocaine abusers: Main and matching effects. *Journal of Consulting and Clinical Psychology, 66*, 832–837.

Neumann, D. A., Houskamp, B. M., Pollock, V. E., & Briere, J. (1996). The long-term sequelae of childhood sexual abuse in women: A meta-analytic review. *Child Maltreatment, 1*, 6–16.

Resick, P. A., & Schnicke, M. K. (1993). *Cognitive processing therapy for rape victims: A treatment manual.* Newbury Park, CA: Sage.

Rotheram-Borus, M. J., Mahler, K. A., Koopman, C., & Langabeer, K. (1996). Sexual abuse history and associated multiple risk behavior in adolescent runaways. *American Journal of Orthopsychiatry, 66*, 390–400.

Russell, D. E. H. (1986). *The secret trauma: Incest in the lives of girls and women.* New York: Basic Books.

Smucker, M. R., Dancu, C. V., Foa, E. B., & Niederee, J. L. (1995). Imagery rescripting: A new treatment for survivors of childhood sexual abuse suffering from post-traumatic stress. *Journal of Cognitive Psychotherapy, 9*, 3–17.

Stice, E., Nemeroff, C., & Shaw, H. E. (1996). Test of the dual pathway model of bulimia nervosa: Evidence for dietary restraint and affect regulation mechanisms. *Journal of Social and Clinical Psychology, 15*, 340–363.

Thompson, N. J., Potter, J. S., Sanderson, C. A., & Maibach, E. W. (1997). The relationship of sexual abuse and HIV risk behaviors among heterosexual adult female STD patients. *Child Abuse and Neglect, 21*, 149–156.

Verheul, R., van den Brink, W., & Geerlings, P. (1999). A three-pathway psycho-biological model of craving for alcohol. *Alcohol & Alcoholism, 34*, 197–222.

Wingood, G. M., & DiClemente, R. J. (1997). Child sexual abuse, HIV sexual risk, and gender relations of African-American women. *American Journal of Preventive Medicine, 13*, 380–384

Wyatt, G. E. (1988). The relationship between child sexual abuse and adolescent sexual functioning in Afro-American and White American women. *Annals of the New York Academy of Sciences, 528*, 111–122.

Zierler, S., Fiengold, L., Laufer, D., Velentgas, P., Kantrowitz-Gordon, I., & Mayer, K. (1991). Adult survivors of childhood sexual abuse and subsequent risk of HIV infection. *American Journal of Public Health, 81*, 572–575.

11

CHILD SEXUAL ABUSE AND HIV: AN INTEGRATIVE RISK-REDUCTION APPROACH

DOROTHY CHIN, GAIL E. WYATT, JENNIFER VARGAS CARMONA, TAMRA BURNS LOEB, AND HECTOR F. MYERS

In recent years, researchers have noted a significant association between child sexual abuse (CSA) and HIV (e.g., Wyatt et al., 2002; see also chap. 3, this volume, for a detailed discussion of this issue). This association has important implications for HIV prevention and intervention. First, the fact that women who contract HIV are more likely to have been sexually abused as children suggests a continuum of victimization, such that early victimization may confer greater sexual risk-taking and likelihood of revictimization, resulting in HIV infection. Thus, the possible pathways between CSA and HIV need to be elucidated to prevent further negative outcomes. Second, the implications for HIV research and intervention are significant. Sexual abuse during childhood is associated with disturbances in the self that pervade an individual's development, and these disturbances are likely to maintain HIV risk behaviors unless ameliorated. Therefore, individuals who are

This chapter was supported in part by National Institute of Mental Health Grant RO1-MH59496. The authors would like to thank Marie Vafors and Elizabeth Robles for assistance with data transcription.

HIV-positive and have a history of CSA may face "double jeopardy" for negative outcomes, including additional risks for reinfection, sexual revictimization, physical impairment, and nonadherence to HIV treatment that are beyond those associated with HIV infection. Intervention approaches for HIV-positive women with sexual abuse histories need to consider pathways of risk, ameliorate the disruptions in development that result from CSA, and address the additive and interactive influences of HIV and CSA on health outcomes. In this chapter, we present an overview of the consequences of CSA that may lead to higher risk for HIV, offer a critique of early intervention paradigms, and present an integrative risk-reduction approach for HIV-positive women with CSA histories, currently in clinical trial, that addresses the link between CSA and HIV in a developmental and cultural context. Finally, preliminary findings from the intervention and implications for future directions are discussed.

CONSEQUENCES OF CHILD SEXUAL ABUSE

The consequences of CSA, manifesting in multiple aspects of the self, have been copiously documented. They include cognitive impairments, affective dysregulation, adverse physical health, and risky behavior, all of which occur in a context of disrupted development. For example, women who experienced early and chronic sexual abuse had a sevenfold increase in HIV risk behavior and markers of risk, such as injection drug use, sexually transmitted diseases (STDs), and engagement in anal sex without condoms (Bensley, Van Eenwyk, & Simmons, 2000). The effects of sexual abuse found in this study appear to be different for men, suggesting a gender-specific, disrupted path of development for women. Other risk behaviors have been associated with CSA, including; earlier onset of sexual activity (Brown & Finkelhor, 1986; Donalson, Whalen, & Anastas, 1989; Riggs, Alario, & McHorney, 1990), greater number of partners (Ganz, Wyatt, & Loeb, 1998), and prostitution (Widom & Kuhns, 1996). The social-affective functioning of women with CSA histories have also been shown to be impaired. Female CSA victims have poorer judgments about people and situations (Smith, 1992) and report more loneliness and less satisfaction with their social support (Gibson & Hartshorne, 1996; Rhodes, Ebert, & Myers, 1993).

Because the relationship of CSA to later functioning in each of these areas is reviewed more comprehensively elsewhere in this volume, we direct the reader to these chapters. For the relation between CSA and HIV risk behavior and health outcomes, see chapter 3 (this volume). For CSA and cognitive processing, see chapter 6 (this volume). For CSA and its effects on social and affective functioning, see chapter 7 (this volume).

On the basis of a review of the literature, the specific mechanisms linking CSA to later HIV infection can be ascertained and posited. That is, the experience of CSA appears to affect the development of girls through a number of vectors, encompassing cognitive, affective, and behavioral factors, often with profound effects. Because of the significant impact of CSA in women, intervention strategies with women dually affected by CSA and HIV must address all of these consequences as well as the interactive, reciprocal effects of CSA and HIV.

EARLY HIV INTERVENTION MODELS

For almost two decades HIV research has been guided primarily by several theories, namely the theory of reasoned action (Albarracin, Johnson, Fishbein, & Muellerleile, 2001; Fishbein, 1980), the theory of planned behaviors (Ajzen, 1991; Ajzen & Fishbein, 1980), the health belief model (Becker, 1974), and the AIDS risk-reduction model (Catania, Kegeles, & Coates, 1990). Upon examination, it may be noted that these theories have several major underlying assumptions that stand counter to much of female socialization and values of a number of ethnic, cultural, and religious groups:

1. Individuals, understanding their personal risks, should prioritize disease transmission and learn the necessary skills.
2. Sex is always planned, anticipated, and consensual.
3. Decisions about sex are made on an individual, rather than interpersonal, basis.
4. If individuals so choose, they have the ability to negotiate issues such as pregnancy, disease prevention, condom use, or sexual practices.
5. Pregnancy is not a wanted outcome.

These major assumptions that underlie earlier intervention approaches may not be applicable to women, particularly ethnic minority women, for several important reasons. First, inherent in these assumptions is the idea that an individual comes with an uncomplicated sexual history. However, the fact that as many as 50% of HIV-positive women have CSA histories (Wyatt et al., 2002) places an ahistorical approach in question. Decisions about sex are often based on past experiences. Previous coercion or pressure from partners, fear of being harmed, or incidents of sexual and physical trauma often complicate decision making in sexual interactions. These factors may encourage individuals to subjugate their personal needs and safety in order to allow partners to make decisions regarding sex.

Sexual abuse before the age of 18 can impair one's sexual autonomy even further. In these cases, sexual contact is often initiated by someone older and with more experience and power. The perpetrator may dictate what kind of sexual experiences should be engaged in, and, as a result, women often fail to develop a sense of their own sexual needs apart from those of their partners. They may gravitate to other partners who make decisions for them and develop a pattern of abdicating control of their sexuality. Therefore, they may not develop the skills to assess their personal risks, allowing role expectations and emotions to predominate decisions regarding pregnancy, contraceptive or condom use, and sexual practices in which they engage (Wyatt, Newcomb, & Riederle, 1993). In addition, in situations in which there is overt coercion and physical threat, disruptions to the development of security and trust can be pervasive and long-lasting.

Second, these theories overlook societal, cultural, gender-specific, and economic factors (Amaro, 1995). For example, among a sample of undocumented Latina immigrants, HIV was considered a concern secondary to finances, even though the women suspected their partners to be nonmonogamous (Romero, Wyatt, Chin, & Rodriguez, 1998). The emotional bond with sexual partners is a factor important to many women and needs to be incorporated into the decision making. This is exemplified by the distinction women make between a partner she has had children with and other partners. That is, if a woman loves and has had children with a partner, she may be less likely to evaluate her risks for disease transmission apart from her commitment to maintain a family. In spite of personal risks, women may be more influenced by their emotional bond with a partner and consequently do not protect themselves from unwanted outcomes. Women are socialized to value love, trust, and intimacy and may be willing to risk personal safety to maintain these values (Chin, 1999). In collectivistic cultures, these values are even more prominent. As evidenced by studies on Latino and Asian women, a collectivistic orientation may lead to greater accommodation of others' desires and the tendency to maintain group harmony at one's personal expense (Chin & Kroesen, 1999). Thus, not only are gender role expectations and values important, but the interaction between gender and culture should also be considered.

The assumptions of the primarily cognitive models have socialized researchers and health care providers to assume that the primary issues related to health promotion and HIV-related risk reduction were relevant for all groups. Consequently, interventions for women were developed on the basis of these theories and these assumptions. Unfortunately, when populations at risk did not make the expected behavior changes or did not sustain them for long periods of time, it was sometimes assumed that they were knowingly engaging in risky behavior and were resistant to change. In other words, victim-blaming occurred. For example, in the Black community, the HIV prevention messages continue to include some of the six assumptions described earlier, but the rates of HIV are still increasing at an alarming rate. Researchers and clinicians may interpret these rates as an indication of risky sexual and drug practices but may not be aware of the history of general, STD-related, and HIV-related health disparities that continue to exist, or the gender-based and cultural values that are in contradiction with the six assumptions.

In an effort to address the deficits of previous models' applicability to women, we developed an intervention specifically for women who are HIV- and CSA-positive, integrating contextual and developmental factors. Below we describe our approach and present some preliminary findings.

THE WOMEN'S HEALTH PROJECT

Conceptual Overview

The Women's Health Project (WHP), a 4-year intervention study funded by the National Institute of Mental Health, was designed to address limitations of contemporary intervention models by incorporating historical and contextual factors that influence women's decision making and risk behaviors. Among current HIV risk-reduction studies, not enough attention has been paid to the role that prior victimization, specifically CSA, has had on the maintenance of high-risk behaviors. The WHP consists of an integrated curriculum that is grounded in key elements of HIV risk reduction (specifically, sex risk and drug risk), adherence interventions that emphasize women's issues, and a focus on increasing self-efficacy to perform lower risk behaviors as well as providing systemic support to sustain change (Sikkema, Winett, & Lombard, 1995; Wingood & DiClemente, 1996; Wong, 1995). It should be noted that in this intervention, HIV risk reduction refers not to the prevention of infection but rather to the prevention of reinfection, particularly by a more virulent or treatment-resistant strain of the virus, as well as to lowering the possibility of transmission to a partner. Concurrently, the WHP incorporates key aspects of treatment for CSA survivors, including short-term, trauma-focused groups that use didactic and group-process format and peer modeling of disclosure (Cole & Barney, 1987; Gold-Steinberg & Buttenheim, 1993; Lundberg-Love, 1990; Roth & Newman, 1991). Components of the engagement model, including using cultural values as motivators for behavior change and peer mentors to model self-disclosure, are utilized as well (Longshore, Grills, & Annon, 1999). The uniqueness of this intervention lies in integrating well-established components of sexual abuse interventions with successful elements of HIV interventions in both content and format.

The intervention targets five areas of outcomes: (a) HIV-related sexual risk behavior, (b) HIV-related drug risk behavior, (c) HIV treatment adherence, (d) interpersonal behaviors, and (e) psychological functioning. Specific outcomes measured in these domains include the frequency of condom use with main and casual sex partners, the use of drugs or alcohol before or during sex, medication regimen adherence, health services utilization, interpersonal conflict and resolution, depression, anxiety, trauma symptoms, self-esteem, and coping.

These outcomes are hypothesized to be proximally influenced by cognitive, affective, and behavioral factors: (a) self-efficacy for each of the five outcome domains (cognitive); (b) sexual health domains consisting of body awareness, sexual socialization, sexual health behaviors, and consequences of trauma (affective); and (c) skills for each of the five outcome domains (behavioral). Thus, these are the vectors of change as conceptualized in the intervention. Concurrently, elements of CSA and trauma interventions relevant to each topic are incorporated, addressing the developmental deficits stemming from CSA that may serve as roadblocks to change. Specifically, cognitive and affective disruptions in the development of the self and their links to behavior are addressed.

Background factors are also assessed and analyzed for their relationship to the proximal factors. These include demographic characteristics (i.e., age, education, marital status, ethnicity, and socioeconomic status), health factors (disease stage, HIV treatment, substance abuse treatment, STD, and pregnancy history), cultural background (acculturation, discrimination history, ethnic identity), psychological history, and trauma history, including the onset, severity, and extent of CSA.

In addition to the developmental context, the participants' social and cultural contexts need to be considered also. To ensure that the curriculum comprehensively addressed the needs of a diverse population of HIV-positive women, pilot groups of Black, Latina, and White women tested the relevance of the information. To offer the groups in Spanish to women who were monolingual or bilingual but preferring to speak Spanish, prior to translation, an advisory committee of Latina professionals in the fields of HIV, child abuse, social work, and public health reviewed and made revisions to the curriculum. The goal of the Spanish translation was to ensure appropriate cultural nuances and language differences across multiple countries of origin, including Mexico, El Salvador, Guatemala, Puerto Rico, and Costa Rica.

The format of the intervention also reflects the developmental context of women with CSA histories. Emphasis is placed on women prioritizing their own goals in a realistic manner set within an accepting environment. For instance, an individual's goal may be to reduce a particular behavior rather than eliminate it. The opportunity to select her own goals, rather than have them outlined for her, results in a personalized treatment program embedded within a standardized curriculum. As such, while addressing those aspects of risk hypothesized to affect HIV-positive women with CSA histories in general, we move away from the "one-size-fits-all" model to a more individually tailored one. Individuals are asked to explicitly grapple with the idea of how reasonable risk reduction is in a given area, given current partners and environmental constraints. Women learn how the decisions they make impact and are affected by important people in their lives. Not meeting goals is viewed as a learning process, and discussion regarding relapses is encouraged to better address barriers to change and prevent setbacks in the future.

The multiethnic composition of the groups requires that the curriculum is culturally sensitive and teaches women to appreciate and understand each other's experiences. Group members struggle with past decisions and experiences; how each woman faces current challenges and perceives her past is unique. The nonjudgmental atmosphere inherent to the groups allows for women who are at different stages of the healing process to feel valued and accepted. This allows women to break the cycle of self-blame by placing their decisions in the context of past life experiences. By increasing understanding of the connection between the past and present, women are able to come to terms with decisions they have made and clear the way for the possibility of change. The stage is then set to change the cognitive, affective, and behavioral patterns that were developmentally constructed.

Many of the WHP participants have never disclosed their experiences with CSA prior to the intervention. Some participants had shared what happened to them, only to be punished or told they were lying about the incident. This isolation serves as a barrier for some women and makes attending the groups and disclosing to group members a daunting task. Some of these women come to group "brimming over," ready to talk about what happened to them, yet feeling intimidated and uncertain. Therefore, to encourage and facilitate participation, we ensured that transportation and child care are provided if needed. Furthermore, for many participants, a nutritious meal serves as an incentive also. Other items (e.g., movie passes, tickets to performing arts and sporting events, cosmetic products) are also provided as reinforcers when available.

Intervention Curriculum

Content

The 11-week intervention addresses HIV risk behaviors, interpersonal behaviors, health behaviors, and psychological status by focusing on the sexual histories of participants and their link to current cognitive, affective, and behavioral patterns. Throughout the sessions, the impact of CSA on women's functioning is emphasized to help survivors make important links between past traumatic experiences, HIV infection, and current functioning. A technique that has been incorporated into the curriculum to emphasize the association between past trauma and abuse, HIV status, and current functioning is a narrative that each woman is asked to write every week about the abuse incident and its consequences (Pennebaker, 1997). The purpose of the narrative is to enable cognitive restructuring of traumatic experiences that may result in positive emotional and physiological results. This technique has been demonstrated to be effective with different groups of trauma victims, including victims of rape and Holocaust survivors (Pennebaker, 1997; see also chap. 9, this volume). Participants are asked to write narratives of the sexual abuse experience and/or being HIV-positive. Women who are not comfortable with writing are given a tape recorder to use to record their most traumatic experiences. The writings are not shared and are kept confidential. Throughout the sessions, the groups are taught and practice a problem-solving technique that is applied to each topic to facilitate decision making. "Keeping females in a healthy place" (KFNHP) is the motto used to aid participants to cue in to the necessary steps in problem solving and decision making when faced with a particular situation or dilemma. For example, the first word, *keeping*, beginning with K, triggers participants to ask themselves about a particular situation, "What do you *know*?" The second word, *females*, beginning with F, refers to the question, "How do you *feel*?" The third word, *in*, cues participants to the question, "What do you *need*?" The fourth word, *healthy*, recalls the question, "What is *holding* you back?" And the final word, *place*, serves as a cue for the question, "What is the *plan*?" Therefore, by continually using the KFNHP technique, the participants learn to approach situations by considering knowledge and information, emotional responses to the problem often stemming from their abuse experiences, what is needed to solve the problem, what obstacles exist, and formulating a plan for resolution.

Another important aspect of the curriculum focuses on enhancing women's support networks. Support is increased using various techniques, including assigning "peer buddies" in the first week, emphasizing interconnectedness among participants, and making relevant community referrals throughout the intervention. Given that the groups are composed of women from a variety of cultural, racial, and religious backgrounds, these issues are directly addressed throughout the curriculum. For instance, during the first session, each participant is asked to talk about what religion she was brought up with and which holidays she celebrated as a child. Participants are also asked to describe where they come from, their cultural heritage, and other past experiences they feel have affected them. These disclosures are thought to broaden understanding of and sensitivity to experiences that differ from one's own. In later sessions, participants discuss how they learned to think about their bodies, which body parts are acceptable to touch, and their feelings about male and female anatomy. Facilitators elicit a list of words participants use for body parts to construct a common terminology for discussions of sexual health. When discussing triggers for risky behaviors, participants are asked to identify historical, cultural, and religious experiences that may prevent a woman from protecting her sexual health (e.g., strong religious beliefs regarding the acceptability of using birth control may trigger anxiety and feelings of guilt when asked to use a condom). Language barriers that impede communication with medical providers are also discussed.

The intervention assists participants' management of psychological status by beginning each session with a 5-minute check-in time comprised of a relaxation technique (a combination of guided imagery, breathing, and thought-stopping) to enhance participants' ability to relax and manage feelings of distress throughout each session. Particularly with CSA survivors, distress may arise from recalling the abuse experience during groups, and stress management and coping is an important component both in and out of these sessions. Each session ends with a 5-minute check-out time in which participants review successful personal coping strategies and positive affirmation techniques to enhance well-being.

The specific order and content of the curriculum is as follows. In Week 1, the participants receive a comprehensive orientation to the intervention, which includes a discussion of ground rules, disclosure issues, spiritual and cultural beliefs, and the 11-week program agenda. Week 2 is devoted to assessment of risky sexual and drug behaviors and identification of myths related to HIV. Weeks 3 through 11 are devoted to the topics of treatment adherence and health behaviors, sexual issues, interpersonal communication, and drug and alcohol use by self or partner, each of which are addressed weekly rather than in a modular approach. This enables the facilitators to address each participant's stage of change (Prochaska & DiClemente, 1982) across topics. Prochaska and DiClemente identified six stages that an individual may go through in the process of changing a problem. These stages include precontemplation (not yet considering the possibility of change), contemplation (awareness of needed change), determination (considering how to change), action, maintenance, and relapse. In using this more integrated approach, continuity and continued impact are ensured, allowing participants who are absent in one or two sessions to still gain information across areas. Each week integrates the past abuse experience with current functioning, emphasizing the relationships among past abuse and sexual and interpersonal functioning, self-concept, and affective status. Finally, Week 11 addresses termination, in which a graduation ceremony takes place with certificates and family members present to celebrate achievements and progress made by the participants.

Format

The format of the curriculum consists of didactic presentations, demonstrations for mastery, role-modeling and role-playing, group discussion, homework assignments, audiovisual stimuli, and health education materials (e.g., condoms, penis models, pill boxes). It is structured, with a balance between psychoeducational content and clinical process. Sessions are held once a week for 2 hours in duration, with a brief 10-minute break in the middle. Participants are asked to arrive a half-hour early for refreshments. This refreshment period enables late arrivals without interfering with group content.

Much thought was also given to the pacing of the presentation and discussion of sexual abuse and other difficult aspects of the curriculum. Because of the highly sensitive nature of the material covered, we took pains to ensure that the most difficult information was embedded in each individual session in a way that allowed the women to begin and end each session with somewhat benign material (i.e., starting with how was their week and progressing toward their goals in a given area). Care was given to place the break at an appropriate time during the session, and facilitators check in with each participant as the session closes. Similarly, the most challenging abuse-related material is placed in the middle sessions, allowing for participants to desensitize to some of the early, more fact-oriented material and begin to learn the tools to disclose past experiences in a comfortable and healthy manner.

Group Facilitation and Training

Each session is conducted by a trained group facilitator in collaboration with a peer mentor. The facilitators have some formal education and clinical training with a female HIV-positive population, as well as knowledge of (and preferably clinical experience with) CSA survivors. However, to realize the goal of eventually transferring the curriculum to HIV service centers, we recognize that the existing staff at these centers may not meet each of our requirements for facilitators. For this reason, we have placed more emphasis on hiring facilitators with extensive clinical experiences with HIV-infected populations and CSA survivors rather than on level of education.

The role of the peer mentor is critical, as she models disclosure and continual development of the self that had been disrupted by CSA to participants. Locating appropriate peer mentors presents unique challenges. It is imperative to have individuals who are at a stage in their healing process in which they could tolerate hearing the stories of other CSA survivors (as well as experiences with HIV infection) without overly internalizing others' trauma and becoming debilitated themselves. The peer mentors must be comfortable with disclosing relevant personal experiences for the benefit of the participants. These women must have enough personal support (whether through individual therapy, other support groups, friends, and family) to be able to share their experiences with others. In addition, because the population of women targeted by the intervention is predominantly women of color (Black and Latina), we recruited women of comparable cultural and language backgrounds for the peer mentor positions.

Supervision is an important component of the intervention. Supervision addresses practical issues involved in facilitating groups as well as processing countertransference issues. Countertransference is a clinical term referring to the process by which personal experiences, cultural biases, and other beliefs or values may hinder facilitators' ability to be effective in group.

Such countertransference issues must be addressed on a consistent basis in supervision. Rescue fantasies among group facilitators are common. Because participants may lead chaotic lives, experience hardships, or engage in high-risk behaviors, facilitators may feel a need to "rescue" participants from these difficult experiences. Further, by being constantly exposed to detailed descriptions of such traumatic experiences from participants, facilitators may experience secondary trauma, an internalization of the participants' trauma, and become overwhelmed and debilitated themselves. Debriefing of secondary trauma may be helpful because of the challenging and sometimes overwhelming task of providing treatment for HIV-positive women who often have chaotic lives, disclose sexual abuse and other traumatic experiences, experience multiple illnesses, and address death.

FINDINGS FROM THE INTERVENTION PILOT

The Women's Health Intervention was piloted on 5 participants prior to its actual start. The curriculum was administered over the course of 11 weeks as designed. At its conclusion, a focus group was conducted to broadly assess the domains of impact as experienced by the participants. The purpose of the focus group was as a manipulation check: to get a sense of whether the curriculum hit the domains of impact as conceptualized. Thus, we assessed the three proximal domains of change as targeted: cognitive, emotional/affective, and behavioral. The focus group lasted 2 hours, and the content was audiotaped and transcribed verbatim. Themes were extracted from the text inductively. Within each domain, several themes emerged inductively in response to open-ended questions, and themes from each domain appeared to interact with one another.

Cognitive Effects

One salient and reliable change described by the participants was how they viewed themselves. In response to an open-ended question about what they learned from the intervention, all of the participants indicated that their "self-worth," "self-esteem," and "regard for myself" increased. They attributed many of their risky behaviors to a lack of self-worth; for example, one participant stated that she did not take medications as instructed because she did not care enough for herself to fight HIV. As a result of an increase in self-worth, she became more active in her treatment:

> This last time I went (to the doctor), I had specific questions to ask and he answered all of them. I wanted my medication reduced, and he said, why don't we change them. . . . I always resisted change, but this time I'm thinking, I want to do this, I am tired of the old ones and all its problems.

Other participants also pointed to greater self-regard as key in changing behavior in other realms. For example, one woman spoke about her inability to refuse sexual advances: "There were a lot of guys and I do not know how to put boundaries up." However, with respect to a recent incident, she reported,

> On this trip there was somebody I really liked, and we kind of hit it off, but I was really proud of myself that I did not let things get further. That is something I would not be able to do before. I guess I see myself as being more important and I do not have to go for everything.

Along with seeing boundaries between the self and others more clearly, the women gained a greater sense of self-worth, which also contributed to increased assertiveness. The participants indicated that "saying no" was something they were doing more often. For instance, one woman stated,

> I must tell you, I always put the grandmother, the aunt who was sick, the kids before myself. Even the dog and the cat. I could be hungry and needy. . . . Not that I wanted to, I just thought that was what I had to do!

Her perspective now is slightly different: "I am not an object and (my partner) can't just pull me and say 'come on'." The realization that one can say no can also assert itself in a revictimization situation. One woman described a recent incident in a hospital: "I was tired and the nurse's aide helped me clean up in bed, but then he starts playing with my . . .[1] and I said 'Stop! What are you doing?'"

It is interesting to note that, in response to a question about what they had learned from the intervention, the participants did not include information about HIV. In fact, when specifically probed about whether they gained knowledge about HIV, they indicated that this was not the most salient or significant. Instead, they pointed to the link between their CSA experience and their current functioning—including drug use, interpersonal and sexual relationships, and treatment adherence—as enlightening, particularly because it was learned and shared in a group format. As one woman stated,

> I learned that there are other women out there that were sexually molested, that I am not the only one. . . . Of course that was something new. We do not normally go around talking about these things (CSA). People would look at you like there was something wrong.

Hearing others' similar experiences and modeling from the peer mentor gave the women a sense of encouragement and empowerment: "I thought, if she did it, I could do it too."

Emotional and Affective Effects

In discussing the impact of the intervention, participants cited some major emotional/affective changes. These themes emerged in response to an

---

[1]The participant trailed off here and did not describe more about this incident.

open-ended question without probes from the focus group leader. Surprisingly, an apparently strong emotional effect was a feeling of freedom and liberation, which was not specifically articulated in the study's aims. For example, one participant stated,

> Not until I came to this group, along with women like myself, and (who) actually had the same type of feelings, was I able to talk about how I really felt about being molested . . . I found some freedom.

The women contrasted this newfound feeling with previous feelings of "stuff being trapped" inside of them. The process of opening up and sharing seemed to lead to feelings of "being free," as another participant stated, helping to "be able to live in every aspect of life, more freely." In turn, the feeling of liberation moderated the level of distress stemming from the HIV and lowered subjective stress in general. A third participant described a feeling very similar to liberation, calling it empowerment.

In addition to freedom and liberation and the concomitant decrease in stress, participants stated that they began to trust more, thus allowing feelings of intimacy to develop with the group facilitator, peer mentor, and other group members. How did trust develop in women who have personal histories that warrant mistrust? In response to a follow-up probe, the participants pointed to the peer mentor as a critical part of the process:

> When I first saw the [peer mentor], my mind said: shit, all they are going to do is suck out our brain one more time. But when she introduced herself and said I am . . . and I have . . . then I went like: Oh, that kind of made all of us one, and we begun to open up.

Thus, having a facilitator with whom group members can identify serves to break down initial barriers to trust, higher in CSA victims and built up over time, and enhances the development of intimacy in the group.

Behavioral Effects

Changes in self-perceptions and affect appeared to lead to behavioral change. One area of specific change voiced by the participants was a difference in their relationships with their partners. They stated that they began to communicate more assertively with their partners, leading to subtle but profound differences. To illustrate, one woman recounted an interaction with her husband:

> The other day I got home a little late, and he said, you were not here when I got home so I thought I had to do all of the dishes. So I said, yes, so what is your problem?

Thus the participant was able to maintain her composure and sense of self-worth instead of feeling diminished by the interaction. Greater assertiveness was also expressed in the sexual realm:

Now I can communicate with my partner about my body, so everything about me changed. When I was really sick and could not do anything, that is when he wanted to have sex with me. And I did not want him to find somebody else. My husband is frisky to the life, but I said, I wish you could find other forms of recreation. And I feel really sorry for him, but you know, when you take those vows, together for better or worse . . . I reminded him of that.

Given that participants were more likely to assert their desires and needs with their sexual partners, especially with regard to sexual practices, their sexual risk is likely to decrease.

Relationships with others were also affected, in particular those with children and treatment providers. The women uniformly expressed that they always took care of others first with great sacrifice to their own well-being. Even while tired or sick, the women still tended to others' needs. However, seeds of change were noted. For example, one woman stated:

I have learned to take a deep breath and say "it's not that serious" and then I am able to respond to whatever that is said to me. Even if it is from my old man, my mom, my kids, anybody. I can say no, I won't do that, or I will do it later.

These changes in interpersonal communication were echoed by the others, for example:

My sister is calling me to ask if I can baby-sit. I love my nephew, but there is no way I can take care of him when I can't even take care of me. And before I would have said okay even though I did not want to. But this here has helped me that I am the one who comes first.

In terms of treatment providers, improved communication with them, stemming from cognitive and affective changes, meant greater engagement in the treatment process and possibly increased treatment adherence. One participant noted that she began to call her physician assistant more often to discuss treatment options. She noted that although she had a good relationship with him, she had greater interest in her health now, and this was reflected in their interaction. Participation in the group spurred interest in nutrition, relaxation techniques, and stress management, suggesting that immediate effects may persist and perhaps lead to even greater change.

Consistent with increased feelings of trust and intimacy with others, greater engagement in social networks was also evident. Participants cited decreased isolation and greater elicitation of support from others.

DISCUSSION AND CONCLUSION

Findings from the intervention pilot confirmed that the targeted domains of change, consist of cognitive, emotional/affective, and behavioral factors, were addressed in the intervention. More specifically, they supported the idea that the developmental disruptions associated with CSA render HIV risk behavior resistant to change, and therefore must be addressed alongside HIV risk. This was demonstrated by participants' reports of feeling unworthy of good health, and therefore having little motivation to engage in self-protective or enhancing behaviors. Once self-regard was increased, engagement in safer behaviors (i.e., not having sex immediately with a new partner) as well as in the treatment process (i.e., communicating with treatment providers more) was evidenced.

In addition, the intervention appeared to begin to restore a sense of boundaries between the self and others, the development of which may have been disrupted by CSA. An appropriate sense of boundaries includes saying no when imposed on as well as being able to trust and be intimate with others when appropriate, both of which participants stated they lacked. After their participation in the intervention, however, the women indicated greater assertion of boundaries in family, treatment, and sexual situations, leading to lower HIV risk and greater health benefits. They also felt a greater sense of trust and intimacy with other group members, owing to the sharing of common experiences and the modeling of the peer mentor. This has led to greater use of social networks to elicit support and decreased isolation.

These initial findings support the integrated intervention as a promising approach for HIV-positive women with CSA histories. Because of the barriers CSA poses to the initiation and maintenance of protective behaviors, they must be addressed concomitantly with HIV risk-reduction strategies that, in the case of HIV-positive individuals, have the ultimate objective of the prevention of reinfection and transmission of the virus to others. In addition to the integrated content, the format of the intervention should also reflect the dual status of the women. Specifically, having a peer model seemed to be critical in catalyzing the development of the participants. The integrated format of the material, which allows for growth to build instead of compartmentalize, was another specific ingredient that appeared effective. We did not specifically anticipate the feelings of liberation that the participants so strongly cited. However, feelings of "being trapped" are consistent with CSA sequelae, and the intervention appears to ameliorate this effect.

FUTURE DIRECTIONS

On the basis of pilot data, the integrated approach as conceptualized and implemented in the Women's Health Project appears promising. Whereas cognitive–behavioral models of intervention may be most efficient and effective for populations less encumbered by developmental disruptions and social considerations, an integrated approach may be the appropriate intervention paradigm for women, particularly those with CSA histories. Obviously, because of the limited sample size in the pilot and the qualitative nature of the data obtained, inferences about the efficacy of the intervention await the conclusion of the study. At the end of the clinical trial, we hope to address the main thesis of whether the intervention was effective, as well as other critical questions such as which subgroups of women are most influenced by the intervention, what components are effective, the degree to which each additional session affects outcomes (dose–response relationship), and the areas of outcomes most affected.

REFERENCES

Ajzen, I. (1991). The theory of planned behavior. *Organizational Behavior and Human Decision Processes, 50*, 179–211.

Ajzen, I., & Fishbein, M. (1980). *Understanding attitudes and predicting social behavior: Attitudes, intentions, and perceived behavioral control.* Englewood Cliffs, NJ: Prentice Hall.

Albarracin, D., Johnson, B. T., Fishbein, M., & Muellerleile, P. A. (2001). Theories of reasoned action and planned behavior as models of condom use: A meta-analysis. *Psychological Bulletin, 127*, 142–161.

Amaro, H. (1995). Love, sex, and power: considering women's realities in HIV prevention. *American Psychologist, 50*, 437–447.

Becker, M. H. (1974). The health belief model and personal health behavior. *Health Education Monographs, 2*, 324–508.

Bensley, L. S., Van Eenwyk, J., & Simmons, K. W. (2000). Self-reported childhood sexual and physical abuse and adult HIV-risk behaviors and heavy drinking. *American Journal of Preventive Medicine, 18*, 151–158.

Brown, A., & Finkelhor, D. (1986). The impact of child sexual abuse: A review of the research. *Psychological Bulletin, 99*, 66–77.

Catania, J. A., Kegeles, S. M., & Coates, T. J. (1990). Towards an understanding of risk behavior: An AIDS risk reduction model (ARRM). *Health Education Quarterly, 17*, 53–72.

Chin, D. (1999). HIV-related sexual risk assessment among Asian/Pacific Islander women: An inductive model. *Social Science and Medicine, 49*, 241–252.

Chin, D., & Kroesen, K. (1999). Disclosure of HIV infection among Asian/Pacific Islander women: Cultural stigma and support. *Cultural Diversity and Ethnic Minority Psychology, 5*, 222–235.

Cole, C. H., & Barney, E. E. (1987). Safeguards and the therapeutic window: A group treatment strategy for adult incest survivors. *American Journal of Orthopsychiatry, 57(4)*, 601–609.

Donalson, P. E., Whalen, M. H., & Anastas, J. W. (1989). Teen pregnancy and sexual abuse: Exploring the connection. *Smith College Studies in Social Work, 59*, 289.

Fishbein, M. (1980). A theory of reasoned action: Some applications and implications. In H. E. Howe, Jr. & M. M. Page (Eds.), *Nebraska symposium on motivation, 1979* (Vol. 27, pp. 65–116). Lincoln: University of Nebraska Press.

Ganz, P., Wyatt, G. E., & Loeb, T. B. (1998). *The prevalence and circumstances of child sexual abuse among breast cancer survivors: Relationship to high risk sexual behaviors.* Manuscript submitted for publication.

Gibson, R. L., & Hartshorne, T. S. (1996). Childhood sexual abuse and adult loneliness and network orientation. *Child Abuse and Neglect, 20,* 1087–1093.

Gold-Steinberg, S., & Buttenheim, M. (1993). Telling one's story in an incest survivor group. *International Journal of Group Psychotherapy, 37,* 173–189.

Longshore, D., Grills, C., & Annon, K. (1999). Effects of a culturally congruent intervention on cognitive factors relevant to drug use recovery. *Substance Use and Misuse, 34,* 1223–1241.

Lundberg-Love, P. (1990). Treatment of adult survivors of incest. In R. Ammerman & M. Herson (Eds.), *Treatment of family violence* (pp. 109–111). New York: Wiley.

National Center for HIV, STD, and TB Prevention, Division of HIV/AIDS Prevention (n.d.). HIV/AIDS among US women: Minority and young women at continuing risk. Available at http://www.cdc.gov/hiv/pubs/facts/women.htm.

Pennebaker, J. W. (1997). *Opening up: The healing power of expressing emotion.* New York: Guilford Press.

Prochaska, J. O., & DiClemente, C. C. (1982). Transtheoretical therapy: Toward a more integrative model of change. *Psychotherapy: Theory, Research, and Practice, 10,* 276–288.

Rhodes, J. E., Ebert, L., & Myers, A. B. (1993). Sexual victimization in young and pregnant and parenting African American women: Psychological and social outcomes. *Violence and Victims, 8,* 153–163.

Riggs, A., Alario, A. J., & McHorney, C. (1990). Health risk behaviors and attempted suicide in adolescents who report prior maltreatment. *Journal of Pediatrics, 116,* 815–821.

Romero, G., Wyatt, G., Chin, D., & Rodriguez, C. (1998). HIV-related behaviors among recently immigrated and undocumented Latinas. *International Quarterly of Community Health Education, 18,* 89–105.

Roth, S., & Newman, E. (1991). The process of coping with sexual trauma. *Journal of Traumatic Stress, 4,* 279–297.

Sikkema, K. J., Winett, R. A., & Lombard, D. N. (1995). Development and evaluation of an HIV-risk reduction program for female college students. *AIDS Education & Prevention, 7,* 145–159.

Smith, G. (1992). The unbearable traumatogenic past: Child sexual abuse. In V. P. Varma, (Ed.), *The secret life of vulnerable children* (pp. 130–156). London: Routledge.

Widom, C. S., & Kuhns, J. B. (1996). Childhood victimization and subsequent risk for promiscuity, prostitution, and teenage pregnancy: A prospective study. *American Journal of Public Health, 86,* 1607–1612.

Wingood, G. M., & DiClemente, R. J. (1996). HIV sexual risk reduction interventions for women: A review. *American Journal of Preventative Medicine, 12,* 209–217.

Wong, M. L. (1995). Behavioral interventions in the control of human immunodeficiency virus and other sexually transmitted diseases—A review. *Annals Academy of Medicine Singapore, 24,* 602–607.

Wyatt, G. E., Myers, H. F., Williams, J. K., Kitchen, C. R., Loeb, T., Carmona, J. V., et al. (2002). Does a history of trauma contribute to HIV risk for women of color? Implications for prevention and policy. *American Journal of Public Health, 92,* 660–665.

Wyatt, G., Newcomb, M. D., & Riederle, M. H. (1993). *Sexual abuse and consensual sex: Women's developmental patterns and outcomes.* Newbury Park, CA: Sage.

12

TRAUMA-FOCUSED VERSUS PRESENT-FOCUSED MODELS OF GROUP THERAPY FOR WOMEN SEXUALLY ABUSED IN CHILDHOOD

DAVID SPIEGEL, CATHERINE CLASSEN,
ELISABETH THURSTON, AND LISA BUTLER

The existing literature on the long-term sequelae of child sexual abuse (CSA) documents a large array of long-term effects (Browne & Finkelhor, 1986; Polusny & Follette, 1995). Long-term effects of CSA can include emotional dysregulation, troubled interpersonal relationships, vulnerability to revictimization, and risk behavior including substance abuse and risk of HIV and other drug-related and sexually mediated infections. Although CSA has come to be recognized as a serious social problem, we are still in the early stages of learning how best to treat CSA survivors. Much remains to be learned about the most effective treatments for these long-term psychological effects and the possible role of such treatments in preventing medical sequelae, including exposure to HIV infection.

This research was supported by Grant No. MH52134 from the National Institute of Mental Health. The authors wish to thank Kirsten Nevill-Manning, Cheryl Koopman, Deborah Rose, Lindsay Picard, Brian Chin, Julia Zarcone, all of the women who participated in this research, and Mount Zion Hospital and the Metropolitan Community Church in San Francisco for providing office space for this research.

In this chapter we describe research we have conducted in an effort to identify effective treatment approaches for CSA survivors. The central question we sought to address is whether it is necessary to help survivors access and process their traumatic memories from childhood in order to decrease CSA-related symptomatology or whether it is sufficient to work on their current problems in living. This chapter begins with a rationale for our program of research. We then describe our pilot study comparing trauma-focused and present-focused group therapies for female CSA survivors. This includes a description of the two group therapy interventions, the population we sampled, and the results of the pilot study. We close the chapter with a description of a large, randomized trial we are currently conducting again comparing trauma-focused and present-focused group therapies for CSA survivors who are also judged to be at risk for HIV infection. Given the higher prevalence of CSA among women, our research has focused on women.

TRAUMA-FOCUSED VERSUS PRESENT-FOCUSED TREATMENT

Despite the prevalence of CSA and its clearly negative effects, there is not yet a clear understanding of how best to treat CSA survivors. Psychotherapy is one way of moderating the negative effects of CSA and potentially of reducing some of the risk factors for contracting HIV infection. In recent years, a consensus has emerged regarding phase-oriented treatment models as the standard of care for working with trauma (Brown, Scheflin, & Hammond, 1998). Phase-oriented treatment models are most often described as consisting of three phases that Brown et al. referred to as (a) stabilization, (b) integration (i.e., trauma-focused memory work), and (c) postintegrative self- and relational development. While the first phase sets the stage for the trauma-focused work and the third phase helps the survivor consolidate and integrate what has been learned, the cornerstone of this treatment model is on processing the traumatic memories. Although a phase-oriented treatment model is now commonly accepted, there has been little controlled, empirical research to examine the importance of the components of the model or its application in a group treatment format.

Much of the literature describing therapeutic interventions with sexual abuse survivors suggests that clinicians treat survivors with the understanding that coming to terms, both affectively and cognitively, with the meaning and impact of traumatic events is a central component of recovery (Coons, Bowman, Pellow, & Schneider, 1989; Herman, 1992; McCann & Pearlman, 1990; Paddison, Einbinder, Maker, & Strain, 1993; Roth, 1993; Spiegel, 1989). This type of intervention allows a survivor to integrate memories of her abuse into her understanding of her life through successive examinations and detailed accounts of specific abuse experiences. Whereas trauma-focused group psychotherapy emphasizes the link between the survivor's symptomatology and the past environment, present-focused group psychotherapy focuses on the link between symptomatology and the immediate environment. Present-focused treatment is designed to help patients reduce distress symptoms by identifying and modifying maladaptive behaviors without revisiting past traumas (Classen, Koopman, Nevill-Manning, & Spiegel, 2001; Yalom, 1980, 1995). In contrast, trauma-focused treatment attenuates distress by retrieving and reinterpreting memories of events that led to the symptoms and formation of the self-structure (Classen, Koopman, et al., 2001; Coons et al., 1989; Herman, 1992; McCann & Pearlman, 1990; Paddison et al., 1993; Roth, 1993; Spiegel, 1989). It also facilitates emotional processing through exposure and desensitization (Foa & Meadows 1997), as well as working through and restructuring traumatic memories (Spiegel, 1997).

Each type of treatment is widely used and has a plausible rationale. However, there is a need for randomized clinical trials comparing these different treatment methods to determine the best course of treatment for survivors of CSA, especially those at high risk of contracting HIV. Currently, there are limited outcome data for group treatment of adult survivors of CSA, and most of these studies are with women. Most reports of group therapy outcomes involve pre- and posttreatment designs without between-treatments comparison or wait-list control groups (Carver, Scheier, & Weintraub, 1989; Hazzard, Rogers, & Angert, 1993; Herman & Schatzow, 1984; Kriedler, Einsporn, Zupancic, & Masterson, 1999; Paddison et al., 1993; Sharpe, Selley, Low, & Hall, 2001; Tsai & Wagner, 1978) or nonrandomized designs (Hall, Mullee, & Thompson, 1995; Morgan & Cummings, 1999; Morrison & Treliving, 2002; Richter, Snider, & Gorey, 1997; Saxe & Johnson, 1999; Talbot et al., 1999; Westbury & Tutty, 1999). In all but two of these studies (Morrison & Treliving, 2002; Sharpe et al., 2001), participants were women.

Of the three randomized clinical studies of group therapy for women sexually abused as children (Alexander, Neimeyer, & Follette, 1991; Stalker & Fry, 1999; Zlotnick et al., 1997), none focused on working specifically with the memories of the traumatic event. Alexander and colleagues compared two time-limited group formats, a process group and a more structured interpersonal transaction group, against a wait-list control condition. Participants in the treatment condition experienced a far greater reduction in depression and distress than did those in the wait-list condition. In addition, participants in the interpersonal transaction group showed greater improvement in distress than the process group, but the process group showed greater improvement in social functioning than the interpersonal transaction group. Zlotnick and colleagues found that posttraumatic stress disorder (PTSD) symptoms and dissociation decreased more for those participants in the affect management group than the wait-list control condition. Stalker and Fry compared 10 sessions of group treatment against 10 sessions of individual treatment. Women benefited from both forms of treatment, but there was no difference in outcome between the two conditions.

Randomized clinical trials comparing different treatment types for CSA survivors are important because of the current climate surrounding abuse. The current focus in literature and society regarding CSA is on the veracity of abuse memories (Butler & Spiegel, 1997; Cicchetti & Rizley, 1981; Gleaves, Smith, Butler, & Spiegel, 2001; Loftus, 1993; Loftus & Hoffman, 1989) and the extent of long-term ill effects (Dallam et al., 2001; Rind, Tromovitch, & Bauserman, 1998; Spiegel 2000a, 2000b). This debate brings up issues regarding the most appropriate method of treatment for women with self-reported histories of CSA. If psychotherapy that focuses on working through memories of sexual abuse is helpful in ameliorating trauma-related symptoms and improving current psychosocial functioning, then clinicians need to learn clinically responsible ways of working with memories. Outside of the current memory debate, memory retrieval carries with it its own risks, including contamination with suggestion and expectancy (Loftus & Hoffman, 1989; Spiegel, 1995). Working with traumatic memory content also needs to be weighed against therapeutic gains, as it can be potentially distressing for patients (Spiegel, 1995). These concerns highlight the need for clinical trials, so therapists can weigh the psychological benefits of working with traumatic memories against the potential risks.

PILOT STUDY

To address this need for empirical data on the relative effectiveness of trauma-focused versus present-focused group therapy, we conducted a pilot study comparing the two against each other and a wait-list control condition. Our aims were to assess (a) whether it was more beneficial for survivors to receive (any) treatment than not to receive treatment and (b) whether the different types of intervention (i.e., trauma-focused vs. present-focused) were associated with different degrees of change in distress and psychosocial functioning.

Method

Participants were assigned to one of three conditions: a trauma-focused psychotherapy group, a present-focused psychotherapy group, or a wait-list, no-treatment control condition. After the screening of more than 300 individuals over the phone and 95 in face-to-face interviews, 55 women met all eligibility criteria and chose to participate in the study.

The inclusion criteria were are as follows:

- The survivor was female.
- The survivor was 18 years of age or older.

- The survivor was English-speaking.
- The survivor had at least two explicit memories of sexual abuse involving genital contact.
- At least two sexual abuse events occurred when the survivor was between 3 and 15 years of age.
- The perpetrator was at least 5 years older than the survivor.
- The survivor knew the perpetrator prior to the sexual abuse.
- The survivor had discussed or attempted to discuss details of the sexual abuse previously with another person (e.g., family member, friend, or therapist) at least 6 months prior to being interviewed for the study.
- The survivor met *Diagnostic and Statistical Manual of Mental Disorders* (4th ed., *DSM–IV*; American Psychiatric Association, 1994) criteria for current PTSD.
- The survivor provided informed consent.

The exclusion criteria were as follows:

- The survivor was diagnosed with conditions that fall into any of the following diagnostic categories: schizophrenia and other psychotic disorders, dementia, delirium, and amnestic or other cognitive disorders.
- The survivor reported ritual abuse.
- The survivor was currently receiving psychotherapy (including individual or group psychotherapy).
- The survivor met *DSM–IV* (American Psychiatric Association, 1994) criteria for alcohol or drug dependence (women were not excluded if they met criteria for alcohol or drug abuse.)
- The survivor was currently suicidal (i.e., within the last month).

Participants in both treatment conditions received 6 months of weekly, 90-minute group therapy sessions led by two experienced group leaders.

Intervention

Each intervention was a manualized group treatment (Classen, Ballinger, & Spiegel, 1993; Henderson, Classen, Ballinger, Spiegel, & Yalom, 1994). Therapists participated in a training workshop and were given weekly supervision by an expert clinician.

Trauma-Focused Therapy

The primary aim of treatment in trauma-focused therapy is to help survivors overcome problems in their current functioning by working through and integrating their traumatic abuse experiences. This process requires survivors to reconstruct their traumatic experiences and integrate the affect associated with the trauma. Through this work, survivors can modify the negative views of self that arose because of the abuse and integrate their traumatic history into their conscious awareness of self and others. Although this clearly entails working with specific memories of abuse and often the context of the abuse, this exploration also requires recognition of how the abuse is connected to the survivor's current emotional and interpersonal functioning. Acknowledging how the abuse has shaped the survivor's beliefs, assumptions, and relationships may help alleviate the power that the traumatic experience has over her current life.

Trauma-focused group leaders are also trained to be aware of occasions when present-day issues are used to avoid addressing the upsetting topic of abuse. In this case, the therapist must redirect the survivor's attention and help her process the feelings that the present-day issue brings up and how those feelings may relate to her trauma history. When current problems in the lives of those in a trauma-focused group require attention, they can be handled with a three-step process. First, the group leaders assess how well the group member is coping and determine if she needs help in dealing with the issue. Then, the member's immediate situation is addressed with either suggestions from the group or support from the group leader. Finally, the leaders return the discussion to a trauma focus, preferably by linking the current-day problem to the survivor's traumatic past.

Most current-day issues that survivors bring to the group are in some way either symptomatic of the childhood trauma or serve to activate issues directly related to the abuse. For instance, one group member began to discuss present substance abuse issues. She wanted the group's support in dealing with those issues, so the therapist linked her current problem to an abuse-related topic. They went on to discuss the depression she feels when she reexperiences the pain of her abuse and how she uses drugs to help alleviate that pain. By demonstrating how the participant's current substance abuse issues are related to her abuse experience, the therapists were able to address her immediate concerns while continuing the group's focus on the trauma.

Present-Focused Therapy

The primary aim of treatment for present-focused therapy is to help survivors address the problems in their daily lives by identifying and modifying the maladaptive patterns of behavior that have arisen as a result of their abuse. This approach is based on the assumption that by focusing on the here-and-now in the group, a survivor can make positive changes in her life, even without understanding how her present problems may be related to the abuse. This approach is commonly used in group therapy with many different populations (Yalom, 1995). In some cases the present-focused approach may be the most appropriate form of treatment, for instance, if current dysfunction is severe.

The first step in a present-focused intervention is for group members to identify the problems they are experiencing in their current lives. The therapists frame this process so that problems that members may not yet have recognized themselves, such as risky behavior, are also identified. Although we did not select our participants on the basis of HIV risk behavior in this pilot study, a number of participants exhibited behaviors that put them at risk for contracting HIV, making those risk factors of primary concern.

As mentioned previously, we learned that participants most likely to have been recently sexually revictimized were women who had problems with being nonassertive, socially avoidant, self-sacrificing, and needy (Classen, Field, Koopman, Nevill-Manning, & Spiegel, 2001). When these problems manifested themselves in the group process or if the group member identifies them as a problem in her outside life, they became a focus of the present-focused group. Another set of problems that are likely to be associated with sexual revictimization and risky sexual behaviors are dissociative experiences. In the present-focused groups, this was addressed by helping the member identify the types of situations that triggered dissociation and helping her problem-solve ways of avoiding such situations or keeping herself grounded if she cannot avoid them. In other cases, a group member's continuation or escalation of use of alcohol or other drugs needed to be addressed. All group members were expected to refrain from showing up to group intoxicated, but the therapists were still asked to be alert to evidence of alcohol or drug use. Intoxication is one way of avoiding full participation in the group by numbing anxiety and dysphoria; ultimately, it slows the process of learning and integrating new information about oneself. All group members were assisted in understanding the role and impact of substance abuse on their lives and the connections between various addictive behaviors.

Despite the present focus of the group, it is not uncommon for group members to spontaneously share their abuse experiences. While this type of sharing may be allowed by the therapists and, in some cases, insisted on by the group members, the focus should be brought back to the present. For example, in one present-focused group, a group member unexpectedly began to describe her abuse history in considerable depth. When she seemed to be done, the group leader paused and gently asked the member, "Can I bring you back to the room? What was it about today's group that made you want to tell your story now? What made you feel safe enough?" Through this redirection, the group member was able to identify intimacy and trust as aspects of her current life that concerned her. The discussion was able to continue from there with a focus on present issues.

Attention to the group process itself is another important component of present-focused therapy. Yalom (1995) explained that attention to the group experience, including the group members and the therapists, "facilitates feedback, catharsis, meaningful self-disclosure, and acquisition of socializing techniques" (p. 136). The group serves as a "laboratory of life," often reflecting members' outside lives as they enact within the group the same behaviors they exhibit in the outside world. As members make these observations of the group dynamics, they can practice more adaptive ways of dealing with them, ultimately modifying their experiences outside of the group.

Clinical Examples

To contrast the trauma-focused and present-focused approaches, consider the following clinical examples. These examples illustrate how present- and trauma-focused treatments can respond to similar issues differently.

During a discussion in the trauma-focused group about the various group members' discomfort with intimacy, one woman gave a powerful description of the first time she was raped by her father at age 8. Three weeks later, this woman complained that she had been experiencing lengthy dissociative episodes and difficulty working since sharing her story. Because it was a trauma-focused group, one of the therapists explained,

> Talking about your memory has stirred up a lot of painful and overwhelming emotions and in order to help you right now we can do one of two things. We can help you to do further work with your traumatic memories so that you can face and handle your emotions, or, if you want, we can help you identify some coping strategies you can use to manage your dissociation so that it does not interfere with your work.

The woman opted to work further with her memory, at which point the therapist took her back to the event and had her describe her thoughts and feelings in detail. The participant was able to identify the specific moment during that experience when she began to dissociate, explaining that she had "no memories" after this event until the age of 14. By discussing the specifics of the abuse, the participant was able to explore how its traumatic elements contribute to her current state, thereby making her current dissociative episodes less alien and frightening. The ultimate goal for this participant is for her to integrate the traumatic event and the associated affect so that she no longer needs to use dissociation as a defense against the memory. If a similar situation occurred in a present-focused group, the therapist would instead help the woman identify the circumstances that trigger her dissociation, identify how she can minimize exposure to those circumstances, and help her to come up with some techniques she can use to ground herself whenever she does dissociate.

In the last few minutes of a present-focused group, one of the members stated that she "loves being raped." She went on to explain that it is familiar to her and reminds her of her childhood, making it somehow pleasurable. Because the group was in its final moments of a session, the therapist acknowledged her comment but had to end the group. At a later session, the therapist brought up the comment to be discussed in more depth. Rather than delving into the specifics of the abuse and in what way it may have been pleasurable for her, as would be done if this were a trauma-focused group, the therapist focused on how the participant can continue her transition from abusive relationships to a healthy relationship with her husband. In this way, present-focused therapy focuses on the consequences of the abuse instead of the abuse itself.

Measures

The Trauma Symptom Checklist–40 (TSC-40; Briere & Runtz, 1989; Elliott & Briere, 1992) is a self-report instrument designed to assess the emotional effects of child or adult traumatic experiences. It consists of 40 items that provide a total score and six subscale scores, including dissociation, anxiety, depression, sexual abuse trauma index, sleep disturbance, and sexual problems. The sexual abuse trauma index of the TSC-40 consists of items that are thought to be characteristic of individuals who have been sexually abused. Respondents rate each item on a scale of 0–4 indicating how often they have experienced each symptom in the last 2 months, with 0 = *never* and 4 = *very often*. This scale has good internal consistency and predictive validity regarding CSA (Elliott & Briere, 1992).

The Inventory of Interpersonal Problems (IIP; Horowitz, Rosenberg, Baer, Ureno, & Villasenor, 1988) is a validated, self-report measure of interpersonal problems. We administered the original version consisting of 127 items, such as items that ask whether it is hard for the respondent to tell a person to stop bothering her and if the respondent fights with other people too much. The respondent indicates the extent to which the item describes something that has been a problem for her and how distressing it is on a scale from 0 (*not at all*) to 4 (*extremely*). Drawing on this original pool of 127 items, a method of scoring the IIP has been validated based on 64 items (Horowitz, Alden, Wiggins, & Pincus, 2000) consisting of eight subscales that represent a circumplex of interpersonal problems based on Wiggins's (1980) interpersonal circle. The circumplex consists of two orthogonal factors—love and dominance—represented on a two-dimensional space. The eight subscales represent varying degrees of interpersonal problems in the areas of love and dominance and include problems in being domineering/controlling, vindictive/self-centered, cold/distant, socially inhibited, nonassertive, overly accommodating, self-sacrificing, and intrusive/needy (Gurtman, 1992).

The Sexual Experiences Survey (SES; Koss & Gidycz, 1985; Koss & Oros, 1982) is a 13-item scale designed to assess a range of sexual experiences, including consensual sex, unwanted sexual contact, attempted rape, and rape. The items begin with low-severity sexual experiences and proceed through a spectrum of aggressive sexual behaviors. The measure has good test–retest reliability and internal consistency. Revictimized participants were those individuals who endorsed any items that indicated unwanted sexual contact (Items 3–7), attempted rape (Items 8 and 9), or rape (Items 10–12).

RESULTS

Comparing Sexually Revictimized and Nonrevictimized Participants at Baseline

Using baseline data from this pilot study, we divided our participants into two groups: those who reported that they had been recently revictimized (i.e., within the past 6 months) and those who reported no revictimization experiences within the past 6 months (Classen, Field, et al., 2001). We hypothesized that women who reported recent revictimization experiences at baseline would also report greater interpersonal problems compared with those who had not been recently revictimized. We found that the recently revictimized women had significantly greater problems by being more nonassertive, self-sacrificing (or overly nurturant), socially inhibited, and responsible. This paints the picture of individuals who tend to put others' needs ahead of their own, who cannot say no, and who are, perhaps, easily exploited.

Results at 6-Month Follow-Up

In a preliminary examination of the data from this pilot study, we combined both the trauma-focused and present-focused groups and compared them with the wait-list condition at the 6-month follow-up. At the 6-month follow-up, 19 women had received group treatment and 33 women had completed the waiting period and were anticipating beginning treatment shortly after the assessment. We found that receiving group therapy resulted in a reduction of two measures of trauma symptoms—dissociation and the sexual trauma index (a composite measure of sexual trauma-related symptoms)—and in three kinds of interpersonal problems—being vindictive/self-centered, nonassertive, and overly accommodating (Classen, Koopman, et al., 2001). For those individuals who when they entered the study reported having been victimized in the past 6 months, only 38% of the women in the treatment group were revictimized again 6 months later, compared with 67% of women in the wait-list condition. Though not statistically significant owing to the small sample size, this reduction in revictimization appears to be clinically meaningful. Given that nearly twice as many women in the wait-list condition endorsed engaging in unwanted sex compared with women who received group therapy, this suggests that group therapy may have helped these women be more assertive with their sexual partners and to exert more control over their own bodies.

Results at 12-Month Follow-Up Comparing Trauma-Focused and Present-Focused Group Therapies

To compare the benefits of the trauma-focused group therapy with the present-focused group therapy condition, we conducted a Time (pretreatment vs. posttreatment) × Group Type (trauma-focused vs. present-focused) × Timing of Intervention (immediate vs. wait-list) repeated measures analysis of variance (ANOVA) on each of the three outcome measures: the TSC-40, IIP, and SES. Pretreatment scores were based on the baseline scores for participants in the immediate treatment condition and the 6-month follow-up scores for women in the wait-list condition. Both assessments were approximately 1 month prior to the beginning of treatment. Posttreatment scores were the 6-month follow-up scores for women in the immediate treatment condition and the 12-month follow-up scores for women in the wait-list condition. The posttreatment assessments occurred within 1 month of completion of the 6-month group therapy intervention.

In Table 12.1 we present the means, standard deviations, and effect sizes for each of the outcome variables by group treatment. In addition, the baseline and 6-month follow-up scores are provided for participants who were assigned to the wait-list condition, along with an effect size. It should be noted that all of the participants in the wait-list condition are also represented in the pretreatment and posttreatment means.

As expected, the repeated measures ANOVA was not significant on any of the outcome variables given the small sample size. An examination of the effect sizes suggests that neither the trauma-focused nor the present-focused group reduced trauma symptoms as measured by the TSC-40. The effect sizes were small and similar to the effect size for the wait-list group.

On the IIP, the trauma-focused group had a moderate effect size compared with small effect sizes in both the present-focused group and wait-list condition. This suggests that the trauma-focused group may be effective in reducing interpersonal problems. Figure 12.1 shows the interpersonal problems at pretreatment and posttreatment for both the trauma-focused group and present-focused group mapped on a circumplex. This finding, however, is interesting in that despite the fact that the present-focused group was specifically focused on dealing with interpersonal problems, it was the trauma-focused intervention that showed the greatest effect on them. This suggests that in this population of abused woman, the path to resolution of interpersonal problems goes through the thicket of traumatic memories.

The SES showed a small effect size for the present-focused group compared with no effect in the trauma-focused group and a negative effect in the wait-list condition. This suggests that the present-focused group may have reduced sexual revictimization, or at least the reporting of sexual revictimization. It should also be noted that except for 1 participant who

TABLE 12.1
Descriptive Statistics on Outcome Measures for Trauma-focused, Present-focused and Wait-list Conditions

Condition	n	Pretreatment Mean (SD)	Posttreatment Mean (SD)	Baseline Mean (SD)	6-Month Follow-up Mean (SD)	Effect Size
Trauma Symptom Checklist—40						
Trauma-focused	24	41.27 (13.8)	37.35 (16.1)			.26
Present-focused	19	40.60 (16.0)	38.0 (15.8)			.15
Wait-list	33			44.80 (20.8)	41.04 (15.4)	.21
Inventory of Interpersonal Problems						
Trauma-focused	21	97.48 (34.5)	78.53 (36.9)			.53
Present-focused	18	86.85 (38.9)	80.63 (44.0)			.15
Wait-list	30			97.77 (37.5)	89.96 (36.3)	.21
Sexual Experiences Survey						
Trauma-focused	25	.48 (.59)	.44 (.58)			.07
Present-focused	18	.35 (.59)	.20 (.41)			.29
Wait-list	32			.25 (.44)	.34 (.55)	-.18

Figure 12.1. Mean subscale scores on the Inventory of Interpersonal Problems circumplex for the trauma-focused and present-focused group therapy condition at pretreatment and posttreatment and for the wait-list control group and 6-month follow-up.

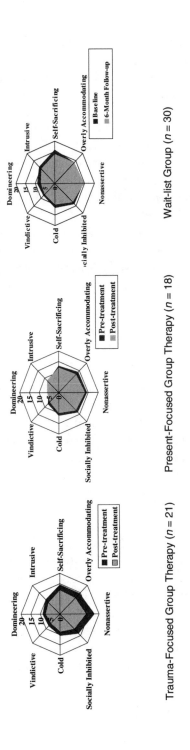

reported having experienced attempted rape, all revictimization experiences involved unwanted sexual contact.

Given our baseline findings that interpersonal problems seemed to be associated with sexual revictimization and given that the trauma-focused group showed a moderate reduction in interpersonal problems, we were surprised to find that the trauma-focused group did not also show a reduction in sexual revictimization. A closer examination of the TSC-40, specifically the reduction in dissociative symptoms, led us to hypothesize that perhaps the women in the trauma-focused condition were simply more in touch with when they were having unwanted sexual contact. We noted that on the dissociation subscale the trauma-focused group had a small effect size (.3) compared with a negligible effect size (.08) in the present-focused group. It is possible that the women in the trauma-focused group, while showing improvement interpersonally, were also dissociating less and therefore were more aware of when they were engaging in unwanted sex. This is, of course, speculation and, as with all the preliminary findings we are reporting, requires rigorous investigation in the future.

CURRENT RESEARCH

On the basis of our pilot study, we were encouraged to hypothesize that a trauma-focused group therapy intervention would reduce the risk for HIV infection in CSA survivors compared with a present-focused group therapy and that both would reduce the risk for HIV infection compared with a wait-list condition. With funding from the National Institute of Mental Health, we have another larger trial currently under way for women with histories of CSA and who are judged to be at risk for HIV infection in which we will compare the two types of group therapy and will be able to confirm or disprove these results more conclusively.

In the present study we are recruiting 192 women with CSA histories and who meet at least one of three risk factors within the previous 12 months: (a) They engage in risky sex, (b) they have been sexually revictimized, and (c) they have problems with drugs or alcohol. Each woman is randomly assigned to one of three conditions: (a) trauma-focused group therapy, (b) present-focused group therapy, and (c) a 12-month wait-list condition. All of the participants will receive 6 months of group therapy (Classen, Butler, & Spiegel, 2001) and will be followed at baseline, 6 months, and 12 months. Our main outcome variables include each of the three risk factors, interpersonal problems, and traumatic stress symptoms. It remains to be seen whether 6 months of group therapy can make a critical difference in reducing the risk for HIV infection in this severely traumatized population. It is our hope that this larger trial will shed some light on how to most effectively help at-risk CSA survivors.

CONCLUSION

Revictimization, risky sexual behavior, and drug- and alcohol-related problems elevate the risk of HIV infection and are serious problems for women survivors of CSA. Effective treatment of the long-term effects of such abuse can serve the secondary and tertiary prevention functions of reducing distress and interpersonal problems. It may also serve as a type of primary prevention, potentially reducing the risk of acquiring and spreading the virus. A crucial question is whether such psychotherapy is more effective if it deals directly with memories of abuse or indirectly through focusing on corrective emotional and interpersonal experiences in the present. Future research is needed to determine those components of psychotherapy that are necessary to or more effective in reducing distress, improving interpersonal functioning, and reducing revictimization and HIV infection risk. Finally, future research should also examine the effectiveness of group psychotherapy for CSA survivors who are male or who belong to minority groups.

REFERENCES

Alexander, P. C., Neimeyer, R. A., & Follette, V. M. (1991). Group therapy for women sexually abused as children: A controlled study and investigation of individual differences. *Journal of Interpersonal Violence, 6,* 218–231.

American Psychiatric Association. (1994). *Diagnostic and statistical manual of mental disorders* (4th ed.). Washington, DC: Author.

Briere, J., & Runtz, M. (1989). The Trauma Symptom Checklist (TSC-33): Early data on a new scale. *Journal of Interpersonal Violence, 4,* 151–163.

Brown, D., Scheflin, A. W., & Hammond, D. C. (1998). *Memory, trauma treatment, and the law.* New York: Norton.

Browne, A., & Finkelhor, D. (1986). Impact of child sexual abuse: A review of the research. *Psychological Bulletin, 99,* 66–77.

Butler, L. D., & Spiegel, D. (1997). Trauma and memory. In L. J. Dickstein, M. B. Riba, & J. O. Oldham (Eds.), *Review of psychiatry* (Vol. 16, pp. II13–II53). Washington, DC: American Psychiatric Press.

Carver, C. S., Scheier, M. F., & Weintraub, J. K. (1989). Assessing coping strategies: A theoretically based approach. *Journal of Personality and Social Psychology, 56,* 267–283.

Cicchetti, D., & Rizley, R. (1981). *Developmental perspectives on the etiology, intergenerational transmission, and sequelae of childhood maltreatment.* San Francisco: Jossey-Bass.

Classen, C., Ballinger, B., & Spiegel, D. (1993). *A trauma-focused group treatment manual for adult survivors of child sexual abuse.* Stanford, CA: Stanford University School of Medicine, Department of Psychiatry and Behavioral Sciences.

Classen, C., Butler, L. D., & Spiegel, D. (2001). *A treatment manual for present-focused and trauma-focused group therapies for sexual abuse survivors at risk for HIV infection.* Stanford, CA: Stanford University School of Medicine, Department of Psychiatry and Behavioral Sciences.

Classen, C., Field, N. P., Koopman, C., Nevill-Manning, K., & Spiegel, D. (2001). Interpersonal problems and their relationship to sexual revictimization in women sexually abused in childhood. *Journal of Interpersonal Violence, 16,* 495–509.

Classen, C., Koopman, C., Nevill-Manning, K., & Spiegel, D. (2001). A preliminary report comparing trauma-focused and present-focused group therapy against a wait-listed condition among childhood sexual abuse survivors with PTSD. *Journal of Aggression, Maltreatment and Trauma, 4,* 265–288.

Coons, C. A., Bowman, P. M., Pellow, E. S., & Schneider, P. (1989). Post-traumatic aspects of the treatment of victims of sexual abuse and incest. *Psychiatric Clinics of North America, 12,* 325–335.

Dallam, S. J., Gleaves, D. H., Cepeda-Benito, A., Silberg, J. L., Kraemer, H. C., & Spiegel , D. (2001). The effects of child sexual abuse: An examination of Rind, Tromovitch and Bauserman (1998). *Psychological Bulletin, 127,* 715–733.

Elliott, D. M., & Briere, J. (1992). Sexual abuse trauma among professional women: Validating the Trauma Symptom Checklist–40 (TSC-40). *Child Abuse and Neglect: The International Journal, 16,* 391–398.

Foa, E. B., & Meadows, E. A. (1997). Psychosocial treatments for posttraumatic stress disorder: A critical review. *Annual Review of Psychology, 48,* 449–480.

Gleaves, D. H., Smith, S. M., Butler, L. D., & Spiegel, D. (2001). *False and recovered memories in the laboratory and clinic: A review of experimental and clinical evidence.* Manuscript in preparation.

Gurtman, M. B. (1992). Trust, distrust, and interpersonal problems: A circumplex analysis. *Journal of Personality and Social Psychology, 62,* 989–1002.

Hall, Z. M., Mullee, M. A., & Thompson, C. (1995). A clinical and service evaluation of group therapy for women survivors of childhood sexual abuse. In M. Aveline & D. Shapiro (Eds.), *Research foundations for psychotherapy practice* (pp. 263–279). New York: Wiley.

Hazzard, A., Rogers, J. H., & Angert, L. (1993). Factors affecting group therapy outcome for adult sexual abuse survivors. *International Journal of Group Psychotherapy, 43,* 453–468.

Henderson, L., Classen, C., Ballinger, B., Spiegel, D., & Yalom, I. (1994). *Present-focused group therapy for sexual abuse survivors: A treatment manual.* Stanford, CA: Stanford University School of Medicine, Department of Psychiatry and Behavioral Sciences.

Herman, J. L. (1992). *Trauma and recovery.* New York: Harper Collins.

Herman, J. L., & Schatzow, E. (1984). Time-limited group therapy for women with a history of incest. *International Journal of Group Psychotherapy, 34,* 605–616.

Horowitz, L. M., Alden, L. E., Wiggins, J. S., & Pincus, A. L. (2000). *IIP: Inventory of Interpersonal Problems manual.* New York: Psychological Corporation.

Horowitz, L. M., Rosenberg, S. E., Baer, B. A., Ureno, G., & Villasenor, V. (1988). Inventory of Interpersonal Problems: Psychometric properties and clinical applications. *Journal of Consulting and Clinical Psychology, 56,* 885–892.

Koss, M. P., & Gidycz, C. A. (1985). Sexual Experiences Survey: Reliability and validity. *Journal of Consulting and Clinical Psychology, 53,* 422–423.

Koss, M. P., & Oros, C. J. (1982). Sexual Experiences Survey: A research instrument investigating sexual aggression and victimization. *Journal of Consulting and Clinical Psychology, 50,* 455–457.

Kriedler, M. C., Einsporn, R. L., Zupancic, M. K., & Masterson, C. (1999). Group therapy for survivors of childhood sexual abuse who are severely and persistently mentally ill. *Journal of the American Psychiatric Nurses Association, 5*(3), 73–79.

Loftus, E. F. (1993). The reality of repressed memories. *American Psychologist, 48,* 518–537.

Loftus, E. F., & Hoffman, H. G. (1989). Misinformation and memory: The creation of new memories. *Journal of Experimental Psychology: General, 118,* 100–104.

McCann, I., & Pearlman, L. (1990). *Psychological trauma and the adult survivor: Therapy, theory, and transformation.* New York: Brunner/Mazel.

Morgan, T., & Cummings, A. L. (1999). Change experienced during group therapy by female survivors of childhood sexual abuse. *Journal of Consulting and Clinical Psychology, 67,* 28–36.

Morrison, A., & Treliving, L. (2002). Evaluation of outcome in a dynamically orientated group for adult males who have been sexually abused in childhood. *British Journal of Psychotherapy, 19,* 59–76.

Paddison, P. L., Einbinder, R. G., Maker, E., & Strain, J. J. (1993). Group treatment with incest survivors. In P. L. Paddison (Ed.), *Treatment of adult survivors of incest* (pp. 35–54). Washington, DC: American Psychiatric Press.

Polusny, M. A., & Follette, V. M. (1995). Long-term correlates of child sexual abuse: Theory and review of the empirical literature. *Applied and Preventative Psychology, 4,* 143–166.

Richter, N. L., Snider, E., & Gorey, K. M. (1997). Group work intervention with female survivors of childhood sexual abuse. *Research on Social Work Practice, 60,* 53–69.

Rind, B., Tromovitch, P., & Bauserman, R. (1998). A meta-analytic examination of assumed properties of child sexual abuse using college samples: Psychological correlates of male child and adolescent sexual experiences with adults: A review of the nonclinical literature. *Psychological Bulletin, 124,* 22–53.

Roth, N. (1993). *Integrating the shattered self: Psychotherapy with adult incest survivors.* Northvale, NJ: Jason Aronson.

Saxe, B. J., & Johnson, S. M. (1999). An empirical investigation of group treatment for a clinical population of adult female incest survivors. *Journal of Child Sexual Abuse, 8,* 67–88.

Sharpe, J., Selley, C., Low, L., & Hall, Z. (2001). Group analytic therapy for male survivors of childhood sexual abuse. *Group Analysis, 34,* 195–209.

Spiegel, D. (1989). Hypnosis in the treatment of victims of sexual abuse. *Psychiatric Clinics of North America, 12,* 295–305.

Spiegel, D. (1995). Hypnosis and suggestion. In D. L. Schacter, J. T. Coyle, G. Fischback, M. M. Mesulam, & L. E. Sullivan (Eds.), *Memory distortion* (pp. 129–149). Cambridge, MA: Harvard University Press.

Spiegel, D. (1997). Trauma, dissociation, and memory. In R. Yehuda & A. McFarlane (Eds.), *Psychobiology of posttraumatic stress disorder* (pp. 225–237). New York: New York Academy of Sciences.

Spiegel, D. (2000a). The price of abusing children and numbers. *Sexuality and Culture, 4*(2), 63–66.

Spiegel, D. (2000b). Suffer the children: Long term effects of sexual abuse. *Society, 37*(4), 18–20.

Stalker, C. A., & Fry, R. (1999). A comparison of short-term group and individual therapy for sexually abused women. *Canadian Journal of Psychiatry, 44,* 168–174.

Talbot, N. L., Houghtalen, R. P., Duberstein, P. R., Cox, C., Giles, D. E., & Wynne, L. C. (1999). Effects of group treatment for women with a history of childhood sexual abuse. *Psychiatric Services, 50,* 686–692.

Tsai, M., & Wagner, N. (1978). Therapy groups for women sexually molested as children. *Archives of Sexual Behavior, 7,* 417–427.

Westbury, E., & Tutty, L. M. (1999). The efficacy of group treatment for survivors of childhood abuse. *Child Abuse and Neglect, 23,* 31–44.

Wiggins, J. S. (1980). Circumplex models of interpersonal behavior. In L. Wheeler (Ed.), *Review of personality and social psychology* (pp. 265–293). Beverly Hills, CA: Sage.

Yalom, I. D. (1980). *Existential psychotherapy.* New York: Basic Books.

Yalom, I. D. (1995). *The theory and practice of group psychotherapy* (4th ed.). New York: Basic Books.

Zlotnick, C., Shea, T., Rosen, K., Simpson, E., Mulrenin, K., Begin, A., & Pearlstein, T. (1997). An affect-management group for women with posttraumatic stress disorder and histories of childhood sexual abuse. *Journal of Traumatic Stress, 10,* 425–436.

13

SEXUAL ASSAULT REVICTIMIZATION: TOWARD EFFECTIVE RISK-REDUCTION PROGRAMS

LISA MARMELSTEIN BLACKWELL, STEVEN JAY LYNN, HOLLY VANDERHOFF, AND CHRISTINE GIDYCZ

In recent years, evidence has accumulated that women who report a history of child sexual abuse (CSA) or victimization appear to be at particular risk for being revictimized (Gidycz, Hanson, & Layman, 1995; Humphrey & White, 2000; Roodman & Clum, 2001). The term *revictimization* refers to the occurrence of a sexual assault in adulthood, following either CSA or an earlier adolescent or adult victimization. Revictimization has emerged as a significant personal problem for many people in society insofar as a history of CSA almost doubles the risk of sexual revictimization occurring during later adolescence and early adulthood (Gidycz et al., 1995; Humphrey & White, 2000). Moreover, a recent meta-analysis of studies that pertain to revictimization (Roodman & Clum, 2001) yielded an effect size of .59, which is indicative of a definite relation between CSA and adult sexual victimization.

The fact that sexual assault revictimization has reached disturbing proportions, and that past behavior and experiences are risk factors for current sexual victimization, constitutes a strong rationale for (a) preventing initial occurrences through programs designed to minimize the risk of initial sexual assault and (b) developing effective programs for individuals who have previously been victims of sexual violence. The need for effective, empirically supported risk-reduction programs is underscored by the following two findings.

First, despite the proliferation of rape prevention programs on college campuses over the past decade, recent national studies found that approximately 15% of female college students reported that they have experienced a rape either during adolescence or early adulthood (Brener, McMahon, Warren, & Douglas, 1999; Fischer, Cullen, & Turner, 2000; Koss, 1998). Second, in the aftermath of sexual assault, many women suffer intense distress and psychological disorders, including posttraumatic stress disorder and depression (Koss, 1993; Resick, 1993). In a study with college students, Brener et al. (1999) found that sexual assault was also associated with a number of prior health risk behaviors, including drug and alcohol use, involvement in sexual activity at an early age, and suicidal ideation. The association between a sexual assault and prior health risk behaviors is particularly noteworthy in that these risky behaviors are likely to perpetuate a cycle of repeated victimizations for women with assault histories (Brener et al., 1999). Accordingly, there is an urgent need to identify interventions that can effectively reduce the alarmingly high rates of sexual assault, particularly among women at greatest risk of assault.

Ideally, the ability to identify high-risk individuals with a history of previous victimization would allow researchers to tailor risk-reduction programs to this population and to focus interventions on those individuals in the population in the direst need of services. This chapter reviews the available literature on sexual assault risk-reduction programs. We highlight studies that address the issue of high-risk women in general, and revictimization in particular, with a focus on college student populations, which have been the target of the majority of interventions to date. Finally, we present a summary and critique of the literature, followed by recommendations for future sexual assault prevention programming for both a general population of women and for women who report a history of sexual victimization.

REVIEW OF SEXUAL ASSAULT RISK-REDUCTION PROGRAMS

We identified 26 studies of sexual assault risk-reduction programs conducted with either women only or a mixed-gender group. We evaluated the methodological rigor of the studies to determine what, if any, conclusions can be drawn from the extant research. Given the diversity of methods used, and the absence of universal standards for evaluating sexual assault prevention research, we examined the available evidence in light of the criteria proposed by Chambless and Hollon (1998) to determine the efficacy of specific treatments for psychological problems.

Chambless and Hollon (1998) recommended that two methodological criteria be met to establish that a psychological treatment is empirically supported. First, the treatment is superior to a no-treatment, alternative treatment, or placebo control group, in a randomized control trial, controlled single-case experiment, or equivalent time-series design; and, second, the study uses a treatment manual or a logical equivalent, a specific population, reliable and valid outcome measures, and appropriate data analysis. When these criteria are met, a treatment may be designated as (a) possibly efficacious if it is shown to be superior to a control treatment in one study, (b) efficacious if it is shown to be superior to a control treatment in at least two independent research settings, and (c) efficacious and specific if shown to be superior to placebo or bona fide alternative treatment in at least two independent research settings.

Our review focused on Chambless and Hollon's (1998) two methodological criteria because our goal was to examine the methodological rigor of the studies in this research area, not to designate a particular program as efficacious per se. Accordingly, Table 13.1 presents a general overview of the methodology and findings of each study, as well as information about how well the study met the criteria of interest.

Studies that randomly assigned participants to conditions were considered to be randomized trials. When studies randomly assigned groups to conditions (in most cases, intact college classes), a superscript in Table 13.1 indicates this. As a rule, risk-reduction programs are not manualized in a strict sense. However, studies that used a standard, planned protocol, a logical equivalent of a treatment manual, were judged to fulfill the "manual" component of the second criterion. Because sexual assault risk-reduction programs are not limited in application to a highly homogeneous audience, we considered the target population of each study (i.e., college students) to qualify as a "specific population," even in the absence of the empirically derived inclusion criterion suggested by Chambless and Hollon (1998).

As Table 13.1 indicates, a number of methodological problems limit the conclusions that can be drawn about the effectiveness of sexual assault prevention programs in general and revictimization in particular. First, most studies lacked a true control group and do not provide meaningful comparisons between treatment and no-treatment groups. Moreover, several studies, especially those completed in the 1980s and early 1990s, do not include a comparison group of any kind, and thereby preclude a rigorous evaluation of the effectiveness of the program. Other studies assigned groups of participants to conditions on the basis of convenience or availability, rather than by way of random individual or group assignment. In fact, only 6 of the 26 studies reviewed were truly randomized controlled trials. Interpretation of any observed differences between treatment and nonrandom comparison groups must be made with caution insofar as apparent treatment effects may be attributed to preexisting group differences. Finally, only 2 studies that

TABLE 13.1
Methodology and Results of Sexual Assault Risk Reduction Programs With College Students

Authors and year	Sample	Conditions	Results	Randomized control group	Treatment group superior to control group	Treatment manual or protocol	Reliable and valid outcome measures
Nonmethodologically Rigorous Studies With Women-Only Groups							
Gray, Lesser, Quinn, and Bounds (1990)	Women; N = 70	Personalized vs. nonpersonalized program of discussion, role-playing, myths, communication, expectations	Women in personalized group show increased perception of vulnerability and increased intention to avoid risk-taking behaviors	No	No (no control group)	Yes	No
Himelein (1999)	High-risk, previously victimized women; N = 7	5 weekly, 90-minute workshops on rape education and strategies to avoid rape	Increased knowledge of sexual assault; increased precautionary dating behaviors	No	No (no control group)	Yes	No
Nonmethodologically Rigorous Studies With Mixed-Gender Groups							
Anderson et al. (1998)	Men and women; N = 215	Interactive mock talk show vs. structured video vs. no-treatment control	Both groups showed reduction in rape-supportive attitudes but effect decreased over time	Yes[a]	Yes	Yes	Yes

Study	Sample	Intervention	Results				
Borden, Karr, and Caldwell-Colbert (1988)	Men and women; N = 50	Lecture on topics including legal terms, trauma syndrome, "typical" rapist description, prevention strategies vs. no-treatment control	No change rape empathy and attitudes toward rape between experimental group and control	No	No	Yes	No
Dallager and Rosen (1993)	Men and women; N = 143	Human sexuality course with 2-class unit on sexual assault/abuse vs. education course	Presentation group showed small decrease in acceptance of rape myth; all participants generally rejected myths	Yes[a]	Yes	Yes	Yes
Ellis, O'Sullivan, and Sowards (1992)	Men and women; N = 151	Contemplation of exposure to rape victim	Women more rejecting of rape myths, men less rejecting unless they knew a rape survivor	No	No (no control group)	No	No
Fischer (1986)	Men and women; N = 822	Lecture (confrontational, nonconfrontational) on rape laws vs. no-treatment control	Experimental group report decreased tolerance for rape, increased ability to identify rape	No	Yes	Yes	No
Fonow, Richardson, and Wemmerus (1992)	Men and women; N = 582	Pretest and no pretest groups seeing videotaped workshop or live workshop vs. no-treatment control	No change in attitudes across groups	Yes[a]	No	Yes	Yes

continues

TABLE 13.1 (Continued)

Authors and year	Sample	Conditions	Results	Randomized control group	Treatment group superior to control group	Treatment manual or protocol	Reliable and valid outcome measures
Frazier, Valtinson, and Candell (1994)	Fraternity and sorority members; $N = 192$	Interactive theatre presentation vs. no-treatment control	Experimental group endorsed fewer rape-supportive attitudes	Yes[a]	Yes	Yes	Yes
Harrison, Downes, and Williams (1991)	Men and women; $N = 96$	Video group vs. video and discussion group vs. no-treatment control	Men in both groups report attitude change; no change for women; no difference between formats	Yes[a]	Yes	Yes	No
Holcomb, Sarvela, Sondag, and Hatton Holcomb (1993)	Men and women; $N = 331$	Workshop on consent and preventions vs. no-treatment control	Experimental group reported less tolerance for date rape; change in attitudes greater for men than women	Yes[a]	Yes	Yes	No
Holcomb, Sondag, and Hatton Holcomb (1993)	Men and women; $N = 654$	Workshop focusing on shared responsibility for rape	Consumer satisfaction only	No	No (no control group)	Yes	No
Lenihan and Rawlins (1994)	Fraternity and sorority members; $N = 636$	Lecture on myths/facts, responsibility; co-ed discussion groups	No change	No	No (no control group)	Yes	Yes

Study	Sample	Manipulation	Findings				
Lenihan, Rawlins, Eberly, Buckley, and Masters (1992)	Men and women; N = 821	Pre- and posttested program group vs. pre- and posttested nonprogram group vs. posttest only group vs. program and posttest group	No change in attitudes beyond pretest differences	Yes[a]	No	Yes	Yes
Lonsway et al. (1998)	Men and women; N = 170	Semester-long course on facilitation of rape education for peers vs. human sexuality course	Attitude change, increased assertion in sexual communication, less acceptance of rape myths in experimental group than in control (but this effect was small and unstable)	Yes[a]	Yes	Yes	No
Malamuth and Check (1984)	Men and women; N = 143	Exposure to consensual sex or rape depictions vs. no-treatment control	Positive attitude change and decrease in myth acceptance in participants in rape condition	Yes[a]	Yes	Yes	No
Mann, Hecht, and Valentine (1988)	Men and women; N = 92	Dramatic presentation vs. discussion group vs. both vs. no-treatment control	No differences in assertiveness; dramatic presentation alone and dramatic presentation plus discussion produced greater change in sexual attitudes than did discussion alone and no-treatment control	Yes[a]	Yes	Yes	Yes
Nelson and Torgler (1990)	Men and women; N = 89	Videotape on acquaintance rape vs. brochure on career planning	Positive, nondifferential change across groups—control group changed as much as both treatment groups	Yes[a]	Yes	Yes	Yes

continues

TABLE 13.1 (Continued)

Methodologically Rigorous Studies With Women-Only Groups

Authors and year	Sample	Conditions	Results	Randomized control group	Treatment group superior to control group	Treatment manual or protocol	Reliable and valid outcome measures
Breitenbecher and Gidycz (1998)	Women; N = 406	Hanson and Bidycz (1993) program modified to include more information on, and attention to, prior victimization as a risk factor for future victimization	No change in sexual communication, knowledge about sexual assault, or dating behavior; no decrease in sexual assault rate treatment group versus control group	Yes	Yes	Yes	Yes
Calhoun et al. (2001)	High-risk, previously victimized women; N = 450	Marx et al.'s (2001) program plus Gidycz rape-survivors video	Decrease in rape rate and increase in self-efficacy and risk-perception in treatment group	Yes	Yes	Yes	Yes
Gidycz, Lynn, et al. (2001)	Women; N = 772	Presentation of statistics, myths/facts, videos of victim stories and dating scenario, practice of assertive behaviors vs. no-treatment control	Women who were victims prior to program showed less victimization at follow-up; no overall assault reduction at follow-up; no effect on dating behavior or sexual communication	Yes	Yes, for subgroup of subjects	Yes	Yes

Study	Sample	Intervention	Outcome				
Hanson and Gidycz (1993)	Women; $N = 360$	Rape myths, facts, statistics, video of events leading to acquaintance rape, discussion vs. no-treatment control	Increased awareness of rape and situational risk factors; no change in sexual communication	Yes	Yes	Yes	Yes
Marx, Calhoun, Wilson, and Meyerson (2001)	High-risk, previously victimized women; $N = 66$	Hanson and Gidycz's (1993) program plus relapse prevention vs. no-treatment control	Decrease in rape rate, increase in self-efficacy in treatment group	Yes	Yes	Yes	Yes
Methodologically Rigorous Studies With Mixed-Gender Groups							
Gidycz, Layman, et al. (2001)	Men and women; $N = 1,136$	Program of statistics, myths/facts, resource identification, safety techniques, description of typical rapist vs. no-treatment control	No decrease in victimization/perpetration rate for program participants; reduction of rape myth acceptance in program participants	Yes	Yes, but for attitudinal variables only	Yes	Yes
Heppner, Humphrey, Debord, and Hillenbrand-Gunn (1995)	Men and women; $N = 258$	Interactional drama vs. didactic/video; elaboration likelihood model vs. no-treatment control	Overall greater change in outcome measures for drama group	Yes	Yes	Yes	Yes
Pinzone-Glover, Gidycz, and Jacobs (1998)	Men and women; $N = 152$	Myths/facts, alcohol use, safety information vs. sexually transmitted disease workshop	Attitude change in men in experimental group greater than women's; differences between men and women's definitions of rape at pretest decreased at posttest	Yes	Yes	Yes	Yes

Note. Random assignment was done by group, not by individual. [a]Treatment was efficacious but was not compared with a truly randomly-assigned control group.

used methodologically rigorous procedures were specifically designed to target women who reported the experience of a sexual assault prior to the study (Calhoun et al., 2001; Marx, Calhoun, Wilson, & Meyerson, 2001).

Conclusions from the research reviewed are also limited by researchers' failure to use reliable and valid assessment measures. If a study used at least one reliable and valid measure, we considered it to have met Chambless and Hollon's (1998) criterion relevant to outcome measures. However, even when this liberal interpretation of the Chambless and Hollon criterion is adopted, it is still possible to identify studies that used measures for which no pertinent reliability or validity information is available. Studies conducted as recently as the mid- and late-1990s were limited in this regard, despite the availability of measures with reasonably sound psychometric properties.

The studies we examined included a wide variety of outcome measures, including but not limited to assertiveness, communication skills, acceptance of rape myths, attitudes about sexual assault, risk-taking behaviors, and information learned. Although all of these variables are potentially important and have been shown to relate to sexual assault risk, the sheer variety of outcome measures and the disparate methods of measurement make cross-study comparisons difficult at best. Accordingly, it is difficult to draw firm conclusions about any one program or even one "genre" of programs, insofar as no two studies examined exactly the same program or measured their outcomes in exactly the same ways. These limitations aside, the following observations represent working hypotheses regarding the elements of effective sexual assault risk-reduction programs.

First, virtually any program appears to be better than no intervention in terms of instigating attitude change. When compared with no-treatment control groups, nearly all of the programs reviewed engendered changes in attitudes, especially regarding the acceptance of rape myths. Often, studies comparing an active control group with an experimental group found equivalent attitudinal and behavioral change in participants across groups. Accordingly, it appears that the simple act of exposing participants to information about sexual assault serves to change attitudes about sexual assault.

Second, programs that consist of multiple formats (i.e., discussion, role-play, didactic presentation) appear to be more effective in changing attitudes than programs that consist of a single method of education. For instance, exposure to general lectures on sexual assault appears to do little to foster attitudinal or behavioral change (Lenihan & Rawlins, 1994). Programs that offer a more interactive or personalized approach are more successful in this regard (e.g., Gray, Lesser, Quinn, & Bounds, 1990; Heppner, Humphrey, Debord, & Hillenbrand-Gunn, 1995), although this is not always the case (Anderson et al., 1998).

As described earlier, the widely disparate outcome measures used preclude any conclusion about what is most effective in targeting specific attitudes or behaviors. Furthermore, few of the studies reviewed examine actual sexual assault rates prior to and following the program. Accordingly, little is known regarding how and under what circumstances prevention programs foster attitudinal and behavioral changes. Insofar as this is the ultimate goal of prevention research, most extant studies have little to contribute to the knowledge base in this area.

On a more positive note, we found that more recent studies are superior to older studies in a number of salient respects. That is, recent studies are more likely to incorporate pre- and posttreatment testing and follow-up evaluations, and they are more likely to use valid and reliable outcome measures and quasi-random control groups. As such practices become more the norm than the exception, the precision and meaning of the outcomes of treatment programs will increase accordingly.

We now turn to more methodologically rigorous and informative studies. To qualify for detailed review in this chapter, a particular study was required to have (a) used a control group, (b) randomly assigned individual participants to conditions, (c) administered reliable and valid assessment instruments, and (d) used a standardized treatment protocol. The studies reviewed below are divided into two sections. Programs involving women only are discussed first, followed by investigations that target a mixed-gender audience.

PROGRAMS WITH WOMEN

Gidycz and her colleagues (Breitenbecher & Gidycz, 1998; Gidycz, Lynn, et al., 2001; Hanson & Gidycz, 1993) have conducted a series of systematic, methodologically rigorous studies of sexual assault risk-reduction programs with women. In their initial study, Hanson and Gidycz (1993) presented their program to 360 undergraduate women. Assessment instruments were administered before the program and during follow-up at the end of the academic quarter. The assessment instruments included the Sexual Experiences Survey (Koss & Oros, 1982), the Dating Behavior Survey (Hanson & Gidycz, 1993), the Sexual Communication Survey (Hanson & Gidycz, 1993), and the Sexual Assault Awareness Survey (SAAS; Hanson & Gidycz, 1993). All of the measures except for the SAAS, for which no data are reported, have demonstrated good psychometric properties. The use of assessment instruments that measure actual behavior, rather than attitudes alone, represents an important advance in the area of sexual assault risk-reduction programming.

The program consisted of the following components: (a) presentation of rape statistics; (b) a discussion of rape myths (e.g., women owe men sex, women who dress provocatively deserve to be raped) and facts; (c) the presentation of two videos, one that portrayed events leading up to an acquaintance rape, and one that showed a woman modeling protective dating behavior; and (d) time for questions and the distribution of resource information.

Results indicated that although there was no difference with regards to sexual communication, the treatment group showed an increased awareness regarding sexual assault, decreased involvement in risky behavior, and a decreased incidence of victimization during the quarter, in comparison with the control group. The last finding, however, has an important qualification: The decreased incidence of victimization applied only to women who did not have a history of sexual abuse or assault. In short, previous victimization appeared to moderate the treatment effect. However, this study did not include materials that specifically targeted the high-risk group of previously victimized women.

Breitenbecher and Gidycz (1998) modified their original program to include more information on, and attention to, prior victimization as a risk factor for future victimization. The program, which included 406 college women, was modified in the following ways: (a) The explicit statement "Having been sexually assaulted in the past increases your risk for being sexually assaulted in the future" was added to the myths and facts sheet; (b) after the women viewed the video that portrayed events leading up to an acquaintance rape, a discussion ensued regarding the psychological impact of sexual assault (e.g., depression, anxiety, dissociation) and the ways in which a prior assault might affect a woman's behavior in a sexual situation; (c) information on risk-reduction strategies included the statement, "Be aware that having been sexually assaulted in the past may affect your thoughts and behavior in ways that you are not fully aware of"; and finally, (d) the presenter emphasized that although psychological effects can follow a sexual assault, no woman is responsible for being assaulted, rather a prior assault can increase vulnerability and necessitate extra vigilance and precautions. Assessment instruments were administered at the beginning and end of the academic quarter.

Despite attempts to increase attention to the potential effects of prior victimization, the program did not significantly affect sexual communication, knowledge about sexual assault, or dating behavior. Perhaps more importantly, the treatment program failed to decrease the rate of sexual assault among treatment-group participants, as compared with a no-treatment control group. That is, unlike the results of Hanson and Gidycz (1993), this program failed to decrease the rate of assault among treated individuals, even for those women who had not been previously sexually assaulted. The introduction of information specific to past abusive experiences may have led women without assault histories to "tune out" the information early on in the program. At the same time, the brevity of the intervention may have precluded meaningful changes in the high-risk group of women. Accordingly, it may be important to ensure that all participants more fully process the information that is conveyed to them and that risk-reduction programs be more extensive and comprehensive in nature.

A later multisite study by Gidycz, Lynn, et al. (2001) contained many of the same components as the previous studies; however, it introduced program components based on two theories of attitude and behavior change: the elaboration likelihood model (ELM; Petty & Cacioppo, 1981, 1986a, 1986b) and the health belief model (Hochman, 1958). The ELM postulates that attitude change can be engendered by way of two separate routes, namely, the peripheral route and the central route. Peripheral route processing occurs when the individual attends to superficial issues (e.g., credibility and expertise of the speaker), whereas central route processing occurs when the individual attends to the core concepts of the message itself. Central route processing has the potential to create attitude change that is likely to persist, resist attack, and influence behavior (Petty, Haugtvedt, & Smith, 1995; Verplanken, 1991).

The tenets of the ELM were incorporated in a number of ways. A video was added to increase the personal relevance of the message and, thereby, increase central route processing. This video depicted a number of female rape victims sharing their stories, discussing the impact the rape had on their lives, and emphasizing how they had thought that they could never be raped. The video was intended to convince participants that sexual assault is something that happens to many women and that they themselves are, in fact, at risk for being assaulted. In addition, to increase attention to, and processing of, risk-reduction information, small- and large-group discussions were incorporated into the design.

The health belief model (Hochman, 1958) postulates that individuals will take action to preserve or improve their health when they perceive that a serious threat to their health exists and they perceive that they have the necessary skills to overcome the threat. Accordingly, the researchers anticipated that discussions on the topics of risky situations, characteristics of sexually aggressive men, and the need for assertive communications and other risk-reduction strategies would increase participants' perceptions of their vulnerability to sexual assault and thereby facilitate central route processing and risk-reduction behaviors.

Despite these efforts to increase the personal salience of the information conveyed, particularly for those with a history of prior victimization, the results of the study were mixed. The program did not have an effect on either dating behavior or sexual communication. At both the 2-month and 6-month follow-up periods, women with a prior history of victimization reported a significantly higher rate of victimization than did women who did not report a history of victimization. Furthermore, there were no differences between the treatment group and the no-treatment control group in the rates of sexual victimization during the 2-month follow-up period. However, in comparison with the control group, women in the treatment group who were moderately victimized (i.e., experienced a nonrape assault) between the time of the program and 2-month follow-up reported a decreased risk of revictimization at 6-month follow-up. In contrast, no decrease in the risk of revictimization at 6-month follow-up was observed for women who had been raped between the two assessment periods.

It is possible to speculate about the reason for the latter finding. The ELM and the health belief model imply that a prerequisite to benefit from the risk-reduction program is the belief that the information presented is personally relevant. Accordingly, those women who experienced a "moderate" sexual assault between the end of the program and the 2-month follow-up might have deemed the information they earlier encountered personally relevant and taken actions that decreased their rate of sexual assault between the 2-month and the 6-month follow-up assessments. However, the fact that women who were raped did not experience a comparable reduction in revictimization rate might indicate that efficient information processing is degraded by the posttraumatic effects of rape—the most severe type of sexual assault reported. It may also be the case that women with histories of rape may be in need of more intensive interventions. Data have consistently underscored the fact that women with histories of rape are at the highest risk for a variety of negative effects including revictimization.

Additional analyses revealed that both central and peripheral measures were related to the risk of being sexually assaulted. More specifically, the greater the amount that the participant reported learning during the program, the greater the expressed interest in the survivor video, and the more helpful and interested the participant perceived the facilitator to be, the less likely the participant was to be assaulted. These results imply that the continued use of the ELM (Petty & Cacioppo, 1986b) is warranted to inform program development.

Gidycz and her colleagues' efforts to improve the methodological rigor of sexual assault risk-reduction programs through the use of (a) psychometrically sound instruments that measure participants' behavior, (b) the inclusion of control groups, (c) strict adherence to treatment protocols, and (d) follow-up assessment are commendable. Furthermore, the inclusion of theory-driven program content and attention to the issue of revictimization are noteworthy.

However, despite these methodological and theoretical improvements, the results of these studies are mixed. Although the initial study (Hanson & Gidycz, 1993) reported decreased rates of assault among women who did not report a sexual assault prior to treatment, the same positive outcome failed to occur among women who were assaulted prior to the study. Moreover, Breitenbacher and Gidycz (1998) failed to replicate the positive finding of Hanson and Gidycz, despite the fact that efforts were made to address the issue of revictimization risk more directly. The third study (Gidycz, Lynn, et al., 2001) found yet another pattern of results. It appeared that being assaulted after the program protected against later revictimization, but only among those women who suffered a less severe form of sexual victimization than rape. Results regarding dating behavior and sexual communication have also been mixed.

Taken together, it seems appropriate to conclude that Gidycz and her colleagues' multifaceted risk-reduction program can reduce the rate of victimization among some women, but the results are neither consistent nor robust. Moreover, the program does not appear to be successful in reducing the risk of revictimization of women who have already been sexually victimized. The results of these studies not only have highlighted the challenges of designing effective risk-reduction programs but also have informed subsequent interventions designed specifically for assault survivors.

Research With Previously Victimized Women

Two recent studies included only participants who reported the experience of a sexual assault prior to the study (Calhoun et al., 2001; Marx et al., 2001). Because the goal was to evaluate programs designed specifically to prevent sexual revictimization, in both studies, women with assault histories were targeted.

Marx et al. (2001) conducted a methodologically rigorous study of a sexual revictimization prevention program. The participants were 66 women who, during the initial session, reported a history of sexual victimization since the age of 14. To minimize potential adverse psychological effects, Marx et al. further screened the women to ensure that any individuals who actively experienced severe psychological symptoms at the time were excluded from the prevention program.

Marx et al.'s (2001) program combined a modified version of Hanson and Gidycz's (1993) program, with a relapse-prevention approach. Hanson and Gidycz's program was modified by deleting the second video, which shows a woman modeling protective dating behaviors, and by adding an exercise in which the participants completed a worksheet listing the perpetrator, as well as situational and personal risk factors that described their victimization histories. The portion of the program adapted from relapse prevention included identification of high-risk situations, problem solving, coping-skills training, assertiveness training, and the development of communication skills. Two 2-hour sessions were held, with no more than 2 days between the sessions. The sessions were run by master's-level, female, graduate research assistants using a standardized manual. Groups were limited to 5–10 participants to facilitate disclosure and group process.

The same questionnaires were administered at an initial session advertised as a study of dating behaviors in college women, and at a follow-up session that was held 2 months after the program was completed. Two of the measures used, the Sexual Experiences Survey (Koss & Oros, 1982) and the Symptom Checklist 90–Revised (Derogatis & Savitz, 1999), have established reliability and validity. However, the psychometric properties of the other two measures—self-efficacy ratings (Hall, 1989) and the response latency measure (Marx & Gross, 1995)—were not mentioned by the authors. The response latency measure consisted of an audiotape presentation of a sexual encounter between a man and a woman that ends in rape. Participants listened to the tape and pressed a button on a computer keyboard when they thought that the man had "gone too far." To prevent biased responding, resulting from knowing that the tape ends with a rape, the measure was administered at posttest only.

The results indicated that there were no significant differences in the rate of overall sexual revictimization (i.e., any type of assault, including, but not limited to, rape) between the treatment (32%) and control (21%) groups. Importantly, however, among the women who were revictimized, the control group members reported being raped at significantly higher rates (30%) than did intervention group members (12%). These reported rapes were the result of either the woman giving in to arguments or pressure or the woman being given alcohol or drugs by the perpetrator. Although none of the women reported a rape resulting from threat or use of force, rapes not involving force may nonetheless constitute unwanted or abusive experiences.

In addition, women who participated in the program had greater increases in self-efficacy for avoiding sexual assault than did women in the control group, regardless of whether they were revictimized. This result pertained to both overall victimization experiences and rape only. Moreover, general psychological functioning improved over time, with greater changes evidenced by the intervention group when all levels of victimization were considered together. Finally, there were no group differences on the measure of risk recognition, an unfortunate outcome given that participants who showed higher levels of risk recognition were less likely to experience a rape during follow-up.

Although Marx et al.'s (2001) study is methodologically rigorous and positive treatment effects were found, including the critically important finding of a decreased rate of rape among the intervention group, the small sample size makes it difficult to draw firm conclusions about the program's effectiveness. Specifically, no women in the study reported rape resulting from force or threat of force. Some of the assaults included as rape occurred when the women gave in to sexual intercourse following pressure and arguments from their partner. Although such experiences may well constitute unwanted experiences, they do not meet the legal definition of rape.

It is possible that training in assertiveness, communication, and problem solving successfully increased women's ability to avoid rape resulting from pressure and use of alcohol. Of course, a program that reduces incidence of any type of unwanted sexual experience, especially with a high-risk sample, represents an important advance in the field.

In an extension of Marx et al.'s (2001) initial study, Calhoun et al. (2001) conducted a multisite investigation of a modified version of Marx et al.'s program. Calhoun et al. added the video of the sexual assault survivors that was used in Gidycz's previous studies. The outcome measures included many of the same instruments that were included in Marx et al.'s study.

The participants were women with assault histories from two large universities, one in the South and the other in the Midwest. Women were assessed at pretest and at a 4-month follow-up session. The results indicated that women in the intervention group displayed greater self-efficacy at the 4-month follow-up than the wait-list control group. Unlike the Marx et al. study, program participants also evidenced shorter latencies on the response latency measure, indicating that they more quickly perceived risk in the audiotaped scenario. Finally, participants were less likely to experience all forms of sexual aggression if they were in the program group (14%) than in the wait-list control group (23%), and all of the forceful rapes that occurred during the 4-month follow-up period (7%) occurred in the control group.

Overall, this study with a much larger sample further supports the efficacy of this intervention for women at high risk for sexual assault. The fact that all of the forceful assaults occurred in the control group indicates that this intervention may be useful for reducing women's risk for the most traumatizing sexual assault experiences. It is noteworthy that the women in this study will be followed for 2 years in order that the long-term effects of the program can be evaluated.

Summary and Recommendations for Future Programming

Marx et al.'s (2001) and Calhoun et al.'s (2001) programs were 4 hours long, compared with the 2-hour program used in the initial studies (Breitenbecher & Gidycz, 1998; Gidycz, Lynn, et al., 2001; Hanson & Gidycz, 1993), and contained components specific to sexual assault education, as well as more general skill building in the areas of assertiveness, communication, and problem solving. The positive results obtained by relatively comprehensive programs that focus on developing component skills imply that intervention programming will need to be both broad in scope and in-depth to maximize treatment gains.

According to the health belief model, to take protective action against a threat, individuals must perceive that they are vulnerable to the threat and believe that they have the ability to overcome the threat. It is noteworthy that in Calhoun et al.'s (2001) study, participants in the program group were better able to identify risk in the audiotaped scenario and also believed that they were better able to avoid a sexual assault than were the control participants. The increased ability to identify the threat coupled with the increase in self-efficacy may be critical components underlying the success of the intervention. Subsequent studies should be directed to dismantling Marx et al.'s (2001) and Calhoun et al.'s (2001) programs and assessing the active role of individual versus combined treatment components.

Hanson and Gidycz's (1993) research implies that it may not be advisable to direct programming to women with a history of child abuse in the context of a more general risk-reduction program. Research that directly compares programs tailored to a wide, unselected audience versus a more select audience of previously victimized women should be a priority.

PROGRAMS WITH MIXED-GENDER AUDIENCES

Of the studies conducted with mixed-gender audiences, only three studies meet the criteria for inclusion in this review (i.e., individual random assignment of participants, inclusion of a control group, use of reliable and valid assessment instruments, and a standardized treatment protocol). Heppner et al. (1995) investigated whether type of programming affects processing of rape prevention messages; attitudes, knowledge, and behaviors related to rape; and stability of change across time. The 258 (50% male and 50% female) participants in the study were randomly assigned to a didactic-video program, an interactive drama program designed to increase the motivation to process information by using a typical dating scenario and brainstorming ideas for clear sexual communication, or a stress-management control program. All of the programs were 90-minutes in length and were facilitated by a male and a female graduate student in counseling psychology. Measures of rape myths (Burt, 1980), social desirability (Hays, Hayashi, & Stewart, 1989), central route processing, and the ability to recognize situations in which a person is coerced to engage in sex (Gibson & Humphrey, 1993) were administered at follow-ups of 1 month, 5 weeks, 4 months, and 5 months after the administration of the pretreatment measures.

The research indicated that the interactive drama program promoted central route processing to a greater extent than did the didactic-video condition, which, in turn, was superior to the control program. In addition, the didactic-video program was more effective than the control program in reducing acceptance of rape myths at 1 month, but the differences were not apparent at later follow-up. Although men in the interactive condition were better able to differentiate coercive and consensual sex than men in the didactic condition, and men in the didactic condition scored better than those in the control condition, the magnitude of the differences were small and probably not meaningful. Moreover, this pattern of differences was not evident in female participants. Finally, the interactive drama group participants scored higher than the didactic video group or the control group on four of the six behavioral indicators (i.e., likelihood of volunteering for a rape project, time spent thinking about the intervention, time spent talking about the intervention, and number of people with whom they discussed the intervention); however, the relation between these behavioral indicators and sexually aggressive behavior had not been validated.

Overall, the results of Heppner et al. (1995) are disappointing. The positive results that were found were unstable, extremely small, or both. Moreover, no measure of actual sexual behavior was used. It appears that although central processing was improved by the inclusion of certain components, this processing was insufficient to produce stable, meaningful change in rape-related attitudes and understanding of coercive behavior. Given these results, actual behavior change would be unlikely.

A second study with a mixed-gender audience was conducted by Pinzone-Glover, Gidycz, and Jacobs (1998). These researchers randomly assigned 152 students to either an acquaintance rape prevention program or a comparison group that consisted of a sexually transmitted disease awareness program. The hour-long rape prevention program was largely the same as the one used by Hanson and Gidycz (1993), with modifications for including male participants. The measures administered were the Rape Myth Acceptance Scale (Burt, 1980), Rape Empathy Scale (Deitz, Blackwell, Daley, & Bentley, 1982), Attitudes Towards Women Scale (Spence, Helmreich, & Stapp, 1973), and questions regarding acquaintance rape scenarios. The first three of these measures have established reliability and validity, whereas no data were provided for the fourth instrument. No measure of the participants' actual sexual behaviors was administered.

To reduce the influence of demand characteristics, Pinzone-Glover et al. (1998) administered the dependent measures as a separate experiment both before and after the programs were presented. In appears that this effort was successful, in that only 2% of participants reported that they suspected the true nature of the experiment. Participants in the rape prevention program became significantly more empathic toward the victim than those in the comparison group. As with the Heppner et al. (1995) study, however, the magnitude of the change in scores was small (e.g., 6 points on a scale with possible scores ranging from 19 to 117). No significant difference was found between the two groups on the measures of rape myth acceptance, and only male program participants (compared with males in the control group) evidenced a significant change in attitudes toward women. Finally, men became more certain of their definition of rape, reaching, by posttest, the range achieved by women at pretest.

However, in a follow-up study using the same outcome measures and program that was used in Pinzone-Glover et al.'s (1998) study, Gidycz, Layman, et al. (2001) did not replicate the findings with the Attitudes Towards Women Scale or the Rape Empathy Scale. Further, in the latter study, Gidycz, Layman, et al. measured self-reported rates of sexual aggression and victimization in men and women, respectively, and found no differences in these rates for the program and control group for either male or female participants. The program evaluation suggested that although the participants indicated that they liked the program, they did not believe that the information applied to them.

Given that only three methodologically rigorous studies with a mixed-gender sample have been conducted, only limited conclusions can be drawn regarding the effectiveness of such programming in reducing rates of sexual victimization. The magnitude of the changes that occurred following the administration of these two programs was small and unlikely to be meaningful. In addition, in the one study that included a measure of sexually aggressive behavior, the results were negative. Based on the small attitude changes that were reported in the two studies that did not assess sexual aggression, it is likely that even if behavior change had been measured, little or no reduction in sexual assault risk would have occurred. Overall, this line of study does not appear promising; however, this conclusion may be premature in that the studies conducted to date have not stratified participants by history of sexual assault.

In addition to limited empirical support for mixed-gender programs, there are some philosophical problems with offering joint programs for men and women (Gidycz, Rich, & Marioni, 2002). We are concerned that in mixed-gender programs, some women who have already been victimized by male sexual violence might be further traumatized by participation in a mixed group. Further, although some of the goals clearly overlap for the sexes, it is difficult to see how some goals that are appropriate for men (e.g., men taking responsibility for other men's behavior) can be fostered when women are also in the room. Further, it has been argued that it is inappropriate to share risk-reduction techniques for women with men because it could provide potential rapists with information that could increase a woman's vulnerability to assault. Finally, an overriding goal of prevention and risk-reduction efforts is to maximize the saliency of the information for participants. The program evaluation for Gidycz, Layman, et al.'s (2001) mixed-gender program clearly indicates that participants in mixed-gender groups do not find the information relevant. Efforts will most likely be better spent on providing programming for single-sexed audiences.

GENERAL CONCLUSION

The studies we reviewed in detail are the most sophisticated and methodologically rigorous interventions to date. Nevertheless, there is considerable room for refinement of the conceptualization and methodology of studies in this research area. For example, little is known about the "clinical significance" of sexual assault programs across a variety of outcome measures. One might ask questions along the lines of whether a 10-point difference on a measure of assertiveness decreases the risk of being revictimized by 1% or by 50%. That is, do differences observed between treatments and control groups, or changes that occur over time, translate into enduring changes in attitudes, behaviors, and sexual victimization rates in the "real world"? Two ways of approaching this question are to report effect sizes and to compare the scores of high- and low-risk participants after interventions or follow-up periods of varying lengths. Only when such information is gleaned will it be possible to determine whether a given program's effectiveness warrants its continued implementation.

Collecting diverse information and using multiple methods of measurement are necessary to capture the complexity of sexual assault prevention. However, broader generalizations and conclusions about prevention effectiveness are nearly impossible to develop when there is no common set of outcome variables measured. To truly advance our knowledge in this area, researchers must establish a well-validated standard battery of attitudinal and behavioral outcome measures relevant to sexual experience that will provide a basis for comparison across studies. Until this occurs, it is unlikely that any program's true efficacy and effectiveness will be demonstrated in a meaningful and convincing manner.

Research on sexual assault and revictimization prevention is founded on the assumption that participants' reports of their sexual experiences are valid and reliable. However, demand characteristics and response sets can influence participants' reports and should be minimized to the fullest possible extent. Accordingly, we recommend that, if resources permit, researchers maintain the contextual independence of the assessment of sexual assault and the prevention program by administering assessment instruments under the guise of one study while the program is presented to participants as a separate study. This design would reduce the likelihood of contamination of the research findings by a carryover of expectations and demand characteristics from the assessment phase of the research to the treatment procedure. However, we also acknowledge that this methodologically rigorous design may not be practical in the context of a large-scale, multiyear study, for example, or in a community-based intervention trial. The fact that the results of risk-reduction programs have been mixed at best implies that demand characteristics, which might be expected to lead to positive results, have not played an influential role in determining the outcomes of research to date.

In addition to the methodological improvements suggested, two concepts require more precise definition. It is important to specify the definition of the terms *rape* and *sexual assault*. Most studies include unwanted sexual contact of any kind, by any means, under the rubric of sexual assault. This broad definition can contribute to the appearance of higher rates of victimization than more restrictive definitions. The definition of rape in at least one study (Marx et al., 2001) included women who reported that they "gave in" to sexual relations because of continual pressure or arguments by their partners. Although pressure and arguments may well be unwanted and have negative psychological repercussions, these behaviors do not meet the legal definition of rape. The results of studies may vary as a function of the definitions of assault and rape that are used. To analyze data in a consistent manner, and to make meaningful comparisons across domains of inquiry (e.g., to use justice-based research) as well as across studies, researchers need to specify how key constructs and behaviors are defined and arrive at agreement in terms of the definitions of sexual assault that are used.

In designing and evaluating programs for women with assault histories, it is particularly important to specify clearly the nature of the past abusive experiences. Women who have had experiences that clearly constitute a rape may be in need of specialized programs. However, it is unclear whether women with more moderate types of abusive experiences, as well as women who have experienced CSA, can best be served in these specialized programs or programs that target a general college student audience. Factors other than the exact nature of the past sexual victimization may need to be taken into consideration when identifying a high-risk group (Himelein, 1999). Although a history of sexual assault constitutes a definite risk factor for subsequent abuse, there is no consensus at this point regarding the constellation of attitudes and behaviors that increase sexual assault risk. Theory-driven operational definitions of the concept of "high risk" are vital to the design and assessment of sexual assault risk-reduction programs.

The extant literature provides support for theory-driven research in general, and the use of the ELM (Petty & Cacioppo, 1986b) in particular, to guide interventions. Although evidence is limited, it appears that the inclusion of treatment components that enhance both peripheral and central route processing (e.g., facilitators perceived by participants as interested in the program and a rape-survivors video) may well augment treatment gains. Additional research to determine ways of increasing information and the depth and efficiency of processing, such as informing individuals they may be tested on material learned and writing statements that elaborate the personal relevance of important information conveyed, could prove useful. We recommend that measures of the degree or depth of processing be included in research designs to examine the possible mediating or moderating role of information elaboration.

Recent research has identified a number of variables that mediate the relation between CSA and adult victimization and provide potentially effective indicators for intervention. Internalized blame for CSA (Arata, 2000; Pope, 2000), presence of posttraumatic stress disorder (Arata, 2000), level of sexual activity (Arata, 2000; Krahe, Scheinberger-Olwig, Waizenhoeffer, & Kolpin, 1999), and alcohol problems (Merrill et al., 1999) may all be subject to modification. In our laboratories, efforts are under way to develop risk-reduction programs that increase women's awareness of the link between drug and alcohol use and sexual assault and that teach women strategies to control drinking in high-risk situations. However, in certain cases, issues and problems may be long-standing, well entrenched, and recalcitrant to brief, single-session interventions. Accordingly, previously victimized women may require more intensive and extensive interventions, which specifically target one or more of these variables, than women who have never been victimized. Such interventions may be more akin to group therapy with a clinical population than to risk-reduction programming with a general student or community population.

The study of sexual assault risk-reduction programs for women, in general, and previous victims of sexual abuse, in particular, has made great strides forward during the last decade. Existing programs are promising; however, much work remains to be done. Most of the studies completed to date have been conducted with college students. However, given the high rates of CSA and adolescent sexual victimization, combined with the imperative to prevent sexual assault before it occurs in the first place, it is likely that programming will need to be conducted with high school, junior high school, and even middle school students. In the quest for a decisive end to sexual assault, it is crucial not to lose sight of the fact that the responsibility for these crimes lies with the perpetrator. Although it is a worthy endeavor to help women to protect themselves, researchers must also strive to prevent victimization at its source by designing programs that decrease the risk of men committing sexual assault.

REFERENCES

Anderson, L. A., Stoelb, M. P., Duggan, P., Hieger, B., Kling, K. H., & Payne, J. P. (1998). The effectiveness of two types of rape prevention programs in changing the rape-supportive attitudes of college students. *Journal of College Student Development, 39,* 131–142.

Arata, C. M. (2000). From child victim to adult victim: A model for predicting sexual revictimization. *Child Maltreatment: Journal of the American Professional Society on the Abuse of Children, 5,* 28–38.

Borden, L. A., Karr, S. K., & Caldwell-Colbert, A. T. (1988). Effects of a university rape prevention program on attitudes and empathy toward rape. *Journal of College Student Development, 29,* 132–136.

Breitenbecher, K. H., & Gidycz, C. A. (1998). An empirical evaluation of a program designed to reduce the risk of multiple sexual victimization. *Journal of Interpersonal Violence, 13,* 472–488.

Brener, N. D., McMahon, P. M., Warren, C. W., & Douglas, K. A. (1999). Forced sexual intercourse and associated health risk behaviors among female college students in the United States. *Journal of Consulting and Clinical Psychology, 67,* 252–259.

Burt, M. R. (1980). Cultural myths and supports for rape. *Journal of Personality and Social Psychology, 38,* 217–230.

Calhoun, K. S., Gidycz, C. A., Loh, C., Wilson, A., Lueken, M., Outman, R. C., & Marioni, N. L. (2001, November). *Sexual assault prevention in high risk women.* Poster presented at the meeting of the Association for the Advancement of Behavior Therapy, Philadelphia, PA.

Chambless, D. L., & Hollon, S. D. (1998). Defining empirically supported therapies. *Journal of Consulting and Clinical Psychology, 66,* 7–18.

Dallager, C., & Rosen, L. A. (1993). Effects of a humans sexuality course on attitudes toward rape and violence. *Journal of Sex Education and Therapy, 19,* 193–199.

Deitz, S. R., Blackwell, K. T., Daley, P. C., & Bentley, B. J. (1982). Measurement of empathy toward rape victims and rapists. *Journal of Personality and Social Psychology. 43,* 372–384.

Derogatis, L. R., & Savitz, K. L. (1999). The SCL-90-R, Brief Symptom Inventory, and matching clinical rating scales. In Mark E. Maruish (Ed.). *The use of psychological testing for treatment planning and outcomes assessment* (2nd ed.; pp. 679–724). Mahwah, NJ: Lawrence Erlbaum Associates.

Ellis, A. L., O'Sullivan, C. S., & Sowards, B. A. (1992). The impact of contemplated exposure to a survivor of rape on attitudes toward rape. *Journal of Applied Social Psychology, 22,* 889–895.

Fischer, B. S., Cullen, F. T., & Turner, M. G. (2000). *The sexual victimization of college women* (U.S. Department of Justice, Publication No. NCJ 182369). Washington, DC: U.S. Government Printing Office.

Fischer, G. J. (1986). College student attitudes toward forcible date rape: I. Cognitive predictors. *Archives of Sexual Behavior, 15,* 457–466.

Fonow, M. M., Richardson, L., & Wemmerus, V. A. (1992). Feminist rape education: Does it work? *Gender and Society, 6,* 108–121.

Frazier, P., Valtinson, G., & Candell, S. (1994). Evaluation of a coeducational interactive rape prevention program. *Journal of Counseling & Development, 73,* 153–158.

Gibson, D. B., & Humphrey, C. F. (1993). *Educating in regards to sexual violence: An interactional dramatic acquaintance rape intervention.* Minneapolis: University of Minnesota, Sexual Violence Program.

Gidycz, C. A., Hanson, K., & Layman, M. J. (1995). A prospective analysis of the relationship among sexual assault experiences: An extension of previous findings. *Psychology of Women Quarterly, 19,* 5–29.

Gidycz, C. A., Layman, M. J., Rich, C. L., Crothers, M., Gylys, J., Matorin, A., & Jacobs, C. D. (2001). An evaluation of an acquaintance rape prevention program: Impact on attitudes and behavior. *Journal of Interpersonal Violence, 16,* 1120–1138.

Gidycz, C. A., Lynn, S. J., Rich, C. L., Marioni, N. L., Loh, C., Blackwell, L. M., et al. (2001). The evaluation of a sexual assault risk reduction program: A multi-site investigation. *Journal of Consulting and Clinical Psychology, 69,* 1073–1078.

Gidycz, C. A., Rich, C. L., & Marioni, N. L. (2002). Interventions to prevent rape and sexual assault. In J. Petrak & B. Hedge (Eds.), *The trauma of adult sexual assault: Treatment, prevention, and policy* (pp. 235–260). New York: Wiley.

Gray, M. D., Lesser, D., Quinn, E., & Bounds, C. (1990). The effectiveness of personalizing acquaintance rape prevention: Programs on perception of vulnerability and on reducing risk-taking behavior. *Journal of College Student Development, 31*, 217–220.

Hall, R. L. (1989). Self-efficacy ratings. In D. R. Laws (Ed.), *Relapse prevention with sex offenders* (pp. 137–146). New York: Guilford.

Hanson, K. A., & Gidycz, C. A. (1993). Evaluation of a sexual assault prevention program. *Journal of Consulting and Clinical Psychology, 61*, 1046–1052.

Harrison, P. J., Downes, J., & Williams, M. D. (1991). Date and acquaintance rape: Perceptions and attitude change strategies. *Journal of College Student Development, 32(2)*, 131–139.

Hays, R. D., Hayashi, T., & Stewart, A. L. (Eds.). (1989). A five item measure of socially desirable response set. *Educational and Psychological Measurement, 49*, 629–636.

Heppner, M. J., Humphrey, C. F., Debord, K. A., & Hillenbrand-Gunn, T. L. (1995). The differential effects of rape prevention programming on attitudes, behavior, and knowledge. *Journal of Counseling Psychology, 42*, 508–518.

Himelein, M. J. (1999). Acquaintance rape prevention with high-risk women: Identification and inoculation. *Journal of College Student Development, 40*, 93–96.

Hochman, M. J. (1958). *Public participation in medical screening programs: A sociopsychological study* (Public Health Service Publication No. 572). Washington, DC: U.S. Government Printing Office.

Holcomb, D. R., Sarvela, P. D., Sondag, A., & Hatton Holcomb, L. C. (1993). An evaluation of a mixed-gender date rape prevention workshop. *College Health, 41*, 159–164.

Holcomb, D. R., Sondag, A., & Hatton Holcomb, L. C. (1993). Healthy dating: A mixed-gender date rape workshop. *College Health, 41*, 155–157.

Humphrey, J. A., & White, J. W. (2000). Women's vulnerability to sexual assault from adolescence to young adulthood. *Journal of Adolescent Health, 27*, 419–424.

Koss, M. P. (1993). Rape: Scope, impact, interventions, and public policy responses. *American Psychologist, 48*, 1062–1069.

Koss, M. P. (1998). Hidden rape: Sexual aggression and victimization in a national sample of students in higher education. In M. E. Odem & J. Clay-Warner (Eds.), *Confronting rape and sexual assault: Worlds of women* (Vol. 3, pp. 51–69). Wilmington, DE: SR Books/Scholarly Resources.

Koss, M. P., & Oros, C. J. (1982). Sexual Experiences Survey: A research instrument investigating sexual aggression and victimization. *Journal of Consulting and Clinical Psychology, 50*, 455–457.

Krahe, B., Scheinberger-Olwig, R., Waizenhoeffer, E., & Kolpin, S. (1999). Childhood sexual abuse and revictimization in adolescence. *Child Abuse and Neglect, 23*, 383–394.

Lenihan, G. O., & Rawlins, M. E. (1994). Rape supportive attitudes among Greek students before and after a date rape prevention program. *Journal of College Student Development, 35*, 450–455.

Lonsway, K. A., Klaw, E. L., Berg, D. R., Waldo, C. R., Kothari, C., Mazurek, C. J., & Hegeman, K. E. (1998). Beyond "no means no": Outcomes of an intensive program to train peer facilitators for campus acquaintance rape education. *Journal of Interpersonal Violence, 13,* 73–92.

Malamuth, N. M., & Check, J. V. (1984). Debriefing effectiveness following exposure to pornographic rape depictions. *Journal of Sex Research, 20,* 1–13.

Mann, C. A., Hecht, M. L., Valentine, K. B. (1988). Performance in a social context: Date rape versus date right. *Central States Speech Journal, 39,* 269–280.

Marx, B. P., Calhoun, K. S., Wilson, A. E., & Meyerson, L. A. (2001). Sexual revictimization prevention: An outcome evaluation. *Journal of Consulting and Clinical Psychology, 69,* 25–32.

Marx, B. P., & Gross, A. M. (1995). Date rape: An analysis of two contextual variables. *Behavior Modification, 19,* 451–463.

Merrill, L. L., Newell, C. E., Thomsen, C. J., Gold, S. R., Milner, J. S., Koss, M. P., & Rosswork, S. G. (1999). Childhood abuse and sexual revictimization in a female navy recruit sample. *Journal of Traumatic Stress, 12,* 211–225.

Nelson, E. S., & Torgler, C. C. (1990). A comparison of strategies for changing college students' attitudes toward acquaintance rape. *Journal of Humanistic Education and Development, 29,* 69–85.

Petty, R. E., & Cacioppo, J. T. (1981). *Attitudes and persuasion: Classic and contemporary approaches.* Dubuque, IA: Brown.

Petty, R. E., & Cacioppo, J. T. (1986a). *Communication and persuasion: Central and peripheral routes to attitude change.* New York: Springer-Verlag.

Petty, R. E., & Cacioppo, J. T. (1986b). The elaboration likelihood model of persuasion. In L. Berkowitz (Ed.), *Advances in experimental social psychology* (Vol. 19, pp. 123–205). San Diego, CA: Academic Press.

Petty, R. E., Haugtvedt, C. P., & Smith, S. M. (1995). Elaboration as a determinant of attitude strength: Creating attitudes that are persistent, resistant, and predictive of behavior. In R. E. Petty, & J. A. Krosnick (Eds.). *Attitude strength: Antecedent and consequences. Ohio State University series on attitudes and persuasion,* Vol. 4. (pp. 93–130). Hillsdale, NJ: Lawrence Erlbaum Associates.

Pinzone-Glover, H. A., Gidycz, C. A., & Jacobs, C. D. (1998). An acquaintance rape prevention program: Effects on attitudes toward women, rape-related attitudes, and perceptions of rape scenarios. *Psychology of Women Quarterly, 22,* 605–621.

Pope, J. A. (2000). Revictimization among female survivors of childhood sexual abuse: Risk and protective factors. *Dissertation Abstracts International: Section B: The Sciences and Engineering, 60,* 4246.

Resick, P. A. (1993). The psychological impact of rape. *Journal of Interpersonal Violence, 8,* 223–255.

Roodman, A. A., & Clum, G. A. (2001). Revictimization rates and method variance: A meta-analysis. *Clinical Psychology Review, 21,* 183–204.

Spence, J. T., Helmreich, R., & Stapp, J. (1973). A short version of the Attitudes Toward Women Scale (AWS). *Bulletin of the Psychonomic Society, 2,* 219–220.

Verplanken, B. (1991). Persuasive communication of risk information: A test of cue versus message processing effects in a field experiment. *Personality and Social Psychology Bulletin, 17,* 188–193.

V

CONCLUSION

CHILD SEXUAL ABUSE AND ADULT SEXUAL RISK: WHERE DO WE GO FROM HERE?

ANN O'LEARY, LINDA J. KOENIG, AND LYNDA S. DOLL

Much has been written about child sexual abuse (CSA) for both lay and professional readers. Indeed, a quick review of the social science database indicates that more than 100 books have been published on the topic in the past decade alone. This volume reviews what we know about associations between CSA and adult sexual risk, possible intermediate outcomes and theoretical mediators for these associations, and cutting-edge interventions to heal the survivor and ameliorate negative effects. This chapter delineates some important directions for future research, based on gaps in the literature suggested by the other chapters in the volume. The first section of this chapter discusses gaps in basic information (i.e., populations and issues); the second section highlights some areas in need of further concept development and supporting data.

This chapter was authored or coauthored by an employee of the United States government as part of official duty and is considered to be in the public domain. Any views expressed herein do not necessarily represent the views of the United States government.

One clear gap is a lack of knowledge about the prevalence of CSA and its sequelae among men, particularly heterosexual men and men from specific ethnic backgrounds and cultures. Heterosexual men who were sexually abused during childhood may be an important source of HIV transmission to women, yet little research has been done in this population. MSM (men who have sex with men) of color, particularly young men, have been disproportionately affected by HIV and AIDS (Valleroy et al., 2000), highlighting the importance of assessing the role of CSA and identifying possible remedies for its sequelae.

The need for cultural specificity is also poorly understood with respect to CSA of women. Cultural definitions of sexuality and acceptable behavior may affect whether particular events are construed as abusive and, thus, whether they are likely to be disclosed and what the parental response will be. Causes of abuse as well as effects of abuse may also vary by culture. Importantly, interventions may require cultural tailoring to be effective.

A fascinating, if somewhat mysterious, sequela of CSA is that of sexual revictimization. As described in chapters 7, and 13 of this volume, it is clear that this phenomenon is robust. However, mechanisms for the effects of CSA on revictimization are poorly understood—although some possibilities are outlined by Lynn, Pintar, Fite, Ecklund, and Stafford (chap. 7, this volume). Of critical importance is the development and evaluation of interventions designed to prevent revictimization for survivors, as few effective interventions have been developed to date (see chap. 13, this volume).

With the exception of alcohol abuse, the potential mediators described in Part II of the book are theoretical and have not been tested empirically. They are, nevertheless, the result of careful analysis of how each pathway might be a consequence of CSA and how it might produce sexual outcomes. We hope that readers will be stimulated to establish these links empirically. Following the statistical approach to testing the effects of mediators (see Baron & Kenny, 1986), examining these mediators involves several steps. The first step involves establishing that the mediators exist at higher levels among survivors of CSA than among individuals with no CSA history. Mediators may be, for example, higher levels of dissociation, different social narratives in sexual situations, different beliefs and feelings, or less adequately integrated linguistic–affective descriptions of traumatic or sexual events. The second step would be to assess whether the putative mechanism predicts or is higher among those with different levels of sexual risk, HIV infection, or other outcomes. The third step should be testing CSA as a predictor of the outcome (much of this work has already been done and is reviewed in Part I). The final step, including the mediator in the predictive model, should reduce the strength of association between CSA and the outcome compared with that association without the mediator included in the model. While several of the chapters in the present volume review intrapersonal factors as potential mediators, more work needs to be done to identify interpersonal and contextual/environmental factors that may directly mediate or moderate the associations between CSA and adult outcomes

The chapter by Pennebaker and Stone (chap. 9, this volume) is unique in that it presents a potential mediator—level of cognitive–affective integration of traumatic experience—in the context of a potentially effective intervention, namely, writing about traumatic experiences. Extending this type of therapy from coping with relatively minor stressors to coping with CSA trauma to evaluate it for possible effects on very consequential life outcomes is an important research direction.

Intervention approaches, described in Part III of the book, remain in need of evaluation. Some have been tested informally, and some are in the process of being tested formally. We hope that by the time this volume becomes available, results of these ongoing studies—by Chin, Wyatt, Vargas Carmona, Loeb, and Myers (chap. 11) and by Spiegel, Classen, Thurston, and Butler (chap. 12)—will have been published. We very much hope that clinicians reading this book will take to heart Briere's information in chapter 10 on incorporating HIV prevention activities into psychotherapy for sexual abuse survivors, many of whom will receive therapy but will not have access to HIV prevention programs. Training mental health care providers in HIV risk reduction is an important goal, one that we hope will be undertaken by professional organizations.

OVERARCHING ISSUES

Several overarching issues—substantive aspects of our ability to conceptualize CSA and its consequences—are controversial or in need of broad theoretical advances and development. These issues are defining CSA, determining the independent effects of CSA, assessing mediators and intermediate outcomes, and evaluating intervention approaches.

Defining Child Sexual Abuse

CSA researchers must come to a common definition of CSA to make study findings comparable. The Centers for Disease Control and Prevention (CDC) is leading an effort to develop a standardized method for assessing CSA (Basile & Saltzman, 2002). Arriving at a common definition may not be easy because defining abuse may vary according to cultural, social, and political contexts. With respect to the specific acts that define abuse, some definitions include behaviors that do not involve touching (e.g., genital exposure, showing photographs, talking about sex), whereas others include only penetrative behaviors. Study definitions often vary with regard to age of the victim, with some defining CSA as occurring before age 12 and others including adolescents up to age 16 or even 18. Some definitions include specific abuse characteristics, such as use of force or length of time over which the abuse occurred; others include perpetrator characteristics, such as age or relationship to the victim. Any comprehensive measure of CSA severity will need to incorporate several factors, particularly those known to be predictive of the severity of outcomes. For example, dissociative processes and forgetting may be related to dependence on the perpetrator, as when the perpetrator is a parent (chap. 6, this volume). Outcomes also tend to be worse the younger the child and the longer the duration of abuse (e.g., Merrill, Thomsen, Sinclair, Gold, & Milner, 2001). There is evidence that outcomes may be worse for women than for men (Rind, Tromovitch, & Bauserman, 1998). Data from gay men abused during childhood indicate substantial variability in how "upsetting" the abuse experience was (Carballo-Diéguez & Dolezal, 1995). Threats and shaming of the child are deleterious; in contrast, disclosure of the abuse is productive and associated with better outcomes, particularly when the listener believes the child and takes steps to end it (Haugaard & Samwel, 1992; Pintello & Zuravin, 2001).

Although not every study of CSA may need a severity measure that takes all of these factors into account, it should be possible to construct a continuous measure of CSA severity that takes some of them into account. An example of such as attempt can be found in Paul, Catania, Pollack, and Stall (2001), in which several severity factors were measured, including number of coercion experiences, number of perpetrators, survivor's age at the time of abuse, duration of abuse, and type of coercion used. Paul and colleagues used these variables to predict outcomes and examined interactions between the variables; however, they did not attempt to construct a single index incorporating all of them. In any case, it does seem likely that more comprehensive measures will yield stronger results and be more effective in predicting relevant outcomes. As noted in the introductory chapter of this volume, analyses to determine which aspects of the abuse are most strongly related to particular outcomes are also needed. However, different ways of assessing CSA may be optimal for answering particular research questions. We recommend that studies of CSA include multiple measures so we can assess the usefulness of each for addressing specific issues.

One definitional issue that may be intrinsically impossible to address is the fact that many claim that memories of CSA can be repressed (Freyd, 1996), contributing "false-negative" data and potentially weakening predictive relationships. It is important to note that the issue of forgetting abuse is controversial (reviewed in Koriat, Goldsmith, & Pansky, 2000). However, if forgetting abuse is indeed possible, these cases may be the most severe, and failure to correctly identify them may distort results more than would random missing data.

Determining Independent Effects of Child Sexual Abuse

One important challenge of linking CSA to outcomes is disentangling effects of CSA from those of other potentially harmful family and community environments that often coexist with CSA (e.g., Browning & Laumann, 1997; Rind et al., 1998). Not only does CSA often occur along with other forms of abuse (physical abuse, emotional abuse, and neglect), but families in which CSA occurs are often dysfunctional in other ways. For example, CSA is more likely to occur in families with marital conflict (Finkelhor & Baron, 1986), substance abuse (Curtis, 1986; Lesniak, 1993), poor interpersonal boundaries (Alexander, 1992), and poor parenting (Burkett, 1991; Zuravin & Fontanella, 1999). Further, the effects of multiple negative experiences in childhood may be additive.

Physical abuse in particular may potentiate effects of sexual abuse. Coid et al. (2001) found a strong association between childhood sexual and physical abuse, confirming that experiences of abuse tend not to occur in isolation. They also confirmed that such CSA is associated with adult abuse and trauma. In their study of women treated in primary care clinics in London, 39% who had experienced unwanted sexual intercourse before 16 years of age had also been beaten on one or more occasions by a parent or caretaker.

Felitti et al. (1998), in the Adverse Childhood Experiences (ACE) study, found a dose–response relationship between exposure to adverse childhood experiences (physical abuse, sexual abuse, neglect, parental violence, and parental criminal behavior) and higher involvement in health risk behaviors (e.g., smoking, poor eating habits, teenage parenthood) during adolescence and adulthood and mortality in adulthood. Thus, in this retrospective cohort study of people treated in an HMO, the greater the exposure to adverse childhood experiences, including sexual and physical abuse, the greater the likelihood of long-term consequences.

One obvious approach to researching this issue is to measure as many of the confounding factors as possible so that they can be adjusted in statistical analyses. Although many aspects of family environment are difficult to assess retrospectively, the effects of sexual abuse in relation to other family variables such as alcohol abuse have been parsed out using advanced statistical methods such as structural equation modeling (see chap. 8, this volume). Alternatively, it may be possible to compare groups of children or adolescents who have been removed from their homes by child welfare services, matched for age of removal, who have or have not been sexually abused. A similar approach was taken by Widom and Kuhns (1996), who used original county court records to compare women who were sexually abused as children with those who were physically abused or neglected. For both of these approaches, one might assume the family environments of these groups to be relatively similar with respect to dysfunction except for the presence of sexual abuse. However, both approaches select for only the most severe cases of abuse that have been reported. Another possibility might be to randomly assign individuals who had suffered CSA to treatment focused solely on the sexual trauma (e.g., exposure therapy) or to treatment focused more broadly on general functioning. Clearly, the best approach would be to assess child and family functioning at the time abuse was reported and to follow these children prospectively. This would, of course, be costly. More important, because all identified children (and perhaps families) would receive treatment, the effects of abuse in the absence of treatment would not be known. Perhaps a more reasonable approach would be that taken by Ferguson, Horwood, and Lynskey (1997), who collected retrospective CSA data from a national cohort study in which family data were assessed from birth and collected prospectively. In this case, the investigators were able to evaluate the relation between abuse and health outcomes adjusting for other aspects of family dysfunction.

For many purposes, it may not matter whether it is sexual abuse per se or other family factors that lead to poor outcomes. Efforts to end each of these exacerbating factors must be made as strongly and as early as possible, as all are unacceptable.

Assessing Mediators and Intermediate Outcomes

Disentangling the differential effects of events occurring between the CSA and later adult sexual health outcomes remains another important goal. The ideas for the chapters in Part III of the book were the result of the editors' reflecting on what we know about trauma and its consequences that may lead to or maintain sexual risk behavior. Although some beginning models have been proposed (Miller, 1999; Whitmire, Harlow, Quina, & Morokoff, 1999), we are far from having an articulated model of how these processes work over time. Further, there may well be other important trauma effects and mediators that are not included here, such as psychobiological processes or family and environmental factors (e.g., runaway, survival sex), but that deserve more attention. It is critically important to bridge trauma sequelae research and risk prevention research to target our interventions most effectively.

Potential mediators of effects of CSA on sexual health and risk behavior are numerous; however, our understanding of their interconnections and causal relationships remains sketchy. The process of mediation analysis can only be interpreted inferentially. While long-term longitudinal research is difficult to conduct and fund, it would increase our understanding of the chain of mediating events linking CSA with more distal outcomes. The cognitive, affective, and behavioral processes of affected children could be studied over time. It may be that certain early processes predict the development of specific later ones; for example, posttraumatic cognitive intrusions in childhood may predict substance abuse in adolescence, which in turn may predict revictimization.

The chapters in Part III of the book suggest numerous possible pathways by which CSA may affect adult sexual risk. Wilsnack and colleagues (chap. 8, this volume) discuss one of the most frequently identified sequelae of CSA, namely, alcohol abuse. Because substance abuse typically does not start until adolescence, it may be a later-stage mediator of the CSA–sexual risk link. Likely to be a common mediator of CSA and substance abuse is psychological depression, as substances are often used to self-medicate psychic pain. Revictimization in adulthood is also a relatively longer term consequence of CSA. Another possible mediator of CSA effects on sexual risk is sexual compulsivity, as promiscuity has been a reported sequela of sexual abuse (Timms & Connors, 1992), and presumably promiscuity would also begin during adolescence or after. Some of the more fundamental and immediate- to short-range mediators may be avoidant cognitive processing such as dissociation and forgetting, as discussed by Zurbriggen and Freyd (chap. 6, this volume). This may in turn be connected with the failure to process affective material in linguistic format, which Pennebaker and Stone (chap. 9, this volume) suggest may be associated with deleterious health consequences. Pennebaker and Stone's work demonstrates that degree of health improvement is predicted by affective–linguistic changes in written text. Some of the effects that, if left uncoded linguistically, may be particularly problematic include many described by Quina, Morokoff, Harlow, and Zurbriggen (chap. 5, this volume), such as terror, self-stigma, powerlessness and helplessness, and betrayal; these affects may occur along with sexual feelings that the events may have evoked. These earlier reactions to abuse may be amenable to early intervention via psychotherapy.

Just as it is important to understand the factors that exacerbate outcomes from CSA and increase risk for adult sexual risk behavior, it is equally important to examine factors that may ameliorate the consequences of CSA. Examples might include family reactions to disclosure, cognitive attributions made by the child, or removal of the child or the perpetrator from the home. If systematic patterns are found for either exacerbating or buffering factors, the implications for intervention through the life span would be significant.

Evaluating Interventions

While not the focus of the present volume, primary prevention deserves mention as the only way to truly address the issue of CSA. Research evaluating awareness-raising interventions has demonstrated their effectiveness in schools (Rispens, Aleman, & Goudena, 1997) and communities (Plummer, 2001). We also need effective interventions for abused children while they are at an age at which they may be more amenable to effective treatment. Also important and relevant to primary prevention is research on and better interventions for perpetrators. In addition to psychotherapeutic approaches, recently developed psychopharmacologic agents such as mood stabilizers and antidepressants may be effective for some perpetrators (Kafka & Hennen, 2000; for reviews, see Kafka, 1997; Suarez, O'Leary, Morgenstern, Hollander, & Allen, 2002).

Effective interventions exist for some of the sequelae of CSA, such as drug and alcohol abuse, posttraumatic stress disorder (PTSD) symptoms, and other psychiatric comorbidities. As described by Blackwell and colleagues (chap. 13, this volume), interventions to prevent revictimization are in their infancy but are being developed. Also, as indicated by Briere (chap. 10, this volume) and Spiegel and colleagues (chap. 12, this volume), traditional individual and group psychotherapy can promote better psychological health among survivors. In addition, effective interventions exist to reduce the risk of HIV and other sexually transmitted diseases (see Peterson & DiClemente, 2000); however, it is still unclear whether such interventions would be more effective for sexual abuse survivors if they dealt in some way with the sexual abuse itself. The work of Pennebaker and Stone (chap. 9, this volume) suggests that they might be. In this work, as described earlier, putting feelings regarding traumatic events into words improves physical and emotional functioning. Psychotherapy, such as that discussed by Briere (chap. 10, this volume), may be effective at least partly through similar processes. Psychotherapy for PTSD (reviewed in Keane, 1998) may effectively reduce some of the cognitive symptoms that CSA survivors display, such as the dissociative tendencies described by Zurbriggen and Freyd (chap. 6, this volume). Evaluations of interventions incorporating CSA material include that described by Chin and colleagues (chap. 11, this volume) and an evaluation in progress by Alex Carballo-Diéguez and colleagues at Columbia University.

One way to shed light on this issue would be to test for CSA moderation of intervention effects, that is, test for treatment condition by CSA interactions in intervention studies. A significant interaction would indicate that CSA survivors responded with less (or more) behavior change to the intervention. The former result would suggest the need for enhanced interventions for sexually abused individuals, possibly including material related to the abuse. We are aware of only one study that attempted anything of this sort (Greenberg, 2001). This study reported that an HIV/STD risk-reduction intervention for women worked as well for CSA survivors as for nonabused participants, in some cases even better, in terms of condom-use skills and communication skills.

The large intervention trial that Spiegel and colleagues (chap. 12, this volume) are beginning will provide useful information regarding this issue. Their study will compare an intervention that focuses on past sexual abuse with one that addresses only present-day issues. This is exactly the type of study that is needed to assess whether CSA survivors require interventions that address the abuse. Similar studies should evaluate interventions targeting different outcomes or different populations. For example, it would also be useful to test these intervention approaches for male survivors; focusing on gay men who are particularly at risk for HIV/STD would be important.

Interventions to prevent negative sexual health outcomes in sexually compulsive individuals may be particularly challenging. Randomized controlled trials of interventions providing cognitive–behavioral therapy for these individuals have not been reported but should be conducted. Also potentially useful are selective serotonin uptake inhibitors for perpetrators (see Suarez et al., 2002).

CONCLUSION

The idea for this volume was prompted by some lively discussions between the editors and a number of trauma researchers, therapists, and HIV prevention interventionists who came together at the CDC to discuss the link between CSA and HIV. We learned a great deal from each other, including that the issue is not limited to HIV and broadly affects a variety of negative sexual health outcomes. The discussions also prompted ideas for research, much of which is now under way, some of it collaborative between trauma researchers and HIV researchers. The synergy produced by the interaction among researchers who otherwise have little contact with each other was exciting and is necessary for progress in understanding and treating the complex issues addressed in this book. We need more venues in which basic and applied scientists can interact. These interactions should include experts on trauma processes and treatment, child development, and prevention and treatment of the myriad consequences of CSA.

REFERENCES

Alexander, P. (1992). Application of attachment theory to the study of sexual abuse. *Journal of Consulting and Clinical Psychology, 60*, 185–195.

Baron, R. M., & Kenny, D. A. (1986). The moderator–mediator variable distinction in social psychological research: Conceptual, strategic, and statistical considerations. *Journal of Personality and Social Psychology, 51*, 1173–1182.

Basile, K. C. & Saltzman, L. E. (2002). *Uniform definitions and recommended data elements for sexual violence*: Version 1.0. Atlanta, GA: National Center for Injury Prevention and Control, Centers for Disease Control and Prevention.

Browning, C. R., & Laumann, E. O. (1997). Sexual contact between children and adults: A life course perspective. *American Sociology Review, 62*, 540–560.

Burkett, L. P. (1991). Parenting behaviors of women who were sexually abused as children in their families of origin. *Family Process, 30*, 421–434.

Carballo-Diéguez, A., & Dolezal, C. (1995). Association between history of childhood sexual abuse and adult HIV-risk sexual behavior in Puerto Rican men who have sex with men. *Child Abuse and Neglect, 19*, 595–605.

Coid, J., Petruckevitch, A., Feder, G., Chung, W., Richardson, J., & Moorey, S. (2001). Relation between childhood sexual and physical abuse and risk of revictimisation in women: A cross-sectional survey. *The Lancet, 358,* 450–454.

Curtis, J. M. (1986). Factors in sexual abuse of children. *Psychological Reports, 58,* 591–597.

Felitti, V. J., Anda, R. F., Nordenberg, D., Williamson, D. F., Spitz, A. M., Edwards, V., et al. (1998). Relationship of childhood abuse and household dysfunction to many of the leading causes of death in adults: The Adverse Childhood Experiences (ACE) study. *American Journal of Preventive Medicine, 14,* 245–258.

Fergusson, D. M., Horwood, L. J., & Lynskey, M. T. (1997). Childhood sexual abuse, adolescent sexual behaviors and sexual revictimization. *Child Abuse and Neglect, 21,* 789–803.

Finkelhor, D., & Baron, L. (1986). Risk factors for child sexual abuse. *Journal of Interpersonal Violence, 1,* 43–71.

Freyd, J. J. (1996). *Betrayal trauma: The logic of forgetting childhood abuse.* Cambridge, MA: Harvard University Press.

Greenberg, J. B. (2001). Childhood sexual abuse and sexually transmitted diseases in adults: A review of and implications for STD/HIV programmes. *International Journal of STD and AIDS, 12,* 777–783.

Haugaard, J. J., & Samwel, C. (1992). Legal and therapeutic interventions with incestuous families. *Medical Law, 11,* 469–484.

Kafka, M. P. (1997). A monoamine hypothesis for the pathophysiology of paraphilic disorders. *Archives of Sexual Behavior, 26,* 343–358.

Kafka, M. P., & Hennen, J. (2000). Psychostimulant augmentation during treatment with selective serotonin reuptake inhibitors in men with paraphilias and paraphilia-related disorders: A case series. *Journal of Clinical Psychiatry, 61,* 664–670.

Keane, T. M. (1998). Psychological and behavioral treatments of post-traumatic stress disorder. In P. E. Nathan & J. M. Gorman (Eds.), *A guide to treatments that work* (pp. 398–407). New York: Oxford University Press.

Koriat, A., Goldsmith, M., & Pansky, A. (2000). Toward a psychology of memory accuracy. *Annual Review of Psychology, 51,* 481–537.

Lesniak, L. P. (1993). Penetrating the conspiracy of silence: Identifying the family at risk for incest. *Family and Community Health, 16,* 66–76.

Merrill, L. L., Thomsen, C. J., Sinclair, B. B., Gold, S. R., & Milner, J. S. (2001). Predicting the impact of child sexual abuse on women: The role of abuse severity, parental support, and coping strategies. *Journal of Consulting and Clinical Psychology, 69,* 992–1006.

Miller, M. (1999). A model to explain the relationship between sexual abuse and HIV risk among women. *AIDS Care, 11,* 3–20.

Paul, J. P., Catania, J., Pollack, L., & Stall, R. (2001). Understanding childhood sexual abuse as a predictor of sexual risk-taking among men who have sex with men: The Urban Men's Health Study. *Child Abuse and Neglect, 25,* 557–584.

Peterson, J. L., & DiClemente, R. J. (Eds.). (2000). *Handbook of HIV prevention.* New York: Plenum/Kluwer Academic.

Pintello, D., & Zuravin, S. (2001). Intrafamilial child sexual abuse: Predictors of postdisclosure maternal belief and protective action. *Child Maltreatment: Journal of the American Professional Society on the Abuse of Children, 6,* 344–352.

Plummer, C. A. (2001). Prevention of child sexual abuse: A survey of 87 programs. *Violence and Victims, 16,* 575–588.

Rind, B., Tromovitch, P., & Bauserman, R. (1998). A meta-analytic examination of assumed properties of child sexual abuse using college samples. *Psychological Bulletin, 124,* 22–53.

Rispens, J., Aleman, A., & Goudena, P. P. (1997). Prevention of child sexual abuse victimization: A meta-analysis of school programs. *Child Abuse and Neglect, 21,* 975–987.

Suarez, T., O'Leary, A., Morgenstern, J., Hollander, E., & Allen, A. (2002). Selective serotonin reuptake inhibitors for the treatment of sexually compulsive behavior. In A. O'Leary (Ed.), *Beyond condoms: Alternative strategies for HIV prevention* (pp. 201–223). New York: Kluwer Academic/Plenum.

Timms, R. J., & Connors, P. (1992). Adult promiscuity following childhood sexual abuse: An introduction. *Psychotherapy Patient, 8,* 19–27.

Valleroy, L. A., Mackellar, D. A., Karon, J. M., Rosen, D. H., McFarland, W., Shehan, D. A., et al. (2000). HIV prevalence and associated risks in young men who have sex with men. *Journal of the American Medical Association, 284,* 198–204.

Whitmire, L. E., Harlow, L. L., Quina, K., Morokoff, P. J. (199). *Childhood trauma and HIV: Women at risk.* New York: Brunner-Routledge.

Widom, C. S., & Kuhns, J. B. (1996). Childhood victimization and subsequent risk for promiscuity, prostitution, and teenage pregnancy. *American Journal of Public Health, 86,* 1607–1612.

Zuravin, S. J., & Fontanella, C. (1999). Parenting behaviors and perceived parenting competence of child sexual abuse survivors. *Child Abuse and Neglect, 23,* 623–632.

AUTHOR INDEX

Numbers in italics refer to listings in the references.

Edgar, M., 32, 36, *46*
Edwards, V., *130, 308*
Ehlers, A., 36, *47*
Ehlert, U., 37, 38, *42, 43*
Ehrhardt, A. A., 118, 121, *130*
Einbinder, R. G., 252, *267*
Einsporn, R. L., 253, *267*
Eisen, M., 169, *177*
El-Bassel, N., 80, 81, 88, 121, 125–127, *130, 133*
Eldridge, G. D., *133*
Elhai, J. D., 99, 104, *111, 112*
Ellen, J. M., 183, *197*
Elliot, D. M., 259, *266*
Elliott, D., 39, *41*
Elliott, D. M., 71, 88, 223, 229, *230*
Ellis, A. L., 273, *292*
Ellis, E. M., 159, *177*
Emerick, C. D., 226, *230*
Emery, R. E., 104, *111*
Emshoff, J., *229*
Enquist, G., 169, *179*
Epstein, J. N., 182, 187, *197*
Esterling, B. A., 211, *214*
Everaerd, W., 204, *216*
Evers, K. E., 125, *130*
Exner, T. M., 118, *130*

Facchin, P., 7, *9*
Faden, R., 72, *89*
Fahey, J. L., 202, *214*
Fairbairn, W. R. D., 162, *177*
Fallot, R. D., 82, 84, 89, 125, *130*, 182, *197*
Fanshel, D., 210, *215*
Fanslow, J. L., 8, *10*
Feder, G., 9, *307*
Fehr, B., 224, *229*
Feigenbaum, J. D., 109, *112*
Feinauer, L. L., 29, *42*
Feingold, L., 92, *200*
Feinman, G., 72, *89*
Feiring, C., 95, 96, 100, 103, *111*
Feldman, H. A., 16, *42*
Feldman-Summers, S., 32, 36, *46*, 140, *155*
Felitti, V. J., 76, 89, *110*, 121, 124, *130*, 303, *308*
Fenaughty, A. M., 183, *197*
Feng, W. Y., *215*
Ferguson, D., *40*
Fergusson, D. M., 22, 33, 35, 38, *42*, 71, 76, 77, 88, 89, 135, *155*, 168, *177*, 182, *197*, 304, *308*

Feske, U., 143, *155*
Festinger, L. A., 172, *177*
Field, N. P., 257, 260, *266*
Fiengold, L., *232*
Figueredo, A. J., 171, *180*
Fincham, F. D., 36, *42*
Fine, D., 82, *88*
Finestone, H. M., 37, *42*
Finkelhor, D., 4, 9, 20, 24, 26, 27, 33, *42*, *44*, 53, 63, 66, 67, 71, 89, 95, 99, 102, 103, *110–112*, 118, 120, 124, *130*, 135, *155*, 163–166, *177, 178*, 219, *231*, 234, 248, 251, *265*
Fischer, B. S., 270, *292*
Fischer, G. J., 273, *292*
Fishbein, M., 235, *248, 249*
Fisher, D. G., 183, *197*
Fisher, P. M., 30, *42*
Fite, R., 164, *177*
Fivush, R., 101, *111*
Flaherty, B. P., 118, *129*
Fleming, J. E., *113*
Fleming, P. L., 71, *90*
Fletcher, M. A., 211, *214*
Flynn, C., *92*
Foa, E. B., 122, *129*, 143, *155*, 161, 169, 171, *176, 177*, 179, 223, *231, 232*, 253, *266*
Foleno, A., 125, *130*
Follette, V. M., 28, 45, 212, *214*, 251, 253, *265, 267*
Foltz, J., 220, *230*
Fong, G. T., 209, *215*
Fonow, M. M., 273, *292*
Fontanella, C., 303, *309*
Fontanilla, I., 211, *214*
Ford, H. H., 123, *129*
Forehand, R., 72, *89*
Forsythe, A. B., *66*
Fourcroy, J., *40*
Foy, D. W., 36, *45*
Francis, M., 207, *215*
Francis, M. E., 207, 208, *216*
Frank, E., 16, *42*
Frazier, P., 274, *292*
Freeman, R. C., 84, *91*
Freshman, M. S., 171, *176*
Freud, S., 137, *155*, 160, *177*
Freyd, J. J., 99, *111*, 120, 124, *130, 134*, 138–141, 143, 144, 149, 150, *155*, 162, 165, 170, *177*, 302, *308*
Friedman, S. R., *90*

Long, P. J., 49, 51, 58, 68, 173, *179*
Longshore, D., 220, *231*, 237, *249*
Lonsway, K. A., 275, *294*
Lopez, P. A., 183, *197*
Losina, E., *10, 112*
Loughlin, M. J., 109, *113*
Lourie, K. J., 123, *129*
Low, G., 135, *156*
Low, L., 253, *267*
Low, N., 127, *129*
Lucenko, B. A., 99, 104, *111, 112*
Lueken, M., 67, *291*
Luke, W., *112*
Lundberg-Love, P., 237, *249*
Lynch, D. A., 72, *90*
Lynn, S. J., 52, 68, 159, 164, 166, 169, 170, *177–180*, 276, 279, 280, 282, 285, *292*
Lynskey, M. T., 22, 33, *42*, 76, 88, 135, *155*, 168, *177*, 182, *197*, 304, *308*
Lyon, M. E., 72, 73, *90*

Mackellar, D. A., *309*
MacLeod, A., 135, *156*
MacLeod, C. M., 143, *156*
Macleod, S., 75, *92*
MacMillan, H. L., 104, *113*
Maddever, H. M., 25, 33, *44*
Madhok, R., 183, *198*
Mahler, K. A., 127, *133*, 220, *232*
Mahoney, M. J., 202, 209, *215*
Maibach, E. W., 75, *91*, 123, *134*, 135, *157*, 181, *199*, 220, *232*
Maker, A. H., 50, 64, 68, 161, 166, 167, *178*
Maker, E., 252, *267*
Malamuth, N. M., 275, *294*
Maltz, W., 123, *131*
Mandoki, C. A., 161, *179*
Mangweth, B., 106, *112*
Manlowe E., 127, *130*
Mannarino, A. P., 96, *114*
March, J. S., *156*
Marchbanks, P. A., 76, *89*
Mardh, P. A., 75, *91*
Margulies, S., 211, *214*
Marin, B. V., 123, 124, 128, *129, 130, 131*
Marioni, N. L., 64, *67*, 288, *291, 292*
Marks, G., 104, *111*
Marquart, J. W., 84, *90*, 127, *132*
Marshall, J. C., 161, *179*
Martin, J., 147, *157*
Martin, J. L., 21, 23, *44*, 120, *133*, 182, *198*

Martin, L., 104, *114*
Martinez, G., *214*
Martinez, L. J., *197*
Martinez-Ramirez, M., 121, *130*
Martino, S., *231*
Martins, P., 127, *132*
Martorello, S. R., 143, *155*
Marx, B. P., 64, 68, 276, 278, 283–285, 289, *294*
Massoth, D., *46*
Masters, B., *294*
Masterson, C., 253, *267*
Masterson, J. F., 162, *179*
Matorin, A. I., 159, 164, 169, *179, 180, 292*
Maude-Griffin, P. M., 226, *231*
Mayall, A., 51, 57, 58, 61, 62, 64, 68
Mayer, K., 92, *131, 200, 232*
Mayer, K. H., *10, 91, 112*
Mayne, T. J., 208, *216*
Mazurek, C. J., *294*
McAuslan, P., 183, *196*
McCabe, M. P., 93, *112*
McCallum, A., 183, *198*
McCann, I., 252, 253, *267*
McCann, I. L., 163, 165, *179*
McCanne, T. R., 167, *180*
McCarthy, P., 143, *155*
McCauley, J., 182, *198*
McClanahan, S. F., 82, *90*
McClelland, G. M., *90*
McCluskey-Fawcett, K., 137, *156*
McDonnell, K. A., 72, *89*
McEwan, R. T., 183, *198*
McFarland, W., *309*
McGlashan, T. H., *231*
McGuigan, S., 38, *42*
McHorney, C., 234, *249*
McKelvie, M., 165, *179*
McKenna, F. P., 143, *156*
McKevitt, C., 127, *129*
McKinlay, J. B., 16, *42*
McKirnan, D., *229*
McLeer, S. V., 121, *129*
McMahon, P. M., 8, *10*, 71, *90*, 270, *291*
McNally, R. J., 143, *156*
McNamara, J., 166, *178*
McRae, B., 220, *230*
McVey, D., 128, *133*
Meadows, E. A., 169, *179*, 253, *266*
Meana, M., 39, *44*
Medrano, M. A., 83–86, *90*
Meichenbaum, D., 209, *215*

SUBJECT INDEX

and present-focused psychotherapy, 257
and rape, 168, 284
and revictimization, 54, 61, 161
and risk behavior, 108, 183–184, 186
sample in studies of, 184–185
studies of, 184–196
and writing exercises, 206
American Academy of Pediatrics, 147
American Indians, 65
Amnesia, 138–140
Anal intercourse, 59, 234
Anal penetration, 100
Anger, 103
Anticipated partner negative response, 125
Antidepressants, 306
Antigay activities, 106
Antisocial personality disorder, 103
Anxiety
    in adult survivors of CSA, 37, 103, 104
    and compulsive sexual repetition, 163
    in CPP patients, 38
    with emotional proximity, 225
    and revictimization, 59
Arousal, 21, 35, 37, 100, 169
ASA. *See* Adult sexual assault
Asian women, 236
Assault
    adult sexual. *See* Adult sexual assault
    physical, 54, 55
    programs for reducing risk of, 279–286
Assertiveness
    and condom use, 125, 126
    female lack of, 257, 260
    male lack of, 103
    and revictimization, 260
    and sexual boundaries, 226–227
    training in, 64, 228–229
    and Women's Health Project, 244–246
Assessment, 278, 304–305
Attachment
    and betrayal trauma, 138, 139
    and cheater detectors, 149
    and incest victims, 162
    issues of, 18
Attachment model, 17
Attention
    divided, 149–150
    and "safe sex" education, 227
    selective, 142–144
Attention-based disorders, 146–147
Attitudes
    about condom use, 128

about sexual assault, 278
change of, 281
Attitudes Toward Women Scale, 124, 287
Attraction/Interest in Sexuality subscale, 164–165
Attraction to risk, 153
Attractiveness, personal, 164–165
Audiotapes, 283–284
Austria, 106
Avoidance, 102, 121–122, 220, 257, 305
Avoidance and Fear of Sexual and Physical Intimacy subscale, 164
Avoidant personality, 162
Awareness
    about sexual assault, 280
    of abuse, 195. *See also* Unawareness of abuse
    of negative assumptions, 222

Babysitters, 98
Bartering of sex, 81–84, 87, 108
Behavioral change, 245–246
Behaviorally phrased questions, 52
Behavioral reenactment, 161
Behavioral responses, 118
"Being present," 150
Bereavement, 212
Betrayal
    as dysfunctional learning, 165
    trauma of, 99
    of trust, 118, 120, 305
Betrayal Trauma Inventory (BTI), 140, 165
Betrayal trauma theory, 137–139
    clinical implications of, 145–147
    and memory impairment, 139–142
    studies of, 138–142
"Beyond the Pleasure Principle" (Sigmund Freud), 160
Binge–purge activities, 223
Birth control, 123
Bisexual men
    CSA prevalence among, 95
    ethnic differences among, 39
    revictimization of, 105
    risk behavior among, 107
Blacks. *See* African Americans
Blame, 100. *See also* Self-blame
"Blaming the victim," 161, 166, 236
Body movement, 206–207
Borderline personality disorder, 36–37, 103, 162
Boundaries, sexual, 18, 226–227, 244, 247

Boys
  characteristics of abused, 98
  CSA effects on, 94
  CSA prevalence among, 4, 71, 95
  sexual abuse of. *See* Sexual abuse of boys
Brief Symptom Inventory, 35
BTI. *See* Betrayal Trauma Inventory
Bulimia, 103

Caregiver abuse. *See also* Family abuse
  and betrayal trauma, 138–141
  and cheater detectors, 149
  clinical implications of, 145–147
  and memory impairment, 165
Caribbeans (people), 120
Causal words, 207
Centers for Disease Control and Prevention
    (CDC), 8, 69, 75, 301, 307
Central route processing, 281, 282, 287, 290
Changing a problem, 241
Cheater detectors, 149
Child care, 239
Childhood, 8
Children
  ADHD in, 147
  pain of, 37
  rape of, 56
Child sexual abuse (CSA), 3–8, 299–307
  adult sequelae of, 5–6, 120–125
  and adult sexual assault, 49–50, 52–53
  and adult sexual functioning, 13
  assessing mediators/intermediate out-
    comes, 304–305
  attachment model of, 17
  and commercial sex workers, 76, 79–84
  common elements of, 14
  consequences of, 234–235
  defining, 14–15, 50, 52, 75, 94–95, 109,
    301–302
  definitions of, 8
  demographics of, 70–71
  determining independent effects of,
    303–304
  developmental model of, 17
  duration of, 99, 121, 140, 141
  evaluating interventions for, 305–307
  evolutionary model of, 17–18
  gender differences in, 19
  and HIV infection, 70, 72–75, 87
  prevalence of, 4–5
  and substance abuse, 182–183
  trauma model of, 16–17

Chronic abdominal pain, 37
Chronic abuse, 99, 106, 234
Chronic pain, 37–38
Chronic pelvic pain (CPP), 37
Coaching, 227
Coercion, 4
  and attachment, 17
  as contextual factor in CSA, 99
  in CSA definitions, 14, 95
  perceptions of, 101
  and revictimization, 226–227
  and risk behavior, 107
Coercive behavior, 106
Cognitions, 117–128
  and attitudinal sequelae in adult survi-
    vors, 120–125
  caveats for model of, 126–128
  and childhood trauma events, 118, 120
  and risk behaviors, 125–126
  Women's Health Project affecting, 243–
    244
Cognitive–behavioral interventions, 18, 223,
    226
Cognitive distortions, 221–222
Cognitive environments, 144–145
Cognitive mechanisms, 147–154
  cheater detectors, 149
  dissociation/divided attention, 149–150
  reality-detecting mechanisms, 148–149
  self-esteem, 147–148
Cognitive operations, 161
Cognitive restructuring, 239
Cognitive therapy, 221–222
Cohabitation, 33
Collectivistic cultures, 236
Combined abuse (sexual and physical), 167–
    168
Commercial sex workers (CSWs)
  and CSA, 76, 79–84, 87, 220
  HIV risk of, 75
  self-esteem of, 148
  and sexual self-image, 125
Communication
  about sex, 161
  in families, 109
  interventions to promote, 306
  with partners, 245–246
  and revictimization, 174
  and sexual functioning, 36
  skills of, 87
  with treatment providers, 240, 246
Communication assertiveness, 126

value of, 302
in Women's Health Project, 239, 240, 242
Disloyalty, 17
Dissatisfaction with life, 121
Dissociation
  and betrayal trauma theory, 137–147
  clinical implications of, 145–147
  as cognitive defense, 168–170
  as cognitive environment, 144–145
  cognitive mechanisms involved in, 136
  as coping measure, 121, 122, 305
  as CSA outcome, 103, 220
  and damaged cognitive mechanisms, 149–150
  as defense mechanism, 153
  and group psychotherapy, 253, 257, 258, 260, 264, 306
  and HIV risk, 122
  and PTSD, 142
  and selective attention, 142–144
  and sexual functioning, 36
  social-narrative model of, 170–176
  and trauma, 137
Dissociative Experiences Scale (DES), 143, 144, 150, 169
Distal outcomes, 107–108
Distorting reality, 148
Distraction, strategic, 224
Distress, 96
  reduction of, 253
  tolerance for, 224
Divided attention, 143, 144, 149–150
Dolls, sexualized play with, 21
Domestic violence, 60
Dominant roles, 106, 124
Dose–response relationship, 303
Drug use
  and adult sexual assault, 49, 270
  and cognitions/attitudes, 125
  as coping measure, 121, 122
  and CSA, 84–86, 220, 234
  and delinquent lifestyles, 168
  and dissociative attachments, 225
  and HIV infection, 71, 75, 108
  intervention in, 226, 290, 306
  and present-focused psychotherapy, 257
  and rape, 168, 284
  recovery from, 120
  and revictimization, 54, 61
DSM–IV. See Diagnostic and Statistical Manual of Mental Disorders

Duration of abuse
  for boys, 99
  and memory impairment, 140, 141
  and well-being, 121
Dysfunctional learning, 163–168
  betrayal as, 165
  powerlessness, 165–166
  stigmatization as, 166–168
  traumatic sexualization as, 163–168

Early drinking syndrome, 192–193
Early onset of sexual activity, 33, 98, 190–194, 234, 270
Eating, 122
Eating disorders, 36
Education
  about abuse, 18, 175
  about HIV/AIDS, 228–229
  level of, 33, 123
Elaboration likelihood model (ELM), 281–282, 290
Emotional abuse, 34
Emotional bonding, 236
Emotional effects, 244–245
Emotional expression, 101
Emotional regulation, 102
Emotional Stroop tasks, 142–143
Emotion-focused coping, 122
Empowerment, 245
Encopresis, 20
Endocrinological factors, 38
Engagement (in treatment), 243, 246
Engagement model, 237
Enuresis, 20
Environment
  cognitive, 144–145
  family. See Family characteristics/environment
Epstein-Barr virus, 211
Erectile dysfunction, 21
Eroticization of risk, 153
Ethnic differences, 4, 39, 235
Evolutionary theory, 17–18
Exhibitionism, 99–100
Exotic dancers, 81
Exposure, 17, 253
Expression, 206
Extrafamilial child sexual abuse, 59, 60

Facilitators, 242, 243
Family abuse, 118, 120
  and alcohol, 185–186

community studies of, 59
and gender role beliefs, 124
Family characteristics/environment, 33
and alcohol, 186, 190, 194, 195, 303
and attachment model, 17
as factor in CSA, 19, 33
and HIV risk behavior, 96
and sexual dysfunction, 106
and stigmatization, 168
and trauma model, 16
Family honor, 109
Family instability, 33, 168
Family response, 100, 109
Fantasies, 34
Fatalism, 121
Fathers, rejection by, 190, 191
Fear
and attachment, 17
and betrayal, 138
as childhood symptom of CSA, 103
effect of, 118
of intimacy, 106, 225
of men, 125
and pregnancy, 38
and sexual function, 20, 37, 38
Stroop studies of, 143
Fearfulness, 102
Feedback, 222, 228
Female abusers, 98, 99, 101
Financial dependence, 127, 236
First sexual contact, 33, 34, 84, 101, 102, 186,
190, 192
Focused cognitive–behavioral interventions,
226
Fondling, 99
Force. *See* Coercion
Freedom, 245
Frequency
of abuse, 99, 107
of intercourse, 34
Freud, Sigmund, 160–161
Friendships (with other men), 106

Gastrointestinal problems, 37
Gay men, 302, 307
adolescent sexual behavior of, 97–98
age of abuse among, 99, 101–102
cognitive/attitudinal predictors in, 117
CSA prevalence among, 4–5, 95
ethnicity of, 39
health of, 202
homophobic behavior of, 106–107

interventions for, 307
revictimization of, 105–106
risky sexual behavior among, 104–108
Gender differences, 302
with CSA, 98–99, 103, 234
in CSA perspectives, 19, 34, 93–94
in lifetime rates of psychopathology, 104
in number of sexual partners, 108
in sexual assertiveness, 126
in socialization, 101
with writing exercises, 205
Gender identity, 106–107
Gender-related behavior, 96
Gender role confusion, 97
Gender roles
beliefs about, 123–124, 236
traditional, 118
Genitalia words, 35–36
Girls, 4, 71
Global Severity Index, 35
Goals, self-selection of, 238
Grade point average, 207
Group facilitators, 242, 243
Group psychotherapy, 251–265
clinical examples of, 258–259
current research on, 264
measures of, 259–260
pilot study of, 254–260
study statistics on, 261–264
trauma-focused vs. present-focused,
252–254
Groups, 239
Guilt, 103, 162, 164, 221

Habituation, 223
Health
physical. *See* Physical health
sexual, 15, 238
Health belief model, 235, 281, 282, 285
Health consciousness, 206
Helplessness, 221, 222, 305
Hepatitis B vaccinations, 211
Heterosexual men, 106, 108, 117, 120, 300
Heterosexual sex, 71, 120
High school students, 85, 108
Hispanic women, 65, 71
HIV Epidemiologic Research Study, 75
HIV infection, 69–88
and CSA consequences, 234–235
and CSA demographics, 70–71
CSA prevalence among women with,
72–75

demographics of, 71–72
from heterosexual men, 300
injection drug use among women with, 85
knowledge about, 244
literature about, 72–85
prevention of. *See* Prevention efforts in U.S., 69
writing exercises affecting, 211
HIV intervention programs, 219–229
and abuse-focused treatment, 225–228
considerations for, 234
delivery of, 87–88
early models of, 235–237
for men, 109–110
and relationship issues, 224–225
response to, 69–70
with self-esteem improvement, 221–222
and tension reduction, 222–224
therapist training for, 228–229
Women's Health Project. *See* Women's Health Project
HIV risk groups, 75–84
Homelessness, 65, 120, 127
Homophobic attitudes, 106–107
Homosexual experiences, 34
Hopefulness, 120
Hopelessness, 121, 220
Hostility, 36, 59
"Hyperfeminine" women, 165
Hypersexuality, 107

Identity
gender, 106–107
sexual, 164
stigmatized, 211–212
IDU. *See* Injection drug use
"If-Then" rules, 136, 151–153
IIP. *See* Inventory of Interpersonal Problems
Immune system, 211
"Improving the moment," 224
Impulsivity, 37
Incentives, 239
Incestuous abuse, 19
and amnesia, 140
community studies of, 59–60
memories of, 165
self-descriptions by survivors of, 162
Individualized counseling, 227–228
Information
about HIV infection, 244
about sexual assault, 278

Information processing, 169–170, 281, 282
Inhibitions, 201–202, 260
Injection drug use, 71, 75, 84–86, 108, 226, 234
Insight words, 207
Instability, family, 33, 168
Institute for Scientific Information, 72
Integration, 252
Interactive drama programs, 286
Intercourse, 35
Internal working models, 17
International Consensus Committee, 15
Interpersonal relationships
and anticipated partner response, 125
and borderline personality disorder, 37
communication in, 246
and CSA, 251
dysfunctional learning in, 163
importance of close, 146
problems with, 103, 259, 260, 264
unhealthy, 162
Interpersonal sensitivity, 59, 104
Interpersonal victimization phenomena, 62
Interventions
in child sexual abuse, 305–307
cognitive, 222
cultural tailoring of, 300
dissociation, 150
and early family experiences, 195
evaluating, 305–307
group psychotherapy, 255–259
HIV. *See* HIV intervention programs
importance of, 128
multimodal, 18
skills-building, 87
social coherence, 175
Women's Health Project. *See* Women's Health Project
Intimacy, 106, 124, 225, 245, 247
Introjection, 162
Inventory of Interpersonal Problems (IIP), 259, 261–263
Isolation, 141–142, 222, 225, 239, 247
Israel, 212

"Keeping females in a healthy place" (KFNHP), 240
Knowledge (about HIV), 244
Knowledge base, gaps in, 300–301
Knowledge isolation, 141–142

Labor, preterm, 38

Language, 206–208, 238, 240, 242, 305
Latinas/Latinos
    family response to CSA among, 100
    financial concerns among, 236
    gay/bisexual, 39, 102
    self-efficacy of, 123
    sexual assertiveness of, 126
    in Women's Health Project, 238
Legal barriers, 18
Legal trouble, 104
Lesbian women, 34
Liberation, 245, 247
Limit-setting, 227
Linguistic coherence, 210
Linguistic Inquiry and Word Count (LIWC), 207–208
Listwise deletion model, 191–192
Living conditions, 127
Localized pelvic pain, 38
Loneliness, 234
Long-term mood effects (of writing), 204
Los Angeles, 60
Lovemaking, 35
Low-income housed women, 65
Lying, 148

Maintenance step (in change process), 241
Male clinicians, 109
Male domination, 124
Male soldiers, 104
Manipulative sexual contact, 14
Manuals, treatment, 271, 283
Marginal living conditions, 127
Marital conflict, 303
"Masochistic tendency," 173
Massachusetts, 108
Masturbation, 21, 34, 163
Meals, 239
Meaning in life, 120, 121
Measures
    in alcohol study, 185–186
    in assault prevention program comparison, 278
    of CSA, 8, 185
    in group psychotherapy study, 259–260
Mediation, 118n
Mediators, effects of, 300–301
Medical disorders, 37
Memories
    describing abuse, 222
    integration of, 252, 253
    repression of, 302

    veracity of abuse, 254
Memory impairment. See also Dissociation
    and betrayal trauma theory, 139–142, 165
    clinical implications of, 145–147
    and group psychotherapy, 258
Men
    bisexual. See Bisexual men
    childhood physical abuse of, 55
    CSA prevalence among, 4, 71, 95
    ethnicity of, 39
    gay. See Gay men
    heterosexual, 106, 108
    interventions for, 306–307
    knowledge about, 300
    sexual assault risk-reduction programs with, 286–288
    sexual problems of, 16
    sexual risk to, 35
    who have sex with men. See Men who have sex with men
Mental illness, 20
Men who have sex with men (MSM), 4, 95, 97, 106
Methadone clinics, 121, 126
Methadone maintenance, 121
Methodological rigor, 5, 7
MI. See Multiple imputation
Middle-class, 121
Minnesota, 108
Minorities. See also African Americans; Latinas/Latinos
    with AIDS, 71
    CSA prevalence among, 95
    female, 65, 71, 120, 123, 235, 242
    and HIV intervention approaches, 235
    male, 95
    rape/stalking reported by, 65
    self-efficacy of, 123
    self-esteem in, 120
    in Women's Health Project, 242
Mixed-gender sexual assault risk-reduction programs, 286–288
Mixed race, 65
Model(s)
    computational, 136
    of CSA/adult drinking/risk behavior, 188, 189
    of CSA–HIV risk behavior for males, 96–97
    of path from CSA to adult HIV risk, 118, 119

perceptions of, 52
reporting of, 65
and response latency measure, 283–285
and revictimization, 5, 50
risk for date, 149
Rape Empathy Scale, 287
Rape Myth Acceptance Scale, 287
Rape myths, 279, 280, 286, 287
Rape narratives, 171
Rape prevention programs, 270. *See also*
Sexual assault risk-reduction programs
Rape-supportive environment, 56
"Reality checks," 146
Reality-detecting mechanisms, 148–149
Reasoned action theory, 235
Recall, errors in, 96
Reenactment, behavioral, 161
Referrals, community, 240
Regulation, affect, 222–224
Rejection by fathers, 190, 191
Relapse-prevention approach, 283
Relapse step (in change process), 241
Relationship(s). *See also* Interpersonal relationships
ability to form/maintain sexual, 36–37
concurrent sexual, 34
durability of, 14
and HIV-prevention programs, 224–225
with important others, 146
internal working models of, 17
parent–child, 33, 103
with partners, 245–246
to perpetrator, 60, 99
and rape, 52
satisfaction with, 33, 35
therapist–client, 145
victim–caretaker, 139, 140, 145
Relaxation techniques, 228–229, 241
Religion, context of, 240
Religious codes
about drinking, 190, 191, 193
about sexual functioning, 18
Repetition, 160–163
Repetition compulsion, 160
Repetitive exposure, 223
Repression, 153
Repressive copers, 208
Rescue fantasies, 243
Respect, 152
Response, family, 100, 109

Response latency measure, 283–285
Responsibility (of perpetrator), 109, 291
Responsiveness, sexual, 35
Revictimization, 33, 49–66, 220, 305
and cognitions/attitudes, 125
college studies of, 56–59
community studies of, 59–61
future research on, 63–66
and group psychotherapy, 260, 264
knowledge about, 300
limitations in literature on, 61–63
of men, 105–106
probability studies of, 53–56
and rape, 5
risk-reduction programs for. *See* Sexual
assault risk-reduction programs
selection criteria for literature on, 52–53
and social narrative, 159–160
vulnerability to, 251
Rights-based approach, 126
Risk behaviors
and age of abused boys, 102
alcohol-related, 186, 188–194
and cognitions/attitudes, 125–126
and coping strategies, 122
and damaged cognitive mechanisms,
147–153
in gay men, 104–108
HIV, 74, 75
injection drug use as, 85
and self-esteem, 120
of sexually abused men, 107–108
and substance use, 183–184
Risk recognition, 49, 169, 170, 236, 284, 285
Risk(s), 8
attraction to, 153
for men, 35
Role expectations, 18
Role of Sex in Relationships subscale, 164
Role-playing, 227
Roles, sexual, 106
Running away, 81

SAAS (Sexual Assault Awareness Survey),
279
"Safe sex" education, 227
Safety
control of personal, 118
willingness to risk, 236
Same-sex attractions, 97
Same-sex behavior, 4, 95, 98, 107

betrayal. *See* Betrayal trauma
    in boys, 94, 99, 105
    confronting, 204
    and dissociation, 137, 144
    impacts of childhood, 118, 120
    and revictimization, 64
    secondary, 243
    and writing exercises, 203, 212–213
Trauma-focused group psychotherapy, 252–
        253, 255–256, 258, 260–264
Trauma model, 16–18
Trauma narratives, 171
Trauma Symptom Checklist–40 (TSC-40),
        259, 261, 262, 264
Traumatic sexualization, 163–165
Traumatic Sexualization Survey (TSS), 164–
        165
Treatment
    client engagement in, 58, 243, 246
    early/ongoing, 109
    importance of, 271, 278
    normalization as, 221–222
    revictimization affected by, 58
Treatment manuals, 271, 283
Treatment providers, 246
Trust, 109
    betrayal of, 118, 120, 305
    development of, 236
    therapist's role in, 146
    and Women's Health Project, 245, 247
Trustworthiness, 149
TSC-40. *See* Trauma Symptom Checklist–
        40
TSS. *See* Traumatic Sexualization Survey
12-step programs, 226
Two-dimensional trauma model, 138, 139

Unawareness of abuse, 136, 139
Unhappiness, 36
Unitization, 169
University of Miami, 205
Unprotected sex, 33, 107, 220
Unresolved conflict, 162
Unrestricted sexual behavior, 34
U.S. Army, 104
U.S. Congress, 94
U.S. Navy, 168

Vaginal discharge, 37
Vaginal intercourse, 59
Vaginal penetration, 100
Veracity of abuse memories, 254

Verbal abuse, 152
Victim–caretaker relationship, 139, 140, 145
Victimization, prior, 280, 283–285
Victim-perpetrator cycle, 19, 20
Videos, 280–284, 286
Violence
    domestic, 60
    from partners, 125, 127, 227
    and power, 128
Violent abuse, 96
Visible stigmatized identity, 211–212
Vulnerability
    of college women, 56
    and CSA, 96
    to hyper-emotionality, 224
    to revictimization, 251
    and substance use, 125
Vulvar vestivulitis, 38

Washington state, 108
Well-being, 120–121
Whites
    AIDS in female, 71
    CSA prevalence among female, 4
    CSA prevalence among male, 95, 98
    rape reported by, 65
    well-being of adult, 120–121
    in Women's Health Project, 238
WHP. *See* Women's Health Project
Wife rape, 60
Withdrawal, 142
Wives, 106
Women
    as abusers, 98, 99, 101
    with AIDS, 71
    childhood physical abuse of, 55
    cognitive/attitudinal paths of. *See* Cog-
        nitions
    CSA prevalence among, 4, 71
    group psychotherapy for. *See* Group psy-
        chotherapy
    HIV infection among. *See* HIV infec-
        tion
    in mixed-gender assault-reduction pro-
        grams, 288
    revictimization of. *See* Revictimization
    sexual assault risk-reduction programs
        with, 279–286
    sexual problems of, 16, 34, 106
Women's Health Project (WHP), 237–248
    behavioral effects of, 245–246
    cognitive effects of, 243–244

ABOUT THE EDITORS

Linda J. Koenig, PhD, is the assistant chief for behavioral science in the Centers for Disease Control and Prevention (CDC) Mother–Child Transmission and Pediatric/Adolescent Studies Section, Division of HIV/AIDS Prevention (DHAP). She received her PhD in clinical psychology from Northwestern University in Evanston, Illinois and completed a National Institute of Mental Health (NIMH) postdoctoral fellowship at Stanford University in Palo Alto, California. Prior to joining the CDC as Chief of the Social and Behavioral Studies Section in the DHAP Epidemiology Branch, Dr. Koenig held academic appointments at Kennesaw State University in Kennesaw, Georgia, and Emory University in Atlanta, Georgia, where she also served as director of clinical training. She has received service commendations for her work on the CDC Violence and Reproductive Health Working Group, and the Anthrax Efficacy, Adverse Events and Adherence Team, for which she received the Secretary's Award for Distinguished Service. Her research addresses the psychosocial aspects of HIV/AIDS among women, children and adolescents, including violence and abuse, risk behavior, and medication adherence.

Lynda S. Doll, PhD, is associate director for science of the National Center for Injury Prevention at the CDC. Prior to taking this position, Dr. Doll held several leadership positions in prevention research at the CDC, including director of the National Center for Chronic Disease Prevention and Health Promotion's Prevention Research Centers, senior behavioral scientist in the CDC Office of Prevention Research, chief of the Behavioral Intervention Research Branch, as well as associate director for Behavioral and Social Science in the Division of HIV/AIDS Prevention. Dr. Doll earned her PhD in developmental psychology from Georgia State University in Atlanta and was among the first psychologists hired at the CDC. She has taken a lead role in developing and managing behavioral and social science research at the CDC. She is a fellow of the American Psychological Association (APA).

Ann O'Leary, PhD, is a senior behavioral scientist and coordinator of women's studies at the CDC Division of HIV/AIDS Prevention, Prevention Research Branch. Her training included a summa cum laude undergraduate degree from the University of Pennsylvania in Philadelphia; a PhD in psychology from Stanford University in Stanford, California, supported by a National Science Foundation fellowship; and one year of postdoctoral training in health psychology at the University of California, San Francisco. She served on the faculty of the Psychology Department at Rutgers University in New Brunswick, New Jersey, from 1986 to 1999. She has conducted research in HIV prevention interventions for the past 15 years and has also published many articles in other aspects of health psychology. Dr. O'Leary has published approximately 100 scientific articles and chapters and has edited three books; *Women at Risk: Issues in the Prevention of AIDS; Women and AIDS: Coping and Care;* and *Beyond Condoms: Alternative Approaches to HIV Prevention.* She is a fellow of the APA and won the inaugural Distinguished Leader award from the APA Committee on Psychology and AIDS. She serves on the editorial boards of several scientific journals and is a frequent consultant to the National Institutes of Health and other scientific organizations.

Willo Pequegnat, PhD, is the associate director for Prevention, Translational, and International Research in the Center for Mental Health Research at the NIMH, where she is the principal investigator on three, HIV-focused, randomized clinical trials. She developed a research program on the role of families in preventing and adapting to HIV/AIDS and chairs the only national annual international research conference on families and HIV/AIDS. She coedited the book on this program, *Working with Families in the Era of AIDS,* as well as the book *How to Write a Successful Research Grant Application: A Guide for Social and Behavioral Scientists.* Dr. Pequegnat is involved in a wide range of national and international research projects. Her areas of expertise include behavioral preventive interventions, neuropsychological assessment, stress and coping, mental and physical functioning, and quality of life. Currently, she is developing a complex set of studies to examine multilevel social organization and complex relationships that include couples, families, communities, society (media, policy), technology (Internet, Web) in national and international settings. She is also studying the issue of social instability, such as the consequences of war, terrorism, migration, and female and drug trafficking on HIV/STD transmission. Dr. Pequegnat earned her PhD in clinical psychology from the State University of New York at Stony Brook. She has lectured, published, and conducted research on a broad range of HIV/STD issues and represents the NIMH on science policy making committees and workgroups.